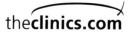

CLINICS IN
CHEST MEDICINE

Pulmonary Arterial Hypertension

GUEST EDITOR
Harold I. Palevsky, MD

March 2007 • Volume 28 • Number 1

SAUNDERS

An Imprint of Elsevier, Inc.
PHILADELPHIA   LONDON   TORONTO   MONTREAL   SYDNEY   TOKYO

W.B. SAUNDERS COMPANY

A Division of Elsevier Inc.

Elsevier Inc. • 1600 John F. Kennedy Boulevard • Suite 1800 • Philadelphia, Pennsylvania 19103-2899

http://www.chestmed.theclinics.com

CLINICS IN CHEST MEDICINE
March 2007
Editor: Sarah E. Barth

Volume 28, Number 1
ISSN 0272-5231
ISBN-13: 978-1-4160-4285-3
ISBN-10: 1-4160-4285-7

Reprints: For copies of 100 or more, of articles in this publication, please contact the Commercial Reprints Department, Elsevier Inc., 360 Park Avenue South, New York, New York 10010-1710. Tel. (212) 633-3813; Fax: (212) 462-1935; e-mail: reprints@elsevier.com.

The ideas and opinions expressed in *Clinics in Chest Medicine* do not necessarily reflect those of the Publisher. The Publisher does not assume any responsibility for any injury and/or damage to persons or property arising out of or related to any use of the material contained in this periodical. The reader is advised to check the appropriate medial literature and the product information currently provided by the manufacturer of each drug to be administered to verify the dosage, the method and duration of administration, or contraindications. It is the responsibility of the treating physician or other health care professional, relying on independent experience and knowledge of the patient, to determine drug dosages and the best treatment for the patient. Mention of any product in this issue should not be construed as endorsement by the contributors, editors, or the Publisher of the product or manufacturers' claims.

Clinics in Chest Medicine (ISSN 0272-5231) is published quarterly by Elsevier Inc., 360 Park Avenue South, New York, NY 10010-1710. Months of issue are March, June, September, and December. Business and Editorial Offices: 1600 John F. Kennedy Blvd., Suite 1800, Philadelphia, PA 19103-2899. Customer Service Office: 6277 Sea Harbor Drive, Orlando, FL 32887-4800. Periodicals postage paid at New York, NY and additional mailing offices. Subscription prices are $211.00 per year (US individuals), $330.00 per year (US institutions), $103.00 per year (US students), $232.00 per year (Canadian individuals), $396.00 per year (Canadian institutions), $135.00 per year (Canadian students), $270.00 per year (international individuals) $396.00 per year (international institutions), and $135.00 per year (international students). International air speed delivery is included in all *Clinics* subscription prices. All prices are subject to change without notice. **POSTMASTER:** Send address changes to *Clinics in Chest Medicine*, Elsevier Periodicals Customer Service, 6277 Sea Harbor Drive, Orlando, FL 32887-4800. Customer Service: 1-800-654-2452 (US). From outside of the US, call 1-407-345-4000.

Clinics in Chest Medicine is covered in *Index Medicus, Current Contents/Clinical Medicine, EMBASE/Excerpta Medica, Science Citation Index,* and *ISI/BIOMED.*

Printed in the United States of America.

GUEST EDITOR

HAROLD I. PALEVSKY, MD, Professor of Medicine, University of Pennsylvania School of Medicine; Chief, Pulmonary, Allergy and Critical Care, Penn Presbyterian Medical Center; and Director, Pulmonary Vascular Disease Program, University of Pennsylvania Medical Center, Philadelphia, Pennsylvania

CONTRIBUTORS

VIVEK N. AHYA, MD, Assistant Professor of Medicine, and Medical Director, Lung Transplantation Program, Pulmonary, Allergy and Critical Care Division, University of Pennsylvania Medical Center, Philadelphia, Pennsylvania

SHOAIB ALAM, MD, Assistant Professor of Medicine, Division of Pulmonary, Allergy and Critical Care Medicine, Penn State University-Hershey Medical Center, Hershey, Pennsylvania

WILLIAM R. AUGER, MD, Professor of Clinical Medicine, Division of Pulmonary and Critical Care Medicine, University of California, San Diego, La Jolla, California

ERIC D. AUSTIN, MD, Pulmonary Fellow, Division of Pediatric Pulmonary Medicine, Department of Pediatrics, Vanderbilt University Medical Center, Nashville, Tennessee

JEFFREY D. EDELMAN, MD, Associate Professor of Medicine, Division of Pulmonary and Critical Care Medicine, Department of Medicine, University of Washington Medical Center, Seattle, Washington

PETER F. FEDULLO, MD, Clinical Professor of Medicine, Division of Pulmonary and Critical Care Medicine, University of California, San Diego, La Jolla, California

IWONA FIJALKOWSKA, PhD, Member, and Research Associate, Division of Cardiopulmonary Pathology, Johns Hopkins University School of Medicine, Baltimore, Maryland

SONIA FLORES, PhD, Associate Professor of Medicine, Division of Pulmonary and Critical Care Medicine, University of Colorado-Denver Health Sciences Center, Denver, Colorado

SEAN P. GAINE, MD, PhD, FRCPI, FCCP, Consultant Respiratory Physician, and Director, National Pulmonary Hypertension Unit, Department of Respiratory Medicine, Mater Misericordiae University Hospital, University College Dublin, Dublin, Ireland

REDA E. GIRGIS, MB, BCh, Associate Professor of Medicine, Division of Pulmonary and Critical Care Medicine, Johns Hopkins University, Baltimore, Maryland

JASON M. GOLBIN, DO, MS, Fellow, Division of Pulmonary and Critical Care Medicine, Mayo Clinic College of Medicine, Rochester, Minnesota

STEVEN M. KAWUT, MD, MS, Assistant Professor of Clinical Medicine and Epidemiology, Division of Pulmonary, Allergy, and Critical Care Medicine, Department of Medicine, College of Physicians and Surgeons, and Department of Epidemiology, Joseph L. Mailman School of Public Health, Columbia University, New York, New York

KIM M. KERR, MD, Associate Clinical Professor of Medicine, Division of Pulmonary and Critical Care Medicine, University of California, San Diego, La Jolla, California

NICK H. KIM, MD, Assistant Clinical Professor of Medicine, Division of Pulmonary and Critical Care Medicine, University of California, San Diego, La Jolla, California

JAMES R. KLINGER, MD, Division of Pulmonary Sleep and Critical Care Medicine, Rhode Island Hospital; and Associate Professor of Medicine, Brown Medical School, Providence, Rhode Island.

MICHAEL J. KROWKA, MD, Professor of Medicine, Division of Pulmonary and Critical Care Medicine, and Division of Gastroenterology and Hepatology, Mayo Clinic College of Medicine, Rochester, Minnesota

DAVID LANGLEBEN, MD, FRCPC, Professor of Medicine, McGill University; Director, Center for Pulmonary Vascular Disease, Division of Cardiology, Sir Mortimer B. Davis Jewish General Hospital, Montreal, Quebec, Canada

MICHAEL J. LANDZBERG, MD, Director, Boston Adult Congenital Heart (BACH) and Pulmonary Hypertension Group, Children's Hospital, Brigham and Women's Hospital, Beth Israel Deaconess Medical Center, Harvard University, Boston, Massachusetts

JAMES E. LOYD, MD, Rudy W. Jacobson Professor in Pulmonary and Critical Care Medicine, Division of Allergy, Pulmonary, and Critical Care Medicine, Department of Medicine, Vanderbilt University Medical Center, Nashville, Tennessee

JESS MANDEL, MD, Associate Professor of Medicine, Associate Dean, University of California, San Diego School of Medicine, La Jolla, California

JOHN C. MARECKI, PhD, Research Associate, Division of Pulmonary and Critical Care Medicine, University of Colorado-Denver Health Sciences Center, Denver, Colorado

STEPHEN C. MATHAI, MD, MHS, Clinical Research Fellow, Division of Pulmonary and Critical Care Medicine, Johns Hopkins University, Baltimore, Maryland

JOHN R. McARDLE, MD, Assistant Professor of Medicine, Section of Pulmonary and Critical Care Medicine, Division of Internal Medicine, and Co-Director, Pulmonary Hypertension Center, Yale University School of Medicine, New Haven, Connecticut

DERMOT O'CALLAGHAN, MB, MRCPI, Specialist Registrar in Respiratory Medicine, Department of Respiratory Medicine, Mater Misericordiae University Hospital, University College Dublin, Dublin, Ireland

RONALD J. OUDIZ, MD, Associate Professor of Medicine, David Geffen School of Medicine at UCLA; and Director, Department of Medicine, Division of Cardiology, Liu Center for Pulmonary Hypertension, Los Angeles Biomedical Research Institute at Harbor-UCLA Medical Center, Torrance, California

HAROLD I. PALEVSKY, MD, Professor of Medicine, University of Pennsylvania School of Medicine; Chief, Pulmonary, Allergy and Critical Care, Penn Presbyterian Medical Center; and Director, Pulmonary Vascular Disease Program, University of Pennsylvania Medical Center, Philadelphia, Pennsylvania

AMY RICHTER, Member, Division of Cardiopulmonary Pathology, Johns Hopkins University School of Medicine, Baltimore, Maryland

JEFFREY S. SAGER, MD, MSCE, Assistant Professor of Medicine, and Associate Medical Director of the Lung Transplantation Program, Pulmonary, Allergy and Critical Care Division, University of Pennsylvania Medical Center, Philadelphia, Pennsylvania

JENNIFER L. SNOW, MD, Fellow, Division of Pulmonary, Allergy, and Critical Care Medicine, Department of Medicine, University of Pennsylvania School of Medicine, Philadelphia, Pennsylvania

WAYNE L. STRAUSS, MD, PhD, Pulmonary Fellow, Division of Pulmonary and Critical Care Medicine, Department of Medicine, Oregon Health and Sciences University, Portland, Oregon

DARREN B. TAICHMAN, MD, PhD, Assistant Professor of Medicine, University of Pennsylvania School of Medicine; Director, Medical Intensive Care Unit, and Associate Director, Pulmonary Vascular Disease Program, Penn Presbyterian Medical Center, Philadelphia, Pennsylvania

VICTOR J. TEST, MD, Assistant Clinical Professor of Medicine, Division of Pulmonary and Critical Care Medicine, University of California, San Diego, La Jolla, California

TERENCE K. TROW, MD, Assistant Professor of Medicine, Section of Pulmonary and Critical Care Medicine, Division of Internal Medicine, and Co-Director, Pulmonary Hypertension Center, Yale University School of Medicine, New Haven, Connecticut

RUBIN M. TUDER, MD, Professor of Pathology and Medicine, and Director, Division of Cardiopulmonary Pathology, Johns Hopkins University School of Medicine, Baltimore, Maryland

CONTENTS

likely related to environmental and genetic modifiers of disease not yet fully elucidated. Although BMPR2-related pathways seem to be pivotal, many other mediator pathways participate in the pathogenesis of different forms of PAH and are being actively investigated, both independently and in combination. As understanding of the molecular basis of this devastating disease improves, opportunities for earlier diagnosis, additional therapeutic regimens, and perhaps disease prevention will emerge.

Accurate diagnosis of pulmonary arterial hypertension is a challenging and complex process that requires a high index of clinical suspicion from even the most astute clinician. This article discusses the use of a variety of noninvasive tests that can help define the population of patients in whom invasive cardiac catheterization should be pursued. It points out the vagaries and limitations of electrocardiography and the radiographic and echocardiographic clues to the diagnosis. Ultimately, right- and, often, concomitant left-heart catheterization is required to establish the diagnosis and distinguish pulmonary arterial hypertension from pulmonary venous hypertension.

Recent discoveries in the disease pathophysiology of pulmonary arterial hypertension have been translated into effective therapies tested in clinical trials. The studies have focused on surrogate and intermediate end points, thought to reflect quantity and quality of life, respectively. The authors present the necessary requirements for establishing the reliability and validity of such end points before they may be used dependably. The authors also review the available data, strengths, and weaknesses of potential end points in pulmonary arterial hypertension.

After half a century of clinical experience and research, management of pulmonary arterial hypertension remains a challenge. Currently, data to support the use of standard therapies for pulmonary arterial hypertension (oxygen supplementation, diuretics, digoxin, anticoagulation, and calcium channel blockers) are mostly retrospective, uncontrolled prospective, or derived from other diseases with similar but not identical manifestations. In the absence of any further prospective, controlled studies, it is reasonable to use these therapies when they are tolerated. When these therapies are poorly tolerated, however, the threshold for discontinuation should be low.

The recognition that endothelin-1 contributes to the pathogenesis of pulmonary arterial hypertension has led to the development of clinically useful endothelin receptor antagonists that improve symptoms and functional capacity and alter the natural history of the disease in a beneficial way. The antagonists have varying degrees of selectivity for the two classes of endothelin receptor, termed ETA and ETB, and the varying degrees may translate into clinical differences. Endothelin receptor antagonists have become an integral part of therapy for pulmonary arterial hypertension, and the indications for their use are expanding.

FORTHCOMING ISSUES

RECENT ISSUES

THE CLINICS ARE NOW AVAILABLE ONLINE!

Access your subscription at:
http://www.theclinics.com

ELSEVIER
SAUNDERS

Clin Chest Med 28 (2007) xiii

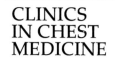

CLINICS
IN CHEST
MEDICINE

Erratum

Pulmonary Artery Catheter and Fluid Management in Acute Lung Injury and the Acute Respiratory Distress Syndrome

Gustavo A. Heresi, MD[a], Alejandro C. Arroliga, MD[b],
Herbert P. Wiedemann, MD[a], Michael A. Matthay, MD[c]

[a]Department of Pulmonary, Allergy and Critical Care Medicine, The Cleveland Clinic Foundation,
9500 Euclid Avenue, A190, Cleveland, OH 44195, USA
[b]Division of Pulmonary and Critical Care Medicine, Scott & White/Texas A&M University System,
2401 South 31st Street, Temple, TX 76508, USA
[c]Cardiovascular Research Institute, University of California in San Francisco, 505 Parnassus Avenue,
M917, San Francisco, CA 94143-0624, USA

In the December 2006 issue (volume 27, number 4), the name of Dr. Herbert P. Wiedemann was misspelled on the cover and on the opening page of the above article (p. 627–635). Dr. Wiedemann's name appears corrected above.

0272-5231/07/$ - see front matter © 2007 Elsevier Inc. All rights reserved.
doi:10.1016/j.ccm.2006.12.005

chestmed.theclinics.com

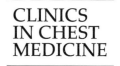

CLINICS
IN CHEST
MEDICINE

Clin Chest Med 28 (2007) xv–xvi

Preface

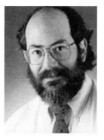

Harold I. Palevsky, MD
Guest Editor

Pulmonary arterial hypertension is the term currently used to describe what previously had been referred to as *precapillary pulmonary hypertension*. Pulmonary arterial hypertension (PAH) as a classification is comprised of idiopathic PAH (formerly referred to as primary pulmonary hypertension [PPH]), familial PAH, and PAH associated with identified conditions. It is distinguished from the pulmonary hypertension consequent to left heart disease, consequent to intrinsic pulmonary disease (obstructive, restrictive, and/or hypoxemia producing conditions), consequent to acute or chronic embolic disorders (eg, primarily thromboembolic disorders), and resulting from disorders directly affecting the pulmonary arterial vasculature (eg, vasculitis and schistosomiasis).

Since pulmonary hypertension was last covered in the *Clinics in Chest Medicine* in September 2001, there have been significant advances in our understanding of the basis for the development of pulmonary arterial vascular disease and in the therapies available for treatment. This issue provides an update of our current understanding of this evolving field.

The contributions to this issue can be viewed in three sections. The first section starts with an article by Darren B. Taichman, MD, PhD, and Jess Mandel, MD, who discuss what is known regarding the epidemiology of PAH. This article is followed by a thorough review of the pathology of

pulmonary hypertension by Rubin M. Tuder, MD, and colleagues. The next contribution, by Eric D. Austin, MD, and James E. Loyd, MD, is an overview of the rapidly advancing understanding of genetics and mediators in PAH. The subsequent contribution by Terrance K. Trow, MD, and John R. McArdle, MD, reviews the evaluation necessary to establish a diagnosis of PAH.

Having laid the groundwork for understanding the pathophysiology and diagnosis of PAH, the next series of articles reviews advances in the treatment of this condition. The first of these, by Jennifer L. Snow, MD, and Steven M. Kawut, MD, MS, reviews how therapies should be evaluated in patients who have PAH. Having established that context, the next article by Shoaib Alam, MD, and me discusses standard (or conventional) therapies for PAH. The next three contributions deal with the specific classes of pharmacologic agents that have been developed to date for the treatment of PAH. The first, by David Langleben, MD, discusses endothelian receptor antagonists. Next, Wayne L. Strauss, MD, PhD, and Jeffrey D. Edelman, MD, discuss prostanoid therapy for PAH. The last, by James R. Klinger, MD, provides a detailed review of the nitric oxide/cGMP signaling pathway in PAH. Following these discussions of monotherapy for PAH, Dermot O'Callaghan, MB, and Sean P. Gaine, MD, PhD, bring us a cutting edge

0272-5231/07/$ - see front matter © 2007 Elsevier Inc. All rights reserved.
doi:10.1016/j.ccm.2007.01.001

discussion of combination therapy and new types of agents for PAH. This section on treatment concludes with a contribution by Jeffrey S. Sager, MD, MSCE, and Vivek N. Ahya, MD, reviewing surgical therapies for PAH.

The last series of articles deals with specific pulmonary hypertension disease states and their evaluation and treatment; several deal with entities that do not fall under the general classification of PAH. The first contribution by Jason M. Golbin, DO, MS, and Michael J. Krowka, MD, covers the diagnosis and treatment of portal pulmonary hypertension. Next, Reda E. Girgis, MD, BCh, and Stephen C. Mathai, MD, MHS, review the unique issues related to pulmonary hypertension due to chronic respiratory disease. Ronald J. Oudiz, MD, then discusses the assessment and management of pulmonary hypertension associated with left heart disease. This is followed by a contribution by Michael J. Landzberg, MD, reviewing the classification, assessment, and therapies for PAH associated with congenital heart disease. The final contribution, by William R. Auger, MD, and colleagues, reviews the evaluation and treatment of chronic thromboembolic pulmonary hypertension.

I trust that the readers of this issue will find these contributions informative, useful, and up-to-date. My sincerest thanks go to each and every one of the authors who contributed their time and effort to this undertaking. I wish to thank Sarah Barth, Editor of the *Clinics in Chest Medicine*, who supported and guided me through the process of preparing this issue despite being out on maternity leave for a portion of the time. I also wish to acknowledge my colleagues at Penn Presbyterian Medical Center, the staff of the Penn Pulmonary Vascular Disease Program, and—most importantly—my family, for their gracious tolerance of yet another demand on my time while this issue was in preparation. Lastly, and I am sure I speak for all of the contributors in this issue, I wish to acknowledge the tremendous courage of our patients in dealing with these conditions and to recognize them for the inspiration and motivation they provide to us to better understand PAH, to develop newer and more effective therapies for it, and to continue working toward a cure.

Harold I. Palevsky, MD
University of Pennsylvania School of Medicine
3400 Spruce Street
Philadelphia, PA 19104, USA

Pulmonary, Allergy and Critical Care
and
Pulmonary Vascular Disease Program
Penn Presbyterian Medical Center
51 N. 39th Street
Philadelphia, PA 19104, USA

E-mail address: harold.palevsky@uphs.upenn.edu

ELSEVIER
SAUNDERS

Clin Chest Med 28 (2007) 1–22

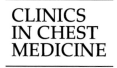

Epidemiology of Pulmonary Arterial Hypertension

Darren B. Taichman, MD, PhD[a],*, Jess Mandel, MD[b]

[a]*University of Pennsylvania School of Medicine, Penn Presbyterian Medical Center,*
51 North 39th Street, 441 PHI Building, Philadelphia, PA 19104, USA
[b]*University of California, San Diego School of Medicine, 9500 Gilman Drive,*
#0729, La Jolla, CA 92093-0729, USA

Advances in the understanding of the basic biology of various forms of pulmonary hypertension (PH) as well as evolution in the therapeutic approach have prompted changes in the manner in which these diseases are classified. These advances have also impacted the prognosis of many patients who have PH. Whereas pursuing an evaluation to determine the presence and cause of PH was once considered a pointless endeavor, with little if any impact on an immutably dismal outcome, a comprehensive evaluation is now the standard of care, because the findings frequently impact choices of therapy and the prognosis.

Changes in the classification of the pulmonary hypertensive diseases

A "sclerosis of the pulmonary arteries" without apparent explanation was first documented in 1891 by Ernst von Romberg [1], and again described as "cardiacos negros" in 1901 by Abel Ayerza of Argentina [2]. Thereafter, his colleagues referred to the entity as "Ayerza's disease," and believed it was a consequence of luetic (syphilitic) vasculitis. Little more was understood until the 1940s, when Oscar Brenner reported the histopathologic changes in the arteries of 100 patients who had PH, notably lacking findings suggestive of syphilis as a cause. In the 1950s, when the advent of cardiac catheterization allowed an investigation of the disease's hemodynamic abnormalities with cardiac catheterization, David

Dresdale and colleagues [3] described a hypertensive vasculopathy of the pulmonary circulation. It was characterized by vasoconstriction, an elevation in pulmonary arterial pressures, and a response to the injection of tolazoline, a vasodilator with both pulmonary and systemic effects. As no cause could be identified for the disease, it was termed "primary pulmonary hypertension" (PPH). Cases of PH for which a cause could be established were thereafter labeled "secondary" PH (eg, PH secondary to left ventricular failure, chronic pulmonary diseases, and hypoxemia) [4]. Later, using acetylcholine, a vasodilator that was cleared exclusively within the pulmonary circulation, Paul Wood demonstrated a pulmonary-specific hemodynamic improvement in patients who had PPH [2]. Intense histologic evaluation led Wagenvoort and Wagenvoort to describe extensive vascular injury and remodeling in a series of 156 patients, which they termed "plexogenic pulmonary arteriopathy," believed to be the pathognomonic hallmark of the disease [5].

Although the terms "primary," "secondary," and "plexogenic" have become a part of the familiar lexicon, an appreciation of important similarities and differences in the histologic and clinical characteristics of varying patient groups has prompted the adoption of more precise terminology. In part to reach consensus on clinically useful classification schemes for the pulmonary hypertensive disorders, there have been three international working groups under the sponsorship of the World Health Organization (WHO) since 1973. These schemes have evolved as new information has emerged regarding both pathophysiologic mechanisms and clinical characteristics. Histologic findings are no

---

* Corresponding author.

E-mail address: darren.taichman@uphs.upenn.edu (D.B. Taichman).

longer the cornerstone of clinical classification, because few of the pathologic patterns observed are truly disease-specific, and biopsies are now only rarely performed. The current approach to classification (Box 1) is based on a hemodynamic definition of PH, coupled with clinical and associated characteristics.

Pulmonary hypertension is deemed present when the mean pulmonary artery pressure exceeds 25 mm Hg at rest, or 30 mm Hg with exercise. The presence of pulmonary arterial hypertension further requires normal left heart filling pressures (ie, a normal left ventricular end diastolic pressure directly measured, or indirectly approximated by a pulmonary artery occlusion pressure less than 15 mm Hg). Classification as PAH further requires the absence of significant chronic respiratory disease or thromboembolic disease.

It is important to recognize the distinction between forms of disease classified as PAH and other known causes of PH (eg, caused by chronic left heart or chronic respiratory disease). This distinction arises from recognition of similarities in the histologic and clinical features of patients who have various forms of PAH. This category (now termed WHO "Group 1" diseases) includes patients who have identifiable genetic causes of PAH (ie, those who have familial PAH), and those who have collagen vascular diseases or other conditions known to be associated with PAH (associated PAH). Patients who have PAH and for whom no known associated disease entity or genetic cause can been found are now classified as having idiopathic PAH (IPAH), in place of the previously used term "primary pulmonary hypertension."

Abandonment of the name "primary pulmonary hypertension" is important as a means of discouraging the confusing and clinically inappropriate term "secondary" PH. Use of such "primary" and "secondary" groupings inappropriately suggests similarities in the pathophysiology and treatment of patients who have many, very different diseases. For example, patients who have COPD, chronic thromboembolic disease, and those who have congenital heart disease might each be loosely labeled as having "secondary" PH, although the pathogenesis is distinct in each category and appropriate therapy is very different. Conceptualizing patients as having either "primary" or "secondary" disease may also obscure important clinical similarities (including appropriate treatment) between what was previously called "primary" PH and other entities labeled "secondary"

(eg, patients who have congenital heart disease or HIV infection).

Although understanding of the basic mechanisms that produce PH remains incomplete, a number of clearly identifiable risk factors for the development of PAH are recognized (Box 2). The causal relationship of some risk factors has been firmly established by controlled epidemiologic studies (eg, exposure to fenfluramine-derived anorectic agents). Others (eg, thyroid disease) are suspected but not definitively established [6,7], and emerging information suggests additional potential risks in need of further study (eg, the use of serotonin receptor reuptake inhibitors during pregnancy and the development of persistent PH in newborns) [8].

Idiopathic pulmonary arterial hypertension

IPAH is a rare disease, with an estimated incidence of one to two cases per million in industrialized countries [9–12] The paucity of patients who have IPAH and the likelihood that diverse causes might produce similar clinical syndromes have complicated descriptions of the natural history of the disease. To overcome the limitations of sporadic reports, National Institutes of Health (NIH) established the prospective National Registry for the Characterization of Primary Pulmonary Hypertension. One hundred eighty-seven patients from 32 centers were enrolled between 1981 and 1985 [13]. The disease affected all ages, both men and women, and many ethnic groups. The mean age of patients in the Registry was 36.4 years, similar for women and men. Women were affected more frequently, however, with a female to male ratio of 1.7:1 (Fig. 1). Nine percent of patients were older than 60. Race and ethnicity of the cohort were similar to those of the general population. Similar demographic trends have been reported in series from France, Israel, Japan, and Mexico [11,14–16]. Dyspnea was the most common presenting symptom, and the mean time from the onset of symptoms to diagnosis among patients in the NIH Registry was 2 years.

In a more recent series, 674 patients referred for treatment of pulmonary arterial hypertension were enrolled in a French national registry over a 1-year period during 2002 and 2003 [12]. Both prevalent and incident patients were evaluated, making up 18% and 82% of the study population respectively. Idiopathic pulmonary arterial hypertension patients accounted for 39% of the

---

Box 1. Classification of the pulmonary hypertensive diseases[a]

Group I. Pulmonary arterial hypertension (PAH)
Idiopathic PAH
Familial PAH
Associated with PAH (APAH):
  Collagen vascular disease
  Congenital systemic to pulmonary shunts (large, small, repaired or nonrepaired)
  Portal hypertension
  HIV infection
  Drugs and toxins
  Other (glycogen storage disease, Gaucher's disease, hereditary hemorrhagic
    telangiectasia, hemoglobinopathies, myeloproliferative disorders, splenectomy)
Associated with significant venous or capillary involvement
  Pulmonary veno-occlusive disease (PVOD)
  Pulmonary capillary hemangiomatosis (PCH)
  Persistent PH of the newborn (PPHN)

Group II. Pulmonary venous hypertension
Left-sided atrial or ventricular heart disease
Left-sided valvular heart disease

Group III. Pulmonary hypertension associated with intrinsic lung disease or hypoxemia
Chronic obstructive pulmonary disease (COPD)
Interstitial lung disease
Sleep-disordered breathing
Alveolar hypoventilation disorders
Chronic exposure to high altitude

Group IV. Pulmonary hypertension caused by chronic thrombotic or embolic disease
Thromboembolic obstruction of proximal pulmonary arteries
Thromboembolic obstruction of distal pulmonary arteries
Pulmonary embolism (tumor, parasites, foreign material)

Group V. Miscellaneous
Sarcoidosis
Histiocytosis X
Lymphangiomatosis
Compression of pulmonary vessels (adenopathy, tumor, fibrosing mediastinitis)

---

[a] Clinical classification of the pulmonary hypertensive states as adapted at the 2003 World Symposium on Pulmonary Arterial Hypertension in Venice, Italy. Note that the diseases are segregated into "groups" (eg, Group 1, being diseases considered forms of pulmonary arterial hypertension, as distinct from Group 3 diseases, being disorders in which PH is associated with hypoxic respiratory states).

Data from Simonneau G, Galie N, Rubin J, et al. Clinical classification of pulmonary hypertension. J Am Coll Cardiol 2004;43:5S–12S; and Rubin LJ. Diagnosis and management of pulmonary arterial hypertension: ACCP evidence-based clinical practice guidelines. Chest 2004;126:7S–10S.

registry, and as in prior studies, disease was seen more commonly in women, with a ratio to men of 1.6:1. The mean age of patients who had IPAH was 52 years, older than that seen in prior series. Although data specific to IPAH were not available, one quarter of patients who had PAH of any form were older than 60 years, and some patients were diagnosed in their 80s. Unfortunately, despite the significant advances in therapy that have occurred since the NIH Registry,

Box 2. Risk factors for the development of pulmonary arterial hypertension

A. *Drugs and toxins*
  1. Definite
     - Aminorex
     - Fenfluramine
     - Dexfenfluramine
     - Toxic rapeseed oil
  2. Very likely
     - Amphetamines
     - L-tryptophan
  3. Possible
     - Meta-amphetamines
     - Cocaine
     - Chemotherapeutic agents
     - Antidepressants
  4. Unlikely
     - Oral contraceptives
     - Estrogen therapy
     - Cigarette smoking

B. *Demographic and medical conditions*
  1. Definite
     - Gender
  2. Possible
     - Pregnancy
     - Systemic hypertension
  3. Unlikely
     - Obesity

C. *Diseases*
  1. Definite
     - HIV infection
  2. Very likely
     - Portal hypertension/liver disease
     - Collagen vascular diseases
     - Congenital systemic-pulmonary-cardiac shunts
     - Splenectomy
  3. Possible
     - Thyroid disorders

Updated from the assessment of risk factors evaluated at the 1998 World Symposium on PH in Evian, France.

Adapted from Simonneau G, et al. Clinical classification of pulmonary hypertension. J Am Coll Cardiol 2004;43(12 Suppl S): 5S–12S.

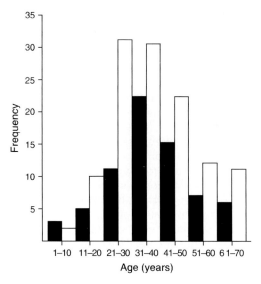

Fig. 1. Distribution of patients with idiopathic pulmonary arterial hypertension entered into the NIH Registry. Patients entered into the National Institutes of Health Registry of the Characterization of Primary Pulmonary Hypertension were most often in their third and fourth decades of life, with a similar ratio of women to men (1.7:1) in all decades. Open bars represent women; shaded bars represent men. (*Adapted from* Rich S, Dantzker DR, Ayres SM, et al. Primary pulmonary hypertension. A national prospective study. Ann Intern Med 1987;107(2):216–23; with permission.)

a significant delay in the diagnosis of IPAH continues. Indeed, 80% of IPAH patients had WHO Functional Class III or IV symptoms (Box 3) at the time of diagnosis. Exercise capacity was severely impaired in these patients, with a mean 6-minute walk distance of only 328 m, and hemodynamic values nearly identical to those of the NIH Registry population.

Prognostic factors in idiopathic pulmonary arterial hypertension

The prognosis of IPAH is very poor in the absence of effective therapy. The median survival of patients in the NIH Registry was 2.8 years, with estimated survival rates of 68% at 1 year, 48% at 3 years, and 34% at 5 years [13]. Similar outcomes have been reported in other series from various countries, [17,18] with the majority of patients dying of right-heart failure.

Demographic factors have not been established as predictors of survival. In a single retrospective study, however, non-white race was

Box 3. World Health Organization functional classification

Class I: Patients who have PH but without resulting limitation of physical activity. Ordinary physical activity does not cause undue dyspnea or fatigue, chest pain, or near syncope.

Class II: Patients who have PH resulting in slight limitation of physical activity. They are comfortable at rest. Ordinary physical activity causes undue dyspnea or fatigue, chest pain, or near syncope.

Class III: Patients who have PH resulting in marked limitation of physical activity. They are comfortable at rest. Less than ordinary activity causes undue dyspnea or fatigue, chest pain, or near syncope.

Class IV: Patients who have PH with inability to carry out any physical activity without symptoms. These patients manifest signs of right-heart failure. Dyspnea or fatigue may even be present at rest. Discomfort is increased by any physical activity.

_____

Adapted from Rubin LJ. Diagnosis and management of pulmonary arterial hypertension: ACCP evidence-based clinical practice guidelines. Chest 2004;126(Suppl 1):9S; with permission.

found to be associated with an increased risk of death, despite the use of similar medications [19]. Neither age nor the duration of symptoms at the time of diagnosis has been found to predict survival. Survival has been similar between men and women in studies both before and since the availability of effective therapies [20–23].

The prognosis is generally worse as symptoms progress. In the NIH Registry, the median survival of patients who had milder symptoms (WHO Functional Classes I or II; see Box 3) was 58.6 months as compared with only 31.5 months for patients who had more severe symptoms (WHO Functional Class III). Patients who had the most severe functional impairment (WHO Functional Class IV) had a median survival of only 6 months [13,20]. Although the outlook has improved with the availability of effective therapy,

functional status remains a highly significant prognostic variable [11,22–25]. Objective measurements of exercise capacity are also predictive of survival. Among 43 patients treated predominantly with infused or oral prostanoids, the pretreatment 6-minute walk distance was independently associated with survival, which was significantly better for those who could walk farther than 332 m (Fig. 2) [26]. Similarly, in randomized trials of epoprostenol therapy, patients who had a lower baseline 6-minute walk distance had poorer survival [23,27]. Maximal oxygen consumption during cardiopulmonary exercise testing also correlates with survival [28].

Findings on echocardiogram, including right atrial enlargement or the presence and size of a pericardial effusion, can be useful in assessing prognosis [29–31]. An index of right ventricular function derived by dividing the combined isovolumetric contraction and relaxation times by the right ventricular ejection time (Tei index) is also predictive of survival, with a higher index associated with a poorer prognosis [32]. Recently, the degree of tricuspid annular displacement during systole was shown to be associated with right ventricular function, hemodynamic measurements, as well as survival in a cohort of patients who had various forms of PAH, and others who had PH associated with chronic respiratory or thromboembolic disease (Fig. 3) [33].

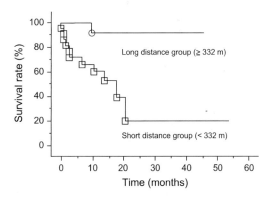

Fig. 2. Survival in IPAH according to 6-minute walk test distance. Kaplan-Meier survival curves according to the median value of distance walked in meters (m) during a 6-minute walk test. Patients unable to walk more than 332 m had a lower survival (P < .001). (*From* Miyamoto S, et al. Clinical correlates and prognostic significance of six-minute walk test in patients with primary pulmonary hypertension. Comparison with cardiopulmonary exercise testing. Am J Respir Crit Care Med 2000;161:487–92; with permission.)

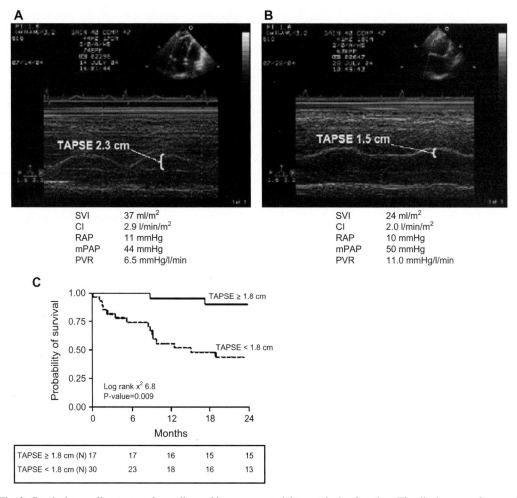

Fig. 3. Survival according to an echocardiographic assessment right ventricular function. The displacement from end-diastole to end-systole of the lateral tricuspic annulus (tricuspid annular plane excursion [TAPSE]) is shown in M-mode views from two patients, one with relatively preserved tricuspid excursion (and right ventricular function) (*Panel A*) as compared with a patient with greater impairment (*Panel B*). Kaplan-Meier estimates of survival in a cohort of patients with PAH (idiopathic or associated with collagen vascular disease) stratified by TAPSE values (*Panels C*). (*From* Forfia P, Fisher MR, Mathei SC, et al. Tricuspid annular displacement predicts survival in pulmonary hypertension. Am J Respir Crit Care Med 2006;14(9):1034–41; with permission.)

Hemodynamic measurements have been predictors of survival in numerous studies, including both observational and clinical trials. Despite isolated differences, overall these studies indicate that values reflecting a declining right ventricular function (eg, an increased right atrial pressure and a decreased cardiac index) are associated with poorer survival [11,15,16,21]. Survival is less consistently linked with mean pulmonary artery pressures (mPAP), and both increasing and decreasing values have been associated with worsened outcomes. This reflects the natural history of

right-heart failure in PAH: mPAP increases progressively as the vascular derangements worsen, only to fall later as the right heart progressively fails and is no longer able to generate an increased pressure (Fig. 4) [34].

Many serum markers are elevated in patients who have IPAH, and are associated with a worse prognosis. Uric acid levels are increased in hypoxic states, and the degree of increase correlates with hemodynamic and functional decline in patients who have IPAH [35]. Levels of B-natriuretic peptide are also increased in patients who

Progression of PAH

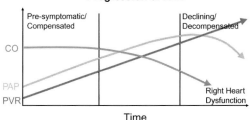

Fig. 4. Hemodynamic changes with progression of pulmonary arterial hypertension. Schematic representation of the changes in cardiac output (CO), mean pulmonary artery pressure (PAP) and pulmonary vascular resistance in the absence of effective therapy. Pulmonary vascular resistance (PVR) rises progressively as the vascular derangements progress, eventually leading to the development of right heart dysfunction. PAPs initially rise as the right ventricle remains capable of generating the increased pressures required to maintain a given degree of cardiac output. Note, however, that with more advanced disease, CO decreases and the PAP falls, because of the inability of the failing right ventricle to generate increased pressures. (*From* Friedman E, Palevsky HI, Taichman DB. Classification and prognosis of pulmonary arterial hypertension. In: J Mandel, Taichman DB, editors. Pulmonary vascular disease. Philadelphia: Elsevier Science; 2006. p. 73; with permission.)

have IPAH, reflective of right-heart failure analogous to that seen in patients who have left-sided heart dysfunction. In one series of 60 patients who had IPAH, serum brain natriuretic peptide (BNP) concentrations were increased versus control, and inversely correlated with both functional status and survival [36]. BNP levels declined as hemodynamic measures improved with therapy, and a persistently elevated BNP (>180 pg/mL) despite therapy predicted a poorer prognosis.

Serum concentrations of endothelin-1, catecholamines, and atrial natriuretic peptide in serum have also been correlated with disease severity. Increases in von Willebrand factor, D-dimer, and troponin-T, or a decrease in the serum albumin level have been individually associated with poorer survival in patients who have IPAH [19,35–42]. None of these putative prognostic markers, however, is routinely incorporated into clinical decision making.

Not surprisingly, the prognosis of patients who have IPAH and who have suffered cardiac arrest is dismal, even when resuscitative efforts are initiated promptly. In one retrospective review of records from over 3000 patients, 132 episodes of attempted cardiopulmonary resuscitation (CPR)

following cardiac arrest were identified. Survival at 90 days following CPR was only 6% [43].

Important caveats in assessing the impact of therapy on prognosis

Whereas a diagnosis of IPAH has been associated with an invariably dismal prognosis, therapies developed in the last decade have significantly improved the prognosis of the condition and yielded many long-term survivors. No currently available medical treatment, however, is considered curative, and lung transplantation continues to be an important therapeutic consideration.

Although multiple studies have evaluated the survival of IPAH patients treated with new therapies, information on patients who have other forms of PAH is sparse. Most subjects in controlled clinical trials of treatment with calcium channel antagonists, prostanoids, endothelin receptor antagonists, or phosphodiesterase inhibitors have had IPAH. Fewer patients who have either familial or various forms of associated PAH have been studied. It is important to bear in mind this paucity of data when informing patients who have some forms of PAH about the expected outcome of treatment. It is also important to acknowledge the limits in understanding the relative efficacy of available agents. Data from head-to-head comparisons are lacking. Most often, patients treated with intravenous epoprostenol have been sicker than those treated with oral therapies, making comparisons between studies problematic.

A regression equation predicting survival on the basis of hemodynamic values was derived using data from the NIH Registry [15,20], and has been used extensively to assess new therapies. Because prognosis in the absence of treatment is dismal, it would be unethical to include long-term, untreated control groups in clinical trials. Instead, survival with new therapies is frequently compared with "expected" outcomes predicted by the NIH Registry equation. Such comparisons have indicated improved survival with the use of prostanoid therapy, calcium channel antagonists, or endothelin receptor antagonists. It must be recognized, however, that the NIH Registry was conducted in an era lacking effective therapy. Because available therapies have since improved dramatically, the NIH Registry equation may no longer be appropriate for predicting survival [19].

The impact of therapy on prognosis

In the French national registry population from 2002 to 2003, the 1-year survival of PAH patients who had either IPAH, familial, or anorexigen-associated PAH was 89.3%. Although information regarding specific treatments involved was not reported, the expected survival on the basis of the NIH Registry equation was 71.8% [12].

The long-term prognosis is good for the small group of IPAH patients who respond acutely to the administration of short-acting pulmonary vasodilators. Testing is performed at the time of right-heart catheterization [44–50]. Although the definition of an acutely responsive patient has varied, a decrease in the mPAP of at least 10 mm Hg to a final value less than 40 mm Hg, with either an increased or unchanged cardiac output, is now generally considered a positive response [51,52]. In one study performed before the availability of other effective treatments [53], the survival rate of acutely responsive patients treated chronically with oral calcium channel antagonists was 94% at 5 years, as compared with only 38% among nonresponders. Unfortunately, only approximately 12% of patients in a recent series demonstrated acute vasoreactivity, and of these only about half experienced a sustained clinical response to oral calcium channel antagonist therapy. For the few acutely vasoreactive patients who do experience a sustained response to oral calcium channel antagonists therapy, the prognosis is excellent. In a retrospective study, Sitbon and colleagues [54] found that among 38 patients who had sustained clinical response (defined as being in WHO Functional Class I or II after 1 year of treatment) survival was 97% in up to 7 years of follow-up; however, oral calcium channel antagonists are of no benefit, and indeed can cause considerable harm when administered to patients who do not display acute pulmonary vasoreactivity.

The prognostic significance of acute pulmonary vasoreactivity is less clear in patients treated with therapies other than oral calcium channel antagonists. The magnitude of improvements in mPAP and cardiac index at the time of acute vasodilator testing correlated with survival in one series of patients treated with long-term epoprostenol infusion; such a correlation was not seen in another group of similarly treated patients [22,23]. A retrospective evaluation of survival in patients treated with calcium channel antagonists, prostanoid therapies, bosentan, warfarin, or a combination of these agents found no correlation between survival and acute vasoreactivity at baseline [19].

Several studies have demonstrated that continuously infused epoprostenol improves survival in patients who have IPAH. In the single randomized study performed, 81 IPAH patients were randomized to treatment with intravenous epoprostenol infusion or "conventional therapy" (which at the time included oral vasodilators, diuretics, cardiac glycosides and anticoagulants). After 12 weeks, only 1 of the 41 epoprostenol treated patients had required lung transplantation, whereas 2 of the 40 patients in the "conventional treatment" group had undergone transplantation and 8 had died [27].

Additional studies have confirmed these favorable findings. In a cohort of 162 IPAH patients, McLaughlin and colleagues [22] observed 1- and 3-year survival rates of 88% and 62% with epoprostenol infusion, compared with rates of 59% and 35% predicted by the NIH Registry equation. Sitbon and colleagues [23] observed remarkably similar results in 178 patients at 1 and 3 years; somewhat lower results were obtained by Kuhn and colleagues [25]. In each study, survival with epoprostenol therapy was improved compared with that predicted by the NIH Registry equation. Indeed, although originally conceived as a "bridge" to lung transplantation, the long-term use of epoprostenol and other treatments has resulted in a decrease in the demand for lung transplantation for patients who have IPAH [55]. In 1998, Robbins and colleagues [56] reported that more than two thirds of their patients treated with epoprostenol were improved sufficiently to be removed from the waiting list for lung transplantation. Despite these encouraging findings, an analysis by McLaughlin and colleagues [17] showed that approximately one third of patients from several series died within 3 years, notwithstanding treatment with epoprostenol, and nearly one half had died within 5 years (Fig. 5).

Comparison to survival predicted by the NIH Registry equation has also been used to assess the efficacy of oral therapy with the endothelin receptor antagonist, bosentan. In an open-label extension of placebo-controlled trials, survival of 169 patients who had IPAH initially treated with bosentan was 96% at 1 year and 89% after 2 years [57]. In a non-inferiority study comparing this same group to historical control patients treated with epoprostenol infusion, outcomes were similar at 1 and 2 years [58]. It must again be noted that,

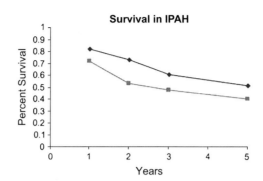

Fig. 5. The effect of chronically infused epoprostenol therapy on survival in patients (N = 431) from multiple series with idiopathic pulmonary hypertension. Survival in the absence of epoprostenol was estimated using a predication equation derived from observations in the NIH registry of primary pulmonary hypertension, at which time effective therapy was not available. ◆—, Epoprostenol Treated; ■—, No Epoprostenol. (*From* McLaughlin VV, et al. Prognosis of pulmonary arterial hypertension: ACCP evidence-based clinical practice guidelines. Chest 2004;126(Suppl 1):78S–92S; with permission.)

in general, patients treated with epoprostenol in clinical trials have been sicker than those enrolled into studies of oral therapies. Given the inconvenience and significant risks of continuously infused therapies, however, randomized trials comparing intravenous with oral treatments have not been performed. It is thus difficult to draw firm conclusions regarding their relative efficacy.

Autopsy studies have revealed in situ thrombosis within venous and arterial vessels in a significant proportion of patients who have PAH, suggesting a potential therapeutic role for systemic anticoagulation [18,59,60]. Warfarin therapy for PAH has not been studied in randomized trials, although observational reports have demonstrated an association between nonrandomized warfarin use and increased survival. As an example, in a prospective study of 64 IPAH patients treated with or without calcium channel antagonists, survival after 5 years was greater among those in either group who had received warfarin at their physician's discretion [53]. Likewise, a retrospective cohort study of idiopathic and aminorex-associated PAH patients reported that treatment with warfarin was associated with improved survival at 5 years [61]. Based upon these data, anticoagulation with warfarin is generally recommended for patients who have significant PAH in the absence of contraindications.

Lung transplantation remains an important option for suitable patients who have IPAH and whose disease fails to respond adequately to medical therapy. Single-lung, double-lung, and heart-lung transplants have been performed, although most centers favor double-lung transplant procedures for this indication when feasible [62]. Although the reported outcome at 5 years for patients who undergo lung transplant for IPAH is similar to those who have other indications, 1-year survival is only approximately 65%, as compared with 74% overall [63]. Fortunately, advances in medical therapies have markedly reduced the need for lung transplantation [64]. Whereas 10% of all lung transplant recipients in 1990 had IPAH, more recently these patients account for only 4% of procedures [65].

Familial pulmonary arterial hypertension

A genetic basis for the development of PAH has been suspected since a family of patients who had IPAH was described by Dresdale [3] in 1951. In the NIH Registry, 6% of patients reported one or more affected family members [13]. Loyd and colleagues [66,67] showed that familial PAH has an autosomal dominant pattern of inheritance, an increased tendency for female carriers to manifest clinical disease, and an earlier onset in successive generations (a phenomenon known as genetic anticipation). Mutations in the gene for a member of the TGF-β superfamily of receptors, the bone morphogenetic protein receptor Type II (*BMP-RII*), have been identified as the major cause of familial PAH [68–71]. More than 140 distinct *BMP-RII* mutations have been identified to date, and disease is believed to occur when haploinsufficiency results in inadequate quantities of protein being produced for normal function [72]. The low penetrance of disease observed in familial PAH suggests that environmental factors likely contribute to disease development in genetically susceptible individuals [73]. Mutations in the gene for another member of the TGF-β superfamily, activin receptor-like kinase-1 (ALK 1), predispose patients who have hereditary hemorrhagic telangiectasia to develop PAH [74–77].

Germline mutations in a *BMP-RII* have been identified in up to 60% of patients who have familial PAH. Some patients who have idiopathic (nonfamilial) and other associated forms of PAH also have *BMPR-II* mutations [70,71,78–83], and common ancestries have been identified in some patients who have PAH previously assumed to be sporadic. Familial cases of PAH might not be recognized because of incomplete family history taking or reporting, as well as low disease penetrance in smaller families [79,84]. Carriers of gene mutations may be asymptomatic despite mild PH documented by echocardiography [85].

Genetic testing of family members can assess the risk of developing PAH. There is a roughly one in five chance of PAH developing in a first-order relative who carries a disease-causing *BMP-RII* mutation. In the absence of genetic testing results, the risk of disease developing in the first-order relative of a patient who has known familial PAH can be approximated as 1 in 10. When testing demonstrates an absence of disease-causing *BMP-RII* mutations, the risk is the same as in the general population (estimated at 1 in 1 million) [73]. Genetic testing should only be performed in conjunction with professional genetic counseling because of the potential interpersonal, psychological, and economic implications of identifying an at-risk genotype.

Pulmonary arterial hypertension associated with specific conditions

Collagen vascular diseases

Among the identifiable risk factors for the development of PAH, the presence of systemic sclerosis is the most commonly reported. In the French national registry, 76% of PAH patients who had collagen vascular disease had scleroderma, accounting for 11.6% of all patients enrolled [12]. PAH occurs most often in patients who have limited disease or the CREST syndrome (calcinosis, Raynaud's phenomenon, esophageal dysmotility, sclerodactyly, telangiectasia). Estimates have varied significantly, but when assessed by right-heart catheterization, PAH has been found in between 7% and 29% of patients [86].

When screening of symptomatic patients is performed by echocardiogram, approximately 13% of patients who had systemic sclerosis were found to have PH in each of two large series [87,88].

The prognosis of patients who have scleroderma and PAH is worse than even those of scleroderma patients who develop severe pulmonary fibrosis. Median survival of patients who have scleroderma and PAH is approximately 1 year, versus 3 years among those who have scleroderma and pulmonary fibrosis alone [89,90]. Even when similar therapies are used (including epoprostenol, calcium channel antagonists, and warfarin) survival of patients who have PAH associated with systemic sclerosis is less favorable than for patients who have IPAH (Fig. 6) [89]. For example, whereas hemodynamic values and exercise capacity improve when patients who have IPAH are treated with bosentan, the benefit observed among similarly treated patients who have scleroderma appears to be primarily a slowing in the rate of deterioration [91].

PAH also occurs in patients who have other forms of collagen vascular disease, including systemic lupus erythematosis (SLE), rheumatoid arthritis, and Sjogren's syndrome. In most studies, pulmonary artery pressures have been estimated by echocardiogram, and thus the true prevalence of PAH is not known. Pulmonary hypertension has been identified by echocardiogram in approximately 10% of patients who have SLE, and in up to 43% of patients who are followed prospectively [92–96]. Estimates are similarly broad among patients who have mixed connective tissue disease, and again lack confirmation by catheterization in most studies. Regardless of the exact frequency, however, the presence of PH appears to be a significant cause of death in these patients. Accordingly, the possibility of PH patients should be considered in all collagen vascular disease patients who have exertional dyspnea or other symptoms, and early evaluation is warranted.

Human immunodeficiency virus

Infection with the HIV increases the risk of developing PAH by unclear mechanisms. The estimated incidence of PAH among HIV-infected patients is 0.5% [9,97]. In one large Swiss cohort of HIV-positive patients, the annual incidence of PH appears to be declining, having peaked at 0.24% in 1993 and decreased to 0.02% in 2001. This reduction has coincided with the

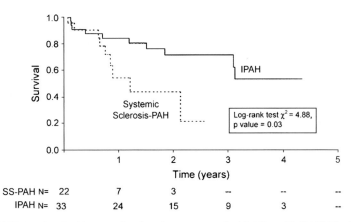

| SS-PAH N= | 22 | 7 | 3 | -- | -- | -- |
| IPAH N= | 33 | 24 | 15 | 9 | 3 | -- |

Fig. 6. Survival in PAH associated with systemic sclerosis as compared with idiopathic PAH. Kaplan-Meier estimates of survival in patients with PAH associated with the systemic sclerosis spectrum of diseases (SS-PAH) and IPAH. (*From* Kawut SM, et al. Hemodynamics and survival in patients with pulmonary arterial hypertension related to systemic sclerosis. Chest 2003;123(2):344–50; with permission.)

introduction of highly active antiretroviral therapies, and it has been postulated that better control of HIV infection might decrease the risk of developing PAH [98]. Whether this is true, or whether therapy for HIV infection in patients who have established PAH will alter the course of the vascular disease remains unknown. The symptoms, hemodynamic findings and survival of PAH associated with HIV are similar to those of IPAH [99]. As with IPAH, the prognosis of patients who have PAH associated with HIV infection is worse when symptoms are more advanced (eg, WHO Functional Class III or IV as compared with either I or II). A CD4 lymphocyte count below $212/mm^3$ is also associated with a poorer prognosis [100]. Mortality is more often directly attributable to PAH and right-heart failure than to infectious complications [99,100].

Portal hypertension

Patients who have chronic liver disease are at risk for the development of pulmonary complications. When portal hypertension and PAH are present, the combination is referred to as portopulmonary hypertension (POPH) [101]. POPH involves vascular derangements that increase pulmonary vascular resistance to produce an increased mPAP, as opposed to increased pulmonary pressures caused solely by the elevated cardiac output that frequently accompanies chronic liver disease. The etiology of PH in these patients may be difficult to unravel because the high cardiac output state may precede or

accompany the development of POPH. Despite similar degrees of clinical impairment, patients who have POPH may manifest numerically smaller increases in pulmonary vascular resistance (PVR) or decreases in cardiac output than those who have IPAH.

The frequency of PAH in patients who have liver disease has not been established. Estimates have ranged from 0.73% in 1241 autopsies from patients who had cirrhosis, to 16% of 62 patients undergoing catheterization during evaluation for transjugular intrahepatic portosystemic shunting [102,103]. In one series of patients evaluated for liver transplantation (and thus who had advanced liver disease and symptoms) the prevalence of POPH was 8.5% [104].

The prognosis of POPH is poor in the absence of effective treatment. In one retrospective series of 78 patients, the mean survival was only 15 months [105]. Little is known regarding the impact of current therapies on survival in POPH, because these patients have been excluded from almost all of the major prospective clinical treatment trials; however, even with the use of such therapies, survival appears to be worse for patients who have POPH than those who have IPAH. In a retrospective cohort of 13 patients who had POPH, survival at 1 and 3 years was 85% and 38%, respectively, as compared with 82% and 72% in 33 patients who had IPAH (Fig. 7) [106].

Many patients who have POPH and advanced hepatic dysfunction require liver transplantation. The presence of PAH, however, increases the

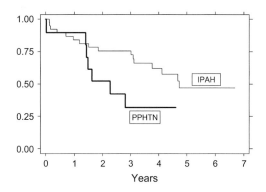

Fig. 7. Survival in patients with PAH associated with chronic liver disease and portal hypertension. Kaplan-Meier estimates of survival in patients with portopulmonary hypertension (PPHTN) as compared with patients with IPAH. (*From* Kawut SM, et al. Hemodynamics and survival of patients with portopulmonary hypertension. Liver Transpl 2005;11(9):1107–11. © 2005 American Association for the Study of Liver Diseases. Reprinted with permission of Wiley-Liss, Inc., a subsidary of John Wiley & Sons, Inc.)

perioperative mortality, and a mPAP above 50 mm Hg generally is considered a contraindication to liver transplantation [107,108]. Although therapy to lower mPAP has permitted successful orthotopic liver transplantation in some patients [109–114], the pulmonary vascular abnormalities of PAH are not consistently reversed by liver transplantation. Although some instances of reversal in patients have been reported, in other patients POPH has progressed despite transplantation [115].

Anorectic agents

The ingestion of certain anorexigens can lead to the development of PAH, possibly by increasing blood levels of the vasoconstrictor serotonin. An epidemic of PAH erupted in Switzerland, Austria, and Germany between 1966 and 1968 when the incidence increased 20 fold following the introduction in those countries of the appetite depressant aminorex fumarate [116]. Although only 2% of those exposed to the drug developed PAH, the relative risk compared with unexposed individuals was 52:1 [117]. The use of fenfluramine derivatives was similarly associated with the development of PAH both in Europe and North America [118]. In a registry of 95 PAH patients in Europe, the odds ratio of PAH was 6.3 after any anorectic agent use, and 23.8 when anorectic agents were taken longer than 3 months [9]. Likewise, a North American registry of 579 patients reported that the

use of fenfluramine was strongly associated with the development of PAH (odds ratio of 7.5 when taken for more than 6 months). The study also identified a high frequency of anorectic agent use among patients who had other associated forms of PAH (eg, collagen vascular disease), suggesting that these drugs might precipitate disease when combined with other risks [119].

In a series of 62 patients evaluated over a 10-year period at a single center in France, the interval between the initial exposure to fenfluramine and the development of dyspnea was approximately 4 years [120]. In the multicenter French national registry from 2002 to 2003, anorexigen-associated PAH was diagnosed within 2 years of drug exposure in 24% of cases, between 2 and 5 years in 32%, and after more than 5 years following drug exposure in 44% [12]. In both series, the baseline hemodynamic values were similar to those of patients who had IPAH, although patients exposed to anorectic-agents were even less likely to demonstrate acute vasoreactivity.

The prognosis of anorectic agent-associated PAH has not been well-established. Data comparing survival with IPAH patients are conflicting. Survival of aminorex-associated PAH patients was better than of those patients who had IPAH in a retrospective study of 104 patients treated with anticoagulation [61]. With additional therapies, including epoprostenol, survival in fenfluramine-exposed patients who had PAH appeared to be similar to that of IPAH patients in one study [120], yet poorer in another series in which patients were matched according to treatments and disease severity [121].

Hemoglobinopathies

The risk of developing PH is increased in patients who have certain chronic hemolytic disorders [122]. Hemolytic states might lead to PAH by releasing both free hemoglobin and arginase into the plasma, where they can reduce the bioavailability of both NO and its substrate, L-arginine [122–124]. Prevalence estimates of PH in patients who have either sickle cell anemia or thalassemia have ranged significantly, according to the age of the population studied, the severity of symptoms, and the method of pulmonary arterial pressure (PAP) assessment used [125–128]. Echocardiographic estimates in 195 adults patients who had sickle cell anemia reported PH in 32%; however, the TR gradient used to define PH was 2.5 m/sec, less than the TR gradient of less than 3.0 m/sec frequently used to suggest the presence of PH [129]. Histologic findings consistent with PAH were noted in 15 of 20 autopsies performed on patients who had sickle cell anemia [130]. Isolated cases of PH with other chronic hemolytic disorders have been reported, including patients who have hereditary spherocytosis and paroxysmal nocturnal hemoglobinuria [131,132].

Patients who have PAH associated with sickle cell anemia tend to have lower mean PAPs and higher cardiac outputs than patients who have idiopathic or other forms of associated PAH. Furthermore, patients who have PAH associated with hemoglobinopathies also have hemodynamic findings consistent with both intrinsic pulmonary vascular disease (ie, an increased PVR) as well as increased pulmonary capillary wedge pressures, suggesting the possibility that left ventricular diastolic dysfunction also plays a role. As an example, in one study of 20 patients who had PH associated with sickle cell anemia [133], the mean PAP was 36 mm Hg, cardiac output 8.6 L/min, and PCWP 16 mm Hg; one half of the patients had PCWP values greater than 15 and the majority had PVR less than three Wood units.

The presence of PH portends a worse prognosis in patients who have sickle cell anemia. Mortality within 2 to 2.5 years of almost 50% of sickle cell patients who have PH has been reported in several series [133–135]. In a prospective NIH registry of 195 adult patients who had sickle cell anemia followed for a mean of 18 months, Gladwin and colleagues [129] found mortality increased when the tricuspid regurgitant velocity was greater than 2.5 m/sec (relative risk 10.1), as compared with death in 2% when the pressures were lower (Fig. 8). Markers of hemolysis, such as plasma arginase, correlate not only with the presence of PH, but also with an increased risk of death [123]. The impact of therapy for PH on patients who have sickle cell anemia (or other forms of hemolytic anemia) has not been studied in a systematic fashion. Because ongoing hemolysis appears to contribute to the increased mortality associated with PH in these patients, therapy to minimize hemolysis is believed to be important in improving survival [123,129]. Although the use of PAH-directed therapies has been reported in patients who have hemolytic anemias [133,136, 137], their impact upon survival has not been adequately studied.

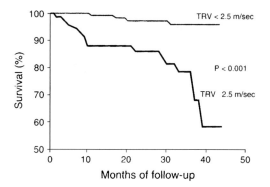

Fig. 8. Survival in patients with sickle cell anemia and pulmonary hypertension. Kaplan-Meier estimates of survival as affected by the presence of pulmonary hypertension as assessed by echocardiogram (defined as a tricuspid regurgitant velocity [TRV] greater than 2.5 m per second). (*From* Machado RF.a.G., M.T. Hemolytic anemia associated pulmonary hypertension. In: Mandel J, Taichman DB, editors. Pulmonary vascular disease. Philadelphia: Elsevier; 2006. p. 170–87; with permission.)

Pulmonary veno-occlusive disease

Pulmonary veno-occlusive disease is a rare form of PH that is characterized by extensive and diffuse obliteration of small pulmonary veins or venules by cellular proliferation, in situ thrombosis, and fibrous tissue [138,139]. In the majority of patients, pulmonary arteriolar changes accompany the venous changes, although it is unclear if arteriolar remodeling develops simultaneously with or as a consequence of progressive venous destruction [140]. PVOD usually presents with dyspnea on exertion and findings of right ventricular failure in a manner similar to IPAH, although subtle differences from IPAH may be present, such as digital clubbing, basilar rales, pleural effusions, and radiographic evidence of pulmonary lymphatic engorgement (eg, Kerley B lines visible on chest radiographs and septal thickening on chest CT) [138,141,142].

Differentiation from other forms of PAH is important, because treatment with prostanoids or other agents that are effective for IPAH may produce pulmonary edema and death in a subset of PVOD patients [143]. Partially because of these difficulties in treatment, the prognosis of PVOD is very poor, with most patients dying within 2 years of diagnosis unless long-term treatment with prostanoids is tolerated [139,141,144]. Immediate consideration of lung transplantation is thus encouraged when the diagnosis of PVOD is established, although recurrence of the condition after transplantation has been reported [145].

The epidemiology of PVOD is not clearly defined. Unlike IPAH, men and women appear equally at risk for PVOD, and the age at diagnosis has ranged from the first weeks through the seventh decade of life [139,146,147]. Because PVOD appears to be approximately one tenth as common as IPAH, the annual incidence of PVOD in the general population has been estimated at 0.1 to 0.2 cases per million persons per year [139]. This may represent an underestimate, however, because many cases are probably misclassified as IPAH, heart failure, or interstitial lung disease. No well-designed studies have adequately examined the magnitude of this likely misclassification phenomenon.

The etiology of PVOD remains unknown, and likely represents a final common clinicopathologic pathway that develops in a susceptible host following exposure to one of a number of different triggers. A *BMP-RII* mutation has been described in one case [83]. A number of factors associated with PVOD have been proposed, but none of these epidemiologic hypotheses have been tested by rigorous methods. Conditions theorized to be associated with an increased risk of PVOD include the development of the condition in a sibling, exposure to antineoplastic chemotherapy, infection with HIV or other agents, or the presence of thrombophilia or autoimmune diseases [59,138, 148–155].

Epidemiologic features of certain non-pulmonary arterial hypertension forms of pulmonary hypertension

Chronic respiratory disease

Parenchymal lung disease and hypoxemia are relatively common, and thus constitute a large proportion of all patients who have PH [156]. In most cases, hypoxia is thought to produce PH via hypoxic vasoconstrictive mechanisms in pulmonary arteriolar smooth muscle, as well as indirectly by stimulating vascular remodeling by changing the balance of endogenous vasoregulators [157].

Chronic obstructive pulmonary disease is epidemiologically the most important cause of PH associated with respiratory disease. Between 12 and 24 million individuals in the United States suffer from COPD, and it is estimated that PH is present in 20% to 35% [158–160]. In most

patients who have COPD, the magnitude of PH is mild (mPAP 35–40 mm Hg), and correlates with the degree of air flow obstruction and hypoxemia [161]. Progression of PH in patients who have COPD at a rate of approximately 0.5 mm Hg in mPAP per year has been described [160,162].

Pulmonary hypertension is associated with decreased survival in COPD. As a dramatic example, a 1971 study reported the 5-year survival rate in patients who had COPD was less than 10% when the mPAP exceeded 45 mm Hg, but was 90% when the mPAP was less than 25 mm Hg [163]. Long-term oxygen therapy is the mainstay of treatment, with benefits in hemodynamics and mortality described in COPD patients in whom PaO_2 is maintained above 55 mm Hg (or greater than 60 mm Hg if evidence of PH is present) [164–166]. There is no established role for prostanoids, endothelin receptor antagonists, or phosphodiesterase inhibitors in the treatment of COPD-associated PH at present [156].

Obstructive sleep apnea (OSA) is another common condition, and results in disordered sleep, hypoventilation, and chronic hypoxemia [167]. It is estimated that in the United States, approximately 3 million men and 1.5 million women suffer from the disorder, and that approximately 20% of these individuals have PH [156,168]. In patients who have concomitant lung disease or extreme obesity, the prevalence of PH is increased further. In most cases, PH associated with OSA is mild, with mPAP remaining below 35 mm Hg [169]. Therapy is based upon relieving sleep-disordered breathing and hypoxia, usually by employing continuous positive airway pressure (CPAP) and supplemental oxygen as necessary.

Interstitial lung disease also may result in PH, both via hypoxic mechanisms and because of compromise of the pulmonary vascular bed by interstitial fibrosis. Unlike in COPD, moderate to severe PH is not unusual in this setting [156]. The contribution of PH to the patient's impaired functional status may be difficult to differentiate from that of restrictive ventilatory physiology, anemia, or muscle weakness related to glucocorticoid therapy. Interstitial lung disease and PH coexist in up to 30% of patients who have progressive systemic sclerosis; the incidence and prevalence of PH in other types of interstitial lung disease are not well-characterized [170]. A negative association of PH with survival has been documented most thoroughly in patients who have the scleroderma spectrum of diseases and in sarcoidosis [171,172].

In treating PH associated with interstitial lung disease, correction of hypoxemia is essential. Clinical trials of prostanoids, endothelin receptor antagonists, or phosphodiesterase inhibitors in patients who have significant interstitial lung disease are ongoing.

Chronic thromboembolic pulmonary hypertension

Chronic thromboembolic pulmonary hypertension (CTEPH) is a clinicopathologic entity characterized by progressive PH and right ventricular failure in the presence of large pulmonary arteries occluded by intraluminal fibrous material that is consistent with organized thromboemboli. The magnitude of hemodynamic abnormalities frequently exceeds the observed degree of large vessel obstruction, suggesting that diffuse pulmonary vascular remodeling in small vessels plays a major role in disease progression. It is generally accepted that the condition results from single or multiple episodes of acute pulmonary thromboembolism that fail to resolve normally via endogenous fibrinolytic mechanisms [173]. Treatment ideally involves surgical pulmonary thromboendarterectomy, with medical therapy playing an adjunctive role in patients who are not surgical candidates, or in patients who fail to improve optimally following the procedure [174].

Between 0.01% and 3.1% of survivors of an episode of acute pulmonary thromboembolism appear to develop CTEPH [175,176]. Among patients who have massive pulmonary embolism, the rate of progression to CTEPH appears significantly higher. As an example, one study of 227 patients who had acute pulmonary embolism and obstruction of at least 50% of the pulmonary vascular bed found that 20% developed CTEPH during a 4- to 8-year follow-up period [177].

It is unclear what mechanisms are culprit in the minority of patients who have acute pulmonary embolism and who develop CTEPH. The only thrombophilic abnormality that has consistently been over-represented among CTEPH patients is the presence of antiphospholipid antibodies, reported in 10% to 20% of CTEPH patients [174,178,179]. Most studies have not found abnormalities of coagulation or fibrinolysis, such as Factor V Leiden or deficiencies of protein C, protein S, or Antithrombin III, to be more common in patients who have CTEPH than the general population. More recently potential roles for elevated Factor VIII or homocysteine levels have been suggested in small series [180,181].

Summary

The epidemiology of PAH is changing. Remarkable advances in understanding the pathobiology and clinical care in PAH have resulted in improved exercise capacity and survival. Despite such important progress, however, neither exercise capacity nor survival is normal. Controlled studies have only just begun to evaluate the role of combinations of therapies, as well as the utility of genetic and other biomarkers to predict a patient's response. It is hoped that such studies will allow for better targeting of therapy to individual patients who have PAH. They may also lead to improvements in the care of patients who have other forms of PH. Expanding therapeutic options might also allow consideration of end points beyond physical function and survival, such as health-related quality of life, when planning care [182–187]. Indeed, the continued suitability of measurements currently used to assess improvement is debated, as is the appropriate duration of these studies [188,189]. Together, these advances in therapy and the end points used to study them will continue to change our assessment of the epidemiology of PAH.

References

[1] Romberg. Uber Sklerose der Lungen Arterie. Dtsch Arch Klin Med 1891;48:197–206 [in German].

[2] Fishman AP. A century of pulmonary hemodynamics. Am J Respir Crit Care Med 2004;170(2):109–13.

[3] Dresdale DT, Schultz M, Michtom RJ. Primary pulmonary hypertension I., clinical and hemodynamic study. Am J Med 1951;11(6):686–705.

[4] Rubin LJ. Diagnosis and management of pulmonary arterial hypertension: ACCP evidence-based clinical practice guidelines. Chest 2004;126(1 Suppl): 7S–10S.

[5] Wagenvoort Ca, Wagenvoort H. Primary pulmonary hypertension: a pathologic study of the lung vessles in 156 classically diagnosed cases. Circulation 1970; 42:1163–84.

[6] Curnock A, Dweik R, Higgins B, et al. High prevalence of hypothyroidism in patients with primary pulmonary hypertension. Am J Med Sci 1999; 318(5):289–92.

[7] Lozano H, Sharma C. Reversible pulmonary hypertension, tricuspid regurgitation and right-sided heart failure associated with hyperthyroidism: case report and review of the literature. Cardiol Rev 2004;12(6):299–305.

[8] Chambers CD, Hernandez-Diaz S, Van Marter LJ, et al. Selective serotonin-reuptake inhibitors and risk of persistent pulmonary hypertension of the newborn. N Engl J Med 2006;354(6):579–87.

[9] Abenhaim L, Moride Y, Brenot F, et al. Appetite-suppressant drugs and the risk of primary pulmonary hypertension. International Primary Pulmonary Hypertension Study Group. N Engl J Med 1996; 335(9):609–16.

[10] Group IPPHS. The International Primary Pulmonary Hypertension Study. Chest Supplement 1994; 105(2):37S–41S.

[11] Appelbaum L, Yigla M, Bendayan D, et al. Primary pulmonary hypertension in Israel: a national survey. Chest 2001;119(6):1801–6.

[12] Humbert M, Sitbon O, Chaouat A, et al. Pulmonary arterial hypertension in France: results from a national registry. Am J Respir Crit Care Med 2006;173(9):1023–30.

[13] Rich S, Dantzker DR, Ayres SM, et al. Primary pulmonary hypertension. A national prospective study. Ann Intern Med 1987;107(2):216–23.

[14] Brenot F. Primary pulmonary hypertension: case series from France. Chest Supplement 1994;105(4): 33S–6S.

[15] Sandoval J, Bauerle O, Palomar A, et al. Survival in primary pulmonary hypertension. Validation of a prognostic equation. Circulation 1994;89(4): 1733–44.

[16] Okada O, Tanabe N, Yasuda J, et al. Prediction of life expectancy in patients with primary pulmonary hypertension. A retrospective nationwide survey from 1980–1990. Intern Med 1999;38(1): 12–6.

[17] McLaughlin VV, Presberg KW, Doyle RL, et al. Prognosis of pulmonary arterial hypertension: ACCP evidence-based clinical practice guidelines. Chest 2004;126(1 Suppl):78S–92S.

[18] Fuster V, Steele PM, Edwards WD, et al. Primary pulmonary hypertension: natural history and the importance of thrombosis. Circulation 1984;70(4): 580–7.

[19] Kawut SM, Horn EM, Berekashvili KK, et al. New predictors of outcome in idiopathic pulmonary arterial hypertension. Am J Cardiol 2005;95(2): 199–203.

[20] D'Alonzo GE, Barst RJ, Ayres SM, et al. Survival in patients with primary pulmonary hypertension. Results from a national prospective registry. Ann Intern Med 1991;115(5):343–9.

[21] Rajasekhar D, Balakrishnan KG, Venkitachalam CG, et al. Primary pulmonary hypertension: natural history and prognostic factors. Indian Heart J 1994;46(3):165–70.

[22] McLaughlin VV, Shillington A, Rich S. Survival in primary pulmonary hypertension: the impact of epoprostenol therapy. Circulation 2002;106(12): 1477–82.

[23] Sitbon O, Humbert M, Nunes H, et al. Long-term intravenous epoprostenol infusion in primary pulmonary hypertension: prognostic factors and survival. J Am Coll Cardiol 2002;40(4):780–8.

[24] Bossone E, Paciocco G, Iarussi D, et al. The prognostic role of the ECG in primary pulmonary hypertension. Chest 2002;121(2):513–8.

[25] Kuhn KP, Byrne DW, Arbogast PG, et al. Outcome in 91 consecutive patients with pulmonary arterial hypertension receiving epoprostenol. Am J Respir Crit Care Med 2003;167(4):580–6.

[26] Miyamoto S, Nagaya N, Satoh T, et al. Clinical correlates and prognostic significance of six-minute walk test in patients with primary pulmonary hypertension. Comparison with cardiopulmonary exercise testing. Am J Respir Crit Care Med 2000; 161(2 Pt 1):487–92.

[27] Barst RJ, Rubin LJ, Long WA, et al. A comparison of continuous intravenous epoprostenol (prostacyclin) with conventional therapy for primary pulmonary hypertension. The Primary Pulmonary Hypertension Study Group. N Engl J Med 1996; 334(5):296–302.

[28] Wensel R, Opitz CF, Anker SD, et al. Assessment of survival in patients with primary pulmonary hypertension: importance of cardiopulmonary exercise testing. Circulation 2002;106(3):319–24.

[29] Raymond RJ, Hinderliter AL, Willis I, et al. Echocardiographic predictors of adverse outcomes in primary pulmonary hypertension. Journal of the American College of Cardiology 2002;39(7): 1214–9.

[30] Hinderliter AL, Willis PWt, Long W, et al. Frequency and prognostic significance of pericardial effusion in primary pulmonary hypertension. PPH Study Group. Primary pulmonary hypertension. Am J Cardiol 1999;84(4):481–4, A10.

[31] Eysmann SB, Palevsky HI, Reichek N, et al. Two-dimensional and Doppler-echocardiographic and cardiac catheterization correlates of survival in primary pulmonary hypertension. Circulation 1989; 80(2):353–60.

[32] Yeo TC, Dujardin KS, Tei C, et al. Value of a Doppler-derived index combining systolic and diastolic time intervals in predicting outcome in primary pulmonary hypertension. Am J Cardiol 1998;81(9):1157–61.

[33] Forfia P, Fisher MR, Mathai SC, et al. Tricuspid annular displacement predicts survival in pulmonary hypertension. Am J Respir Crit Care Med 2006; 174(9):1034–41.

[34] Friedman E, Palevsky HI, Taichman DB. Classification and prognosis of pulmonary arterial hypertension. In: Mandel J, Taichman DB, editors. Pulmonary vascular disease. Philadelphia: Elsevier Science; 2006. p. 66–82.

[35] Nagaya N, Uematsu M, Satoh T, et al. Serum uric acid levels correlate with the severity and the mortality of primary pulmonary hypertension. Am J Respir Crit Care Med 1999;160(2):487–92.

[36] Nagaya N, Nishikimi T, Uematsu M, et al. Plasma brain natriuretic peptide as a prognostic indicator

in patients with primary pulmonary hypertension. Circulation 2000;102(8):865–70.

[37] Voelkel MA, Wynne KM, Badesch DB, et al. Hyperuricemia in severe pulmonary hypertension. Chest 2000;117(1):19–24.

[38] Lopes AA, Maeda NY, Goncalves RC, et al. Endothelial cell dysfunction correlates differentially with survival in primary and secondary pulmonary hypertension. Am Heart J 2000;139(4):618–23.

[39] Shitrit D, Bendayan D, Bar-Gil-Shitrit A, et al. Significance of a plasma D-dimer test in patients with primary pulmonary hypertension. Chest 2002; 122(5):1674–8.

[40] Torbicki A, Kurzyna M, Kuca P, et al. Detectable serum cardiac troponin T as a marker of poor prognosis among patients with chronic precapillary pulmonary hypertension. Circulation 2003;108(7):844–8.

[41] Nootens M, Kaufmann E, Rector T, et al. Neurohormonal activation in patients with right ventricular failure from pulmonary hypertension: relation to hemodynamic variables and endothelin levels. J Am Coll Cardiol 1995;26(7):1581–5.

[42] Nagaya N, Nishikimi T, Uematsu M, et al. Plasma brain natriuretic peptide as a prognostic indicator in patients with primary pulmonary hypertension. J Cardiol 2001;37(2):110–1.

[43] Hoeper MM, Galie N, Murali S, et al. Outcome after cardiopulmonary resuscitation in patients with pulmonary arterial hypertension. Am J Respir Crit Care Med 2002;165(3):341–4.

[44] Morgan JM, Griffiths M, du Bois RM, et al. Hypoxic pulmonary vasoconstriction in systemic sclerosis and primary pulmonary hypertension. Chest 1991;99(3):551–6.

[45] Krasuski RA, Warner JJ, Wang A, et al. Inhaled nitric oxide selectively dilates pulmonary vasculature in adult patients with pulmonary hypertension, irrespective of etiology. J Am Coll Cardiol 2000;36(7):2204–11.

[46] Rubin LJ, Groves BM, Reeves JT, et al. Prostacyclin-induced acute pulmonary vasodilation in primary pulmonary hypertension. Circulation 1982; 66(2):334–8.

[47] Sitbon O, Brenot F, Denjean A, et al. Inhaled nitric oxide as a screening vasodilator agent in primary pulmonary hypertension. A dose-response study and comparison with prostacyclin. Am J Respir Crit Care Med 1995;151(2 Pt 1):384–9.

[48] Galie N, Ussia G, Passarelli P, et al. Role of pharmacologic tests in the treatment of primary pulmonary hypertension. Am J Cardiol 1995;75:55A–62A.

[49] Nootens M, Schrader B, Kaufmann E, et al. Comparative acute effects of adenosine and prostacyclin in primary pulmonary hypertension. Chest 1995; 107(1):54–7.

[50] Palevsky HI, Long W, Crow J, et al. Prostacyclin and acetylcholine as screening agents for acute pulmonary vasodilator responsiveness in primary pulmonary hypertension. Circulation 1990;82(6): 2018–26.

[51] Barst RJ, McGoon M, Torbicki A, et al. Diagnosis and differential assessment of pulmonary arterial hypertension. J Am Coll Cardiol 2004;43(12 Suppl S):40S–7S.

[52] Badesch DB, Abman SH, Ahearn GS, et al. Medical therapy for pulmonary arterial hypertension: ACCP evidence-based clinical practice guidelines. Chest 2004;126(1 Suppl):35S–62S.

[53] Rich S, Kaufmann E, Levy PS. The effect of high doses of calcium-channel blockers on survival in primary pulmonary hypertension. N Engl J Med 1992;327(2):76–81.

[54] Sitbon O, Humbert M, Jais X, et al. Long-term response to calcium channel blockers in idiopathic pulmonary arterial hypertension. Circulation 2005;111(23):3105–11.

[55] Lang G, Klepetko W. Lung transplantation for end-stage primary pulmonary hypertension. Ann Transplant 2004;9(3):25–32.

[56] Robbins IM, Christman BW, Newman JH, et al. A survey of diagnostic practices and the use of epoprostenol in patients with primary pulmonary hypertension. Chest 1998;114(5):1269–75.

[57] McLaughlin VV, Sitbon O, Badesch DB, et al. Survival with first-line bosentan in patients with primary pulmonary hypertension. Eur Respir J 2005; 25(2):244–9.

[58] Sitbon O, et al. Survival in patients with class III idiopathic pulmonary arterial hypertension treated with first-line oral bosentan compared with an historical cohort of patients started on i.v. epoprostenol. Thorax 2005;60:1025–30.

[59] Bjornsson J, Edwards WD. Primary pulmonary hypertension: a histopathologic study of 80 cases. Mayo Clin Proc 1985;60(1):16–25.

[60] Cohen M, Fuster V, Edwards WD. Anticoagulation in the treatment of pulmonary hypertension. In: Fishman AP, editor. The pulmonary circulation: normal and abnormal. mechanisms, management, and the national registry. Philadelphia: University of Pennsylvania Press; 1990. p. 501–10.

[61] Frank H, Mlczoch J, Huber K, et al. The effect of anticoagulant therapy in primary and anorectic drug-induced pulmonary hypertension. Chest 1997; 112(3):714–21.

[62] Doyle RL, McCrory D, Channick RN, et al. Surgical treatments/interventions for pulmonary arterial hypertension: ACCP evidence-based clinical practice guidelines. Chest 2004;126(1 Suppl):63S–71S.

[63] Trulock EP, Edwards LB, Taylor DO, et al. The Registry of the International Society for Heart and Lung Transplantation: twenty-first official adult lung and heart-lung transplant report–2004. J Heart Lung Transplant 2004;23(7):804–15.

[64] Edelman J, Palevsky HI. Has prostacyclin replaced transplantation as the treatment for primary

pulmonary hypertension. Clinical Pulmonary Medicine 2000;7(2):90–6.

[65] Ahya V, Sager JS. Lung transplantation for pulmonary arterial hypertension. In: Mandel J, Taichman DB, editors. Pulmonary vascular disease. Philadelphia: Elsevier Science; 2006. p. 119–31.

[66] Loyd JE, Primm RK, Newman JH. Familial primary pulmonary hypertension: clinical patterns. Am Rev Respir Dis 1984;129(1):194–7.

[67] Loyd JE, Butler MG, Foroud TM, et al. Genetic anticipation and abnormal gender ratio at birth in familial primary pulmonary hypertension. Am J Respir Crit Care Med 1995;152(1):93–7.

[68] Nichols WC, Koller DL, Slovis B, et al. Localization of the gene for familial primary pulmonary hypertension to chromosome 2q31-q32. Nat Genet 1997;15(3):277–80.

[69] Morse JH, Jones AC, Barst RJ, et al. Mapping of familial primary pulmonary hypertension locus (PPH1) to chromosome 2q31-q32. Circulation 1997; 95(12):2603–6.

[70] Deng Z, Morse JH, Slager SL, et al. Familial primary pulmonary hypertension (gene PPH1) is caused by mutations in the bone morphogenetic protein receptor-II gene. Am J Hum Genet 2000; 67(3):737–44.

[71] Lane KB, Machado RD, Pauciulo MW, et al. Heterozygous germline mutations in BMPR2, encoding a TGF-beta receptor, cause familial primary pulmonary hypertension. The International PPH Consortium. Nat Genet 2000;26(1):81–4.

[72] Machado RD, Aldred MA, James V, et al. Mutations of the TGF-beta type II receptor BMPR2 in pulmonary arterial hypertension. Hum Mutat 2006; 27(2):121–32.

[73] Elliott CG. Genetics of pulmonary arterial hypertension. In: Mandel J, Taichman DB, editors. Pulmonary vascular disease. Philadelphia: Elsevier Science; 2006. p. 50–65.

[74] Trembath RC, Thomson JR, Machado RD, et al. Clinical and molecular genetic features of pulmonary hypertension in patients with hereditary hemorrhagic telangiectasia. N Engl J Med 2001;345(5): 325–34.

[75] Chaouat A, Coulet F, Favre C, et al. Endoglin germline mutation in a patient with hereditary haemorrhagic telangiectasia and dexfenfluramine associated pulmonary arterial hypertension. Thorax 2004;59(5):446–8.

[76] Harrison RE, Flanagan JA, Sankelo M, et al. Molecular and functional analysis identifies ALK-1 as the predominant cause of pulmonary hypertension related to hereditary haemorrhagic telangiectasia. J Med Genet 2003;40(12):865–71.

[77] Abdalla SA, Gallione CJ, Barst RJ, et al. Primary pulmonary hypertension in families with hereditary haemorrhagic telangiectasia. Eur Respir J 2004; 23(3):373–7.

[78] Thomson JR, Machado RD, Pauciulo MW, et al. Sporadic primary pulmonary hypertension is associated with germline mutations of the gene encoding BMPR-II, a receptor member of the TGF-beta family. J Med Genet 2000;37(10): 741–5.

[79] Newman JH, Wheeler L, Lane KB, et al. Mutation in the gene for bone morphogenetic protein receptor II as a cause of primary pulmonary hypertension in a large kindred. N Engl J Med 2001; 345(5):319–24.

[80] Newman JH, Trembath RC, Morse JA, et al. Genetic basis of pulmonary arterial hypertension: current understanding and future directions. J Am Coll Cardiol 2004;43(12 Suppl S):33S–9S.

[81] Humbert M, Deng Z, Simonneau G, et al. BMPR2 germline mutations in pulmonary hypertension associated with fenfluramine derivatives. Eur Respir J 2002;20(3):518–23.

[82] Roberts KE, McElroy JJ, Wong WP, et al. BMPR2 mutations in pulmonary arterial hypertension with congenital heart disease. Eur Respir J 2004;24(3): 371–4.

[83] Runo JR, Vnencak-Jones CL, Prince M, et al. Pulmonary veno-occlusive disease caused by an inherited mutation in bone morphogenetic protein receptor II. Am J Respir Crit Care Med 2003; 167(6):889–94.

[84] Elliott G, Alexander G, Leppert M, et al. Coancestry in apparently sporadic primary pulmonary hypertension. Chest 1995;108(4):973–7.

[85] Grunig E, Janssen B, Mereles D, et al. Abnormal pulmonary artery pressure response in asymptomatic carriers of primary pulmonary hypertension gene. Circulation 2000;102(10):1145–50.

[86] Mukerjee D, St George D, Coleiro B, et al. Prevalence and outcome in systemic sclerosis associated pulmonary arterial hypertension: application of a registry approach. Ann Rheum Dis 2003;62(11): 1088–93.

[87] Stupi AM, Steen VD, Owens GR, et al. Pulmonary hypertension in the CREST syndrome variant of systemic sclerosis. Arthritis Rheum 1986;29(4): 515–24.

[88] MacGregor AJ, Canavan R, Knight C, et al. Pulmonary hypertension in systemic sclerosis: risk factors for progression and consequences for survival. Rheumatology (Oxford) 2001;40(4):453–9.

[89] Kawut SM, Taichman DB, Archer-Chicko CL, et al. Hemodynamics and survival in patients with pulmonary arterial hypertension related to systemic sclerosis. Chest 2003;123(2):344–50.

[90] Steen VD, Medsger TA Jr. Severe organ involvement in systemic sclerosis with diffuse scleroderma. Arthritis Rheum 2000;43(11):2437–44.

[91] Rubin LJ, Badesch DB, Barst RJ, et al. Bosentan therapy for pulmonary arterial hypertension. N Engl J Med 2002;346(12):896–903.

[92] Shen JY, Chen SL, Wu YX, et al. Pulmonary hypertension in systemic lupus erythematosus. Rheumatol Int 1999;18(4):147–51.

[93] Badui E, Garcia-Rubi D, Robles E, et al. Cardiovascular manifestations in systemic lupus erythematosus. Prospective study of 100 patients. Angiology 1985;36(7):431–41.

[94] Li EK, Tam LS. Pulmonary hypertension in systemic lupus erythematosus: clinical association and survival in 18 patients. J Rheumatol 1999; 26(9):1923–9.

[95] Simonson JS, Schiller NB, Petri M, et al. Pulmonary hypertension in systemic lupus erythematosus. J Rheumatol 1989;16(7):918–25.

[96] Winslow TM, Ossipov MA, Fazio GP, et al. Five-year follow-up study of the prevalence and progression of pulmonary hypertension in systemic lupus erythematosus. Am Heart J 1995;129(3):510–5.

[97] Speich R, Jenni R, Opravil M, et al. Primary pulmonary hypertension in HIV infection. Chest 1991;100(5):1268–71.

[98] Zuber JP, Calmy A, Evison JM, et al. Pulmonary arterial hypertension related to HIV infection: improved hemodynamics and survival associated with antiretroviral therapy. Clin Infect Dis 2004; 38(8):1178–85.

[99] Petitpretz P, Brenot F, Azarian R, et al. Pulmonary hypertension in patients with human immunodeficiency virus infection. Comparison with primary pulmonary hypertension. Circulation 1994;89(6): 2722–7.

[100] Nunes H, Humbert M, Sitbon O, et al. Prognostic factors for survival in human immunodeficiency virus-associated pulmonary arterial hypertension. Am J Respir Crit Care Med 2003;167(10):1433–9.

[101] Swanson K, Krowka M. Portopulmonary hypertension. In: Mandel J, Taichman DB, editors. Pulmonary vascular disease. Philadelphia: Elsevier Science; 2006. p. 132–42.

[102] Benjaminov FS, Prentice M, Sniderman KW, et al. Portopulmonary hypertension in decompensated cirrhosis with refractory ascites. Gut 2003;52(9): 1355–62.

[103] McDonnell PJ, Toye PA, Hutchins GM. Primary pulmonary hypertension and cirrhosis: are they related? Am Rev Respir Dis 1983;127(4):437–41.

[104] Ramsay MA, Simpson BR, Nguyen AT, et al. Severe pulmonary hypertension in liver transplant candidates. Liver Transplantation & Surgery 1997; 3(5):494–500.

[105] Robalino BD, Moodie DS. Association between primary pulmonary hypertension and portal hypertension: analysis of its pathophysiology and clinical, laboratory and hemodynamic manifestations. Journal of the American College of Cardiology 1991;17(2):492–8.

[106] Kawut SM, Taichman DB, Ahya VN, et al. Hemodynamics and survival of patients with portopulmonary hypertension. Liver Transpl 2005;11(9):1107–1011.

[107] Krowka MJ, Mandell MS, Ramsay MA, et al. Hepatopulmonary syndrome and portopulmonary hypertension: a report of the multicenter liver transplant database. Liver Transplantation 2004; 10(2):174–82.

[108] Krowka MJ, Plevak DJ, Findlay JY, et al. Pulmonary hemodynamics and perioperative cardiopulmonary-related mortality in patients with portopulmonary hypertension undergoing liver transplantation. Liver Transplantation 2000;6(4): 443–50.

[109] Kuo PC, Johnson LB, Plotkin JS, et al. Continuous intravenous infusion of epoprostenol for the treatment of portopulmonary hypertension. Transplantation 1997;63:604–16.

[110] Findlay JY, Plevak DJ, Krowka MJ, et al. Progressive splenomegaly after epoprostenol therapy in portopulmonary hypertension. Liver Transplantation & Surgery 1999;5(5):381–7.

[111] Krowka MJ, Frantz RP, McGoon MD, et al. Improvement in pulmonary hemodynamics during intravenous epoprostenol (prostacyclin): a study of 15 patients with moderate to severe portopulmonary hypertension. Hepatology 1999;30(3):641–8.

[112] Kahler CM, Graziadei I, Wiedermann CJ, et al. Successful use of continuous intravenous prostacyclin in a patient with severe portopulmonary hypertension. Wien Klin Wochenschr 2000;112(14): 637–40.

[113] Makisalo H, Koivusalo A, Vakkuri A, et al. Sildenafil for portopulmonary hypertension in a patient undergoing liver transplantation. Liver Transplantation 2004;10(7):945–50.

[114] Minder S, Fischler M, Muellhaupt B, et al. Intravenous iloprost bridging to orthotopic liver transplantation in portopulmonary hypertension. Eur Respir J 2004;24(4):703–7.

[115] Rodriguez-Roisin R, Krowka MJ, Herve P, et al. Pulmonary-Hepatic Vascular Disorders Scientific Committee ERS Task Force. Eur Respir J 2004; 24:861–80.

[116] Gurtner HP. Aminorex pulmonary hypertension. In: Fishman AP, editor. The pulmonary circulation: normal and abnormal. Philadelphia: University of Pennsylvania Press; 1990. p. 397–411.

[117] Brenot F. Risk factors for primary pulmonary hypertension. In: Rubin LJ, Rich S, editors. Primary pulmonary hypertension. New York: Marcel Dekker; 1996. p. 131–49.

[118] Brenot F, Herve P, Petitpretz P, et al. Primary pulmonary hypertension and fenfluramine use. Br Heart J 1993;70(6):537–41.

[119] Rich S, Rubin LJ, Walker AM, et al. Anorexigens and pulmonary hypertension in the United States: results from the surveillance of North American pulmonary hypertension. Chest 2000;117(3):870–4.

[120] Simonneau G, Fartoukh M, Sitbon O, et al. Primary pulmonary hypertension associated with the use of fenfluramine derivatives. Chest 1998;114 (3 Suppl):195S–9S.

[121] Rich S, Shillington A, McLaughlin V. Comparison of survival in patients with pulmonary hypertension associated with fenfluramine to patients with primary pulmonary hypertension. Am J Cardiol 2003;92(11):1366–8.

[122] Machado RF, Gladwin MT. Hemolytic anemia associated pulmonary hypertension. In: Mandel J, Taichman DB, editors. Pulmonary vascular disease. Philaelphia: Elsevier; 2006. p. 170–87.

[123] Morris CR, Kato GJ, Poljakovic M, et al. Dysregulated arginine metabolism, hemolysis-associated pulmonary hypertension, and mortality in sickle cell disease. JAMA 2005;294(1):81–90.

[124] Castro O. Pulmonary hypertension in sickle cell disease and thalassemia. In: Peacock AJ, Rubin L, editors. Pulmonary circulation: diseases and their treatment. London: Arnold Publishers; 2004. p. 237–43.

[125] Jootar P, Fucharoen S. Cardiac involvement in beta-thalassemia/hemoglobin E disease: clinical and hemodynamic findings. Southeast Asian J Trop Med Public Health 1990;21(2):269–73.

[126] Du Z, Roguin N, Milgram E, et al. Pulmonary hypertension in patients with thalassemia major. Am Heart J 1997;134(3):532–7.

[127] Aessopos A, Farmakis D, Deftereos S, et al. Thalassemia heart disease: a comparative evaluation of thalassemia major and thalassemia intermedia. Chest 2005;127(5):1523–30.

[128] Aessopos A, Farmakis D. Pulmonary hypertension in {beta}-thalassemia. Ann N Y Acad Sci 2005; 1054:342–9.

[129] Gladwin MT, Sachdev V, Jison ML, et al. Pulmonary hypertension as a risk factor for death in patients with sickle cell disease. N Engl J Med 2004; 350(9):886–95.

[130] Haque AK, Gokhale S, Rampy BA, et al. Pulmonary hypertension in sickle cell hemoglobinopathy: a clinicopathologic study of 20 cases. Hum Pathol 2002;33(10):1037–43.

[131] Verresen D, De Backer W, Van Meerbeeck J, et al. Spherocytosis and pulmonary hypertension coincidental occurrence or causal relationship? Eur Respir J 1991;4(5):629–31.

[132] Heller PG, Grinberg AR, Lencioni M, et al. Pulmonary hypertension in paroxysmal nocturnal hemoglobinuria. Chest 1992;102(2):642–3.

[133] Castro O, Hoque M, Brown BD. Pulmonary hypertension in sickle cell disease: cardiac catheterization results and survival. Blood 2003;101(4): 1257–61.

[134] Powars D, Weidman JA, Odom-Maryon T, et al. Sickle cell chronic lung disease: prior morbidity and the risk of pulmonary failure. Medicine (Baltimore) 1988;67(1):66–76.

[135] Sutton LL, Castro O, Cross DJ, et al. Pulmonary hypertension in sickle cell disease. Am J Cardiol 1994;74(6):626–8.

[136] Machado RF, Martyr S, Kato GJ, et al. Sildenafil therapy in patients with sickle cell disease and pulmonary hypertension. Br J Haematol 2005;130(3): 445–53.

[137] Derchi G, Forni GL, Formisano F, et al. Efficacy and safety of sildenafil in the treatment of severe pulmonary hypertension in patients with hemoglobinopathies. Haematologica 2005;90(4): 452–8.

[138] Mandel J. Pulmonary veno-occlusive disease. In: Mandel J, Taichman DB, editors. Pulmonary vascular disease. Philadelphia: Elsevier Science; 2006. p. 157–69.

[139] Mandel J, Mark EJ, Hales CA. Pulmonary veno-occlusive disease. Am J Respir Crit Care Med 2000;162(5):1964–73.

[140] Simonneau G, Galie N, Rubin LJ, et al. Clinical classification of pulmonary hypertension. J Am Coll Cardiol 2004;43(12 Suppl S):5S–12S.

[141] Holcomb BW Jr, Loyd JE, Ely EW, et al. Pulmonary veno-occlusive disease: a case series and new observations. Chest 2000;118(6):1671–9.

[142] Swensen SJ, Tashjian JH, Myers JL, et al. Pulmonary venooclusive disease: CT findings in eight patients. AJR Am J Roentgenol 1996;167(4): 937–40.

[143] Palmer S, Robinson L, Wang A, et al. Massive pulmonary edema and death after prostacyclin infusion in a patient with pulmonary veno-occlusive disease. Chest 1998;113:237.

[144] Okumura H, Nagaya N, Kyotani S, et al. Effects of continuous IV prostacyclin in a patient with pulmonary veno-occlusive disease. Chest 2002;122(3): 1096–8.

[145] Izbicki G, Shitrit D, Schechtman I, et al. Recurrence of pulmonary veno-occlusive disease after heart-lung transplantation. J Heart Lung Transplant 2005;24(5):635–7.

[146] Thadani U, Burrow C, Whitaker W, et al. Pulmonary veno-occlusive disease. Q J Med 1975; 44(173):133–59.

[147] Wagenvoort CA. Pulmonary veno-occlusive disease. Entity or syndrome? Chest 1976;69(1):82–6.

[148] Davies P, Reid L. Pulmonary veno-occlusive disease in siblings: case reports and morphometric study. Hum Pathol 1982;13(10):911–5.

[149] Devereux G, Evans MJ, Kerr KM, et al. Pulmonary veno-occlusive disease complicating Felty's syndrome. Respir Med 1998;92(8):1089–91.

[150] Hourseau M, Capron F, Nunes H, et al. Pulmonary veno-occlusive disease in a patient with HIV infection. A case report with autopsy findings. Ann Pathol 2002;22(6):472–5.

[151] Joselson R, Warnock M. Pulmonary veno-occlusive disease after chemotherapy. Hum Pathol 1983;14(1):88–91.

[152] Knight BK, Rose AG. Pulmonary veno-occlusive disease after chemotherapy. Thorax 1985;40(11): 874–5.

[153] Townend JN, Roberts DH, Jones EL, et al. Fatal pulmonary venoocclusive disease after use of oral contraceptives. Am Heart J 1992;124(6):1643–4.

[154] Voordes C, Kuipers J, Elema J. Familial pulmonary veno-occlusive disease: a case report. Thorax 1977;32(6):763–6.

[155] Williams L, Fussell S, Veith R, et al. Pulmonary veno-occlusive disease in an adult following bone marrow transplantation. Case report and review of the literature. Chest 1996;109(5):1388–91.

[156] Gerke A, Mandel J. Pulmonary hypertension secondary to chronic respiratory disease. In: Mandel J, Taichman DB, editors. Pulmonary vascular disease. Philadelphia: Elsevier Science; 2006. p. 143–56.

[157] Shimoda L, Sham J, Sylvester J. Altered pulmonary vasoreactivity in the chronically hypoxic lung. Physiol Res 2000;49(5):549–60.

[158] Burrows B, Kettel LJ, Niden AH, et al. Patterns of cardiovascular dysfunction in chronic obstructive lung disease. N Engl J Med 1972;286(17):912–8.

[159] Weitzenblum E, Hirth C, Ducolone A, et al. Prognostic value of pulmonary artery pressure in chronic obstructive pulmonary disease. Thorax 1981;36(10): 752–8.

[160] Weitzenblum E, Sautegeau A, Ehrhart M, et al. Long-term course of pulmonary arterial pressure in chronic obstructive pulmonary disease. Am Rev Respir Dis 1984;130(6):993–8.

[161] Doi M, Nakano K, Hiramoto T, et al. Significance of pulmonary artery pressure in emphysema patients with mild-to-moderate hypoxemia. Respir Med 2003;97(8):915–20.

[162] Kessler R, Faller M, Weitzenblum E, et al. "Natural history" of pulmonary hypertension in a series of 131 patients with chronic obstructive lung disease. Am J Respir Crit Care Med 2001;164(2):219–24.

[163] Bishop J. Role of hypoxia in the pulmonary hypertension of chronic bronchitis and emphysema. Scand J Respir Dis Suppl 1971;77:61–5.

[164] Continuous or nocturnal oxygen therapy in hypoxemic chronic obstructive lung disease: a clinical trial. Nocturnal Oxygen Therapy Trial Group. Ann Intern Med 1980;93:391–8.

[165] Long term domiciliary oxygen therapy in chronic hypoxic cor pulmonale complicating chronic bronchitis and emphysema. Report of the Medical Research Council Working Party. Lancet 1981; 1:681–6.

[166] Zielinski J, Tobiasz M, Hawrylkiewicz I, et al. Effects of long-term oxygen therapy on pulmonary hemodynamics in COPD patients: a 6-year prospective study. Chest 1998;113(1):65–70.

[167] White D. Sleep apnea. Proc Am Thorac Soc 2006; 3(1):124–8.

[168] Namen A, Dunagan D, Fleischer A, et al. Increased physician-reported sleep apnea: the National Ambulatory Medical Care Survey. Chest 2002; 121(6):1741–7.

[169] Laks L, Lehrhaft B, Grunstein RR, et al. Pulmonary hypertension in obstructive sleep apnoea. Eur Respir J 1995;8(4):537–41.

[170] Ungerer R, Tashkin D, Furst D, et al. Prevalence and clinical correlates of pulmonary arterial hypertension in progressive systemic sclerosis. Am J Med 1983;75(1):65–74.

[171] Shorr A, Davies D, Nathan S. Predicting mortality in patients with sarcoidosis awaiting lung transplantation. Chest 2003;124(3):922–88.

[172] Trad S, Amoura Z, Beigelman C, et al. Pulmonary arterial hypertension is a major mortality factor in diffuse systemic sclerosis, independent of interstitial lung disease. Arthritis Rheum 2006;54(1):184–91.

[173] Fedullo P, Rubin L, Kerr K, et al. The natural history of acute and chronic thromboembolic disease: the search for the missing link. Eur Respir J 2000; 15(3):435–7.

[174] Chin K, Fedullo PF. Chronic thromboembolic pulmonary hypertension. In: Mandel J, Taichman DB, editors. Pulmonary vascular disease. Philadelphia: Elsevier Science; 2006. p. 188–209.

[175] Moser K, Auger W, Fedullo P. Chronic major-vessel thromboembolic pulmonary hypertension. Circulation 1990;81(6):1735–43.

[176] Pengo V, Lensing AW, Prins MH, et al. Incidence of chronic thromboembolic pulmonary hypertension after pulmonary embolism. N Engl J Med 2004;350(22):2257–64.

[177] Liu P, Meneveau N, Schiele F, et al. Predictors of long-term clinical outcome of patients with acute massive pulmonary embolism after thrombolytic therapy. Chin Med J (Engl) 2003;116(4):503–9.

[178] Auger W, Permpikul P, Moser K. Lupus anticoagulant, heparin use, and thrombocytopenia in patients with chronic thromboembolic pulmonary hypertension: a preliminary report. Am J Med 1995;99(4):392–6.

[179] Wolf M, Boyer-Neumann C, Parent F, et al. Thrombotic risk factors in pulmonary hypertension. Eur Respir J 2000;15(2):395–9.

[180] Bonderman D, Turecek P, Jakowitsch J, et al. High prevalence of elevated clotting factor VIII in chronic thromboembolic pulmonary hypertension. Thromb Haemost 2003;90(3):372–6.

[181] Colorio C, Martinuzzo M, Forastiero R, et al. Thrombophilic factors in chronic thromboembolic pulmonary hypertension. Blood Coagul Fibrinolysis 2001;12(6):427–32.

[182] Highland KB, Strange C, Mazur J, et al. Treatment of pulmonary arterial hypertension: a preliminary decision analysis. Chest 2003;124(6):2087–92.

[183] Hoeper MM, Oudiz RJ, Peacock A, et al. End points and clinical trial designs in pulmonary arterial hypertension: clinical and regulatory perspectives. J Am Coll Cardiol 2004;43(12 Suppl S): 48S–55S.

[184] Rubin LJ, Galie N. Pulmonary arterial hypertension: a look to the future. J Am Coll Cardiol 2004;43(12 Suppl S):89S–90S.

[185] Taichman DB, Christie J, Biester R, et al. Validation of a brief telephone battery for neurocognitive assessment of patients with pulmonary arterial hypertension. Respir Res 2005;6(1):39.

[186] Taichman DB, Shin J, Hud L, et al. Health-related quality of life in patients with pulmonary arterial hypertension. Respir Res 2005;6(1):92.

[187] White J, Hopkins Ramona O, Glissmeyer Eric W, et al. Cognitive, emotional, and quality of life outcomes in patients with pulmonary arterial hypertension. Respir Res 2006;7(1):55.

[188] Rich S. The current treatment of pulmonary arterial hypertension: time to redefine success. Chest 2006;130(4):1198–202.

[189] Roberts K, Preston I, Hill NS. Pulmonary hypertension trials: current end points are flawed, but what are the alternatives? Chest 2006;130(4):934–6.

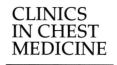

CLINICS
IN CHEST
MEDICINE

Clin Chest Med 28 (2007) 23–42

Pathology of Pulmonary Hypertension

Rubin M. Tuder, MD[a],*, John C. Marecki, PhD[b],
Amy Richter[a], Iwona Fijalkowska, PhD[a],
Sonia Flores, PhD[b]

[a]*Division of Cardiopulmonary Pathology, Johns Hopkins University School of Medicine, 720 Rutland Avenue,
Ross Research Building, Baltimore, MD 21217, USA*
[b]*Division of Pulmonary and Critical Care Medicine, University of Colorado-Denver Health Sciences Center,
4200 East Ninth Avenue, Box C272, Denver, CO 80262, USA*

Focus on the pathologic changes underlying pulmonary hypertension (PH) dominated the early investigations of this disease, which was first described late in the nineteenth century. Pulmonary vascular pathology continues to play an important role in the present age of cell and molecular investigation of the pathogenesis of PH. This importance stems from the permanent quest to correlate pulmonary vascular remodeling with the altered pulmonary vascular hemodynamics, a critical advancement in the late 1940s and early 1950s with a wide impact on the present understanding of the disease. However, as occurs with most descriptive tools applied to medical sciences, the pathologic insight into the extent and type of a particular form of pulmonary vascular remodeling has failed to establish cause-and-effect relationships in the natural history of PH, and has had a limited impact on diagnosis and therapy. These limitations derive largely from the reliance of current knowledge on studies of autopsies, because lung tissue is rarely available for histopathology during the course of the disease.

The pathologic diagnosis of pulmonary vascular remodeling depends on the histologic assessment of the cellular composition of pulmonary vascular walls, which, if abnormal, is described as pulmonary vascular *lesions*. Although it most relies on examination of histologic slides stained with hematoxylin and eosin stains, the pathologic interpretation of PH has benefited from the progressive use of cell-specific immunohistochemical markers to better define the structure and cellular composition of the pulmonary vascular lesions. Despite the advances in the understanding and treatments targeting the disease, the pathology of PH clearly lags behind the comprehensive approach used by pathologists in their assessment of other diseases, such as cancer. This approach presently includes the screening for abnormal expression of the p53 tumor suppressor or adenomatous polyposis coli (APC) genes, abnormal expression of cytokeratins in breast adenocarcinomas, and markers of cell proliferation in sarcomas, among several tissue markers that help in the final diagnosis, staging prognosis, and treatment. By comparison, the histopathologic diagnosis of PH infrequently fulfills some or all of these important tasks of the pathologic workup aimed at clinical management.

The functional status of the pulmonary circulation and the levels of pulmonary vascular resistance and pulmonary artery pressures ultimately determine the outcome and treatment of patients who have PH. The authors have proposed that the functional status of the hypertensive pulmonary circulation could be broadly correlated with a specific type of pulmonary vascular remodeling present at pathologic evaluation of the pulmonary arteries [1]. This article on the pathology of PH is framed within these

This work was supported by the grant P01HL66254 to RMT and grant R01 1HL083491 to SCF, from the National Institutes of Health.

* Corresponding author.

E-mail address: rtuder@jhmi.edu (R.M. Tuder).

Table 1
Intima remodeling

Cell	Smooth muscle cells		Extracellular matrix	Endothelial cells		
Lesion	Eccentric	Concentric	Fibrotic	Plexiform	Concentric	Dilation/Angiomatoid
Normal pulmonary artery pressure	Yes	No	No	No	No	No
Mild/moderate pulmonary hypertension	Yes	No	Yes	No	No	No
Severe pulmonary hypertension	Yes	Yes	Yes	Yes	Yes	Yes

functional categories, which are that PH can be broadly divided into mild-to-moderate versus severe based on pulmonary artery pressures, their impact on right ventricular performance, and overall mortality (Tables 1 and 2) [1]. Many non–neoplastic lung diseases with intima thickening or medial hypertrophy, such as idiopathic interstitial pneumonias (IPF) [2] and chronic obstructive pulmonary diseases (COPD) [3], present with mild-to-moderate PH. However, conditions associated with endothelial cell proliferative lesions (including plexiform lesions), marked intima fibrosis (eg, idiopathic pulmonary arterial hypertension [IPAH], and scleroderma), or medial and intimal smooth muscle cell growth (as observed in a fraction of IPF or COPD lungs) cause severe PH. As this article shows, the ability to relate the mode of pulmonary vascular remodeling to the severity of disease is rather limited. This article highlights the changes associated with IPAH as those that are paradigmatic of the pathology of severe PH.

To highlight the pathology of PH, this article follows the recommendations of the Evian meeting on pulmonary hypertension in 1998, which

Table 2
Medial remodeling

Cell	Smooth muscle cells	Extracellular matrix
Normal pulmonary artery pressure	Yes[a]	No
Mild/moderate pulmonary hypertension	Yes	Yes
Severe pulmonary hypertension	Yes	Yes

[a] Medial hypertrophy is localized and restricted to some pulmonary arteries.

supported a more descriptive approach to the pulmonary vascular changes in PH [4]. Recent findings related to the pathogenesis of human PH are also reviewed (Table 3). Their translation into the pathologic diagnosis of PH may eventually lead to a more refined and clinically useful approach toward diagnosis and staging. The latest reorganization of the pathologic nomenclature of PH by the international meeting in Venice in 2004 provides a useful framework of reference to the diagnosis of pulmonary vascular lesions in PH [5]. Reviews on normal histology of pulmonary arteries [6,7] and a historical perspective of the research accomplishments in the past 100 years of studies of the pulmonary circulation [8] provide a valuable background to this article.

Intima lesions

Pathology

Intimal lesions account for most of the reduction of luminal area of small pulmonary arteries and potentially largely influence the overall pulmonary vascular resistance. Intimal lesions consist of eccentric intima thickening, and fibrotic, plexiform, concentric, and dilation or angiomatoid lesions (Figs. 1–4; see Table 1). Focal eccentric lesions can be detected in normal lungs, but these lesions are more widespread and, to a larger extent, impinge on the vascular lumen in PH. Some of these lesions may result from the organization (ie, lysis of fibrin, recanalization by newly formed blood vessels, or ingrowth of myofibroblasts) of localized thrombi, which form the nidus for a localized growth of smooth muscle cells. More advanced lesions acquire a fibrotic pattern, with interspersed myofibroblasts and marked accumulation of mucopolysaccharides

Table 3
Molecular mediators involved in pulmonary vascular remodeling

Molecules	Up or down	Pathways affected[a]	Vascular cells affected
TGF-β receptor type 2	Down	B, E	EC, SMC
BMPR2	Down	B, E	EC, SMC
Nitric oxide	Down	A, C, E	EC, SMC
Prostacyclin	Down	A, C	EC, SMC
Caveolin-1	Down	A	EC
BAX	Down	B	EC
[K+] channels	Down	B, D	SMC
Thrombomodulin	Down	C	EC
Endothelin-1	Up	A, B, C, D, E	EC, SMC, AF
Tissue factor	Up	A, C, E	EC
von Willebrand factor	Up	C, E	EC, SMC
5-Lipoxygenase	Up	A, D, E	E
VEGF	Up	A, B, C, E	EC, SMC
VEGF receptors	Up	A, B, C, E	EC, SMC
HIF-1α	Up	A, B	EC, SMC, AF
Serotonin transporter	Up	A, D	SMC
Serotonin receptor	Up	A, D	SMC
RANTES	Up	E	Mφ
IL-6	Up	E	EC
MIP-1α	Up	E	Mφ
Fractalkine	Up	E	T cells
PDGF	Up	A	EC, SMC, AF
TGF-β	Up	A	SMC, AF
Tenascin	Up	A, B	SMC
MMP-2	Up	A	SMC
TIMP-1	Up	A	SMC
MT-MMP1	Up	A	SMC

Abbreviations: AF, adventitial fibroblast; BMPR2, bone morphogenetic protei receptor 2; EC, endothelial cells; HIF, hypoxia inducible factor; IL, interleukin; Mφ, Macrophages; MIP, macrophage inflammatory protein; MMP, matrix metalloprotease; MT, membrane-type; PDGF, platelet-derived growth factor; RANTES, regulated on activation, normal T-cell expressed and secreted; SMC, smooth muscle cells, TGF, transforming growth factor; TIMP, tissue inhibitor of metalloprotease; VEGF, vascular endothelial growth factor.

[a] Pathobiologic processes: A, increased cell proliferation; B, decreased cell apoptosis; C, increased clotting; D, increased vasoconstriction; E, inflammation.

(see Fig. 3). These fibrotic lesions are widely present in explanted lungs of patients who have severe PH, including lungs with IPAH or PAH associated with the CREST syndrome [9]. However, the lungs of cigarette smokers show variable degrees of eccentric thickening associated with pulmonary endothelial cell dysfunction, with or without evidence of PH [10].

The organization of myofibroblasts or endothelial cells in "onion-skin" layers underlies the presentation of concentric lesions (see Figs. 1 and 2). These lesions are characteristic of severe PH, because they significantly reduce the luminal area. The authors documented the presence of concentric lesions in vascular segments proximal

to plexiform lesions [11], suggesting that the concentric lesions arise from remodeled plexiform lesions. Concentric lesions composed of smooth muscle cells have also been described [12]. Whether endothelial- or smooth muscle–based lesions have a similar impact on the course of PH is unclear. However, these lesions may arise from similar progenitors, because endothelial cells can transdifferentiate into smooth muscle cells when stimulated with platelet-derived growth factor (PDGF)-BB [13] or transforming growth factor (TGF)-β [14]. Pulmonary arteries may also become almost occluded by the accumulation of acellular matrix, suggesting a terminal scarring process (Fig. 3A). Approximately 20% to 25%

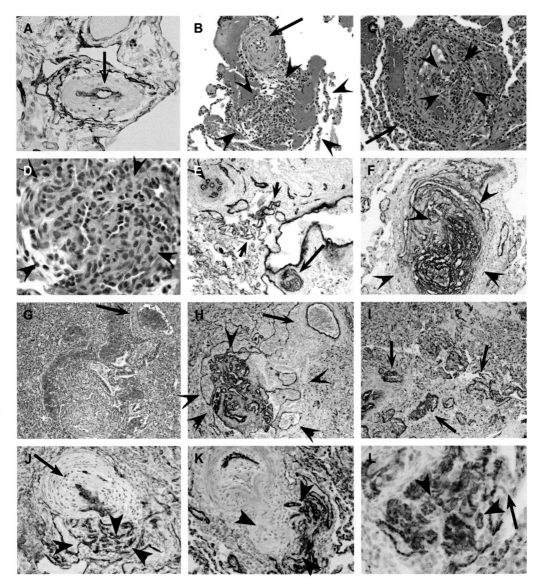

Fig. 1. Histopathology of endothelial cell lesions in IPAH. (*A*) Pulmonary artery showing medial hypertrophy and lined by a single layer of endothelial cells, as outlined by factor VIII–related antigen immunostaining (*arrow*). (*B*) Plexiform lesion, outlined with the rim of arrowheads, with the proximal vascular arterial segment with marked intimal and medial thickening by smooth muscle cells (*arrow*). Note the proliferation of endothelial cells with the outer edge (*arrowheads located from 3 5 o'clock*) occupied by dilated blood vessel–like structures. (*C*) Cross-section of a plexiform lesion, outlined with arrowheads. Note perilesional inflammatory infiltrate (*arrow*). (*D*) High-magnification histology of plexiform lesions showing slit-like vascular channels lined with hyperchromatic and cuboidal endothelial cells. Cells in the core do not display distinct cytoplasmic borders. (*E*) Low-magnification immunohistology with factor VIII–related antigen immunohistochemistry of different endothelial cell–based vascular lesions. This area has revascularized lesions (possibly an organized thrombus), with well-formed and distinct small capillaries and vessels (*large arrowhead*), a plexiform lesion (*arrow*), and dilated and angiomatoid lesions (*between arrowheads*). (*F*) High-magnification immunohistology of cellular plexiform lesion stained with factor VIII–related antigen (*small arrowheads*). (*G, H*) Histologic identification of plexiform and dilation lesions (*G*) is markedly improved by factor VIII–related antigen immunohistochemistry (*H*) (*arrowheads*), whereas the parent vessel (*arrow*) shows mild medial remodeling. (*I*) Highlight of vascular dilation and angiomatoid lesions with factor VIII–related antigen immunohistochemistry. (*J*) Endothelial cells in plexiform lesion highlighted with CD34 immunohistochemistry (*arrowheads*). Proximal pulmonary artery with marked intima and medial thickening is highlighted by the arrow. (*K, L*) Endothelial cells are highlighted by CD31 immunohistochemistry (*arrowheads*). (*L*) Note that capillary endothelial cells also express CD31 (*arrow*).

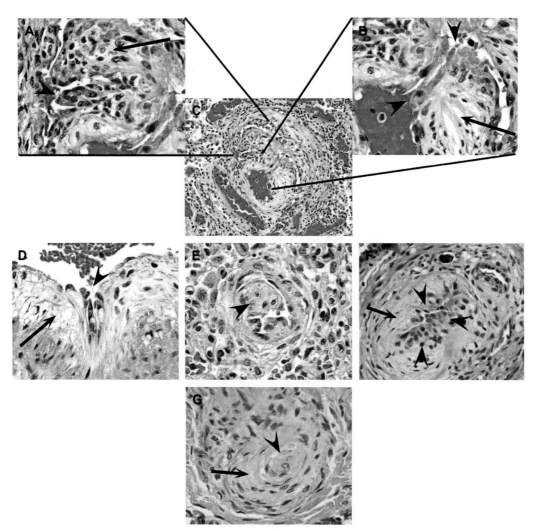

Fig. 2. Histologic patterns of endothelial cell injury and lesions in IPAH. (*A–C*). Plexiform lesion (*B*) with high magnification of proliferated endothelial cells in *A*. A luminal projection of endothelial cells is highlighted with an arrowhead, whereas cells in cellular core are marked with an arrow. In *B*, the proximal segment is shown in high magnification, highlighting the atypical endothelial cell (*arrowheads*) facing the vascular lumen, whereas a myxoid component organized as concentric layers of smooth muscle cells is highlighted with the arrow. (*D*) A similar pattern of abnormal endothelial cells (*arrowhead*) and the myxoid subendothelial layer (*arrow*) are highlighted. (*E*) An intimal projection is highlighted (*arrowhead*). (*F*) Increased number of endothelial cells (*arrowheads*) in the intima, whereas the myxoid subintimal layer is highlighted with the arrow. These lesions (*B, D–F*) usually contain endothelial cells that can be highlighted with factor VIII–related antigen immunohistochemistry. The cluster of endothelial cells possibly represents early plexiform lesions. (*G*) A concentric lesion (*arrowhead*) with adjacent smooth muscle–like cells (*arrow*).

of pulmonary arteries between 25 and 200 μm in diameter are compromised by intima occlusion or concentric lesions [15]. These two patterns of luminal obliteration might represent temporally related lesions, which start as an abnormal proliferation of endothelial or smooth muscle cells, progress into an "onion-skin" lesion, and then become acellular with abundant extracellular matrix deposition (see Fig. 4).

Plexiform lesions, typically located in branching pointes of muscular arteries [11], consist of a network of vascular channels lined up by endothelial cells (see Figs. 1 and 2) [16] and a core of myofibroblastic or less well-differentiated cells

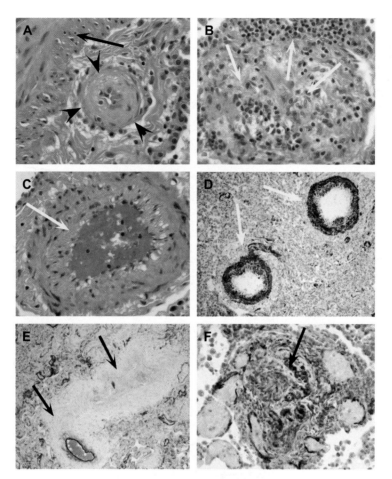

Fig. 3. (*A*) Fibrotic, relatively paucicellular intima thickening (*outlined with arrowheads*) in a pulmonary artery with the media highlighted with the arrow. (*B*) Marked intima remodeling with almost complete obliteration by fibrous tissue with a marked intravascular and perivascular inflammatory infiltrate (*arrows*). (*C*) Smooth muscle cell hypertrophy, with prominent thickening of medial layer (*arrow*). (*D*) Highlight of medial hypertrophy with smooth muscle α actin immunohistochemistry. (*E*) Markedly remodeled pulmonary artery with endothelial cell layer highlighted with factor VIII–related antigen immunohistochemistry. Note that the intima and medial smooth muscle cells are negative for factor VIII–related antigen reactivity. (*F*) Ingrowth of smooth muscle cells in a plexiform lesions, highlighted with smooth muscle cell α actin immunohistochemistry (*arrow*).

(see Fig. 3) [17]. The authors have found that these lesions are characteristically found in cases of severe PH, including IPAH, and PH associated with HIV infection, liver cirrhosis, CREST syndrome, congenital heart malformations, and schistosomiasis. Because endothelial cells contribute significantly to concentric and plexiform lesions, endothelial-cell immunostaining with factor VIII–related antigen or CD31 may help identify the different stages of endothelial cell proliferation (see Figs. 1 and 2) [6]. These stains can help detect small clusters of endothelial cells [18], and cell

proliferation markers such as MIB-1 may also contribute to the identification of proliferating endothelial cells (normal pulmonary endothelial cells have a very low proliferation rate) [19]. Dilation lesions represent another potential endothelial cell lesion, with the formation of a rosary of dilated channels (also known as *angiomatoid lesions*), often distally to a plexiform lesion (see Fig. 2) [6]. As with plexiform lesions, the authors observed dilation lesions in severe PH (see Table 1). These lesions containing endothelial cells have abundant collagen IV expression, which is

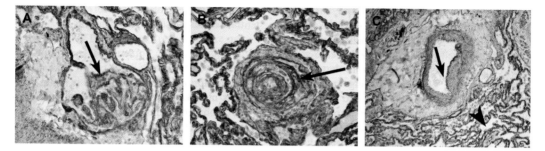

Fig. 4. Distribution of collagen IV, a component of basement membrane of endothelial cells (*arrows*) in PH pulmonary arteries. (*A, B*) Plexiform lesion. (*C*) Pulmonary artery with medial thickening. The collagen IV basement membrane of alveolar capillaries shows the clear demarcation of capillary basement membrane.

a component of basement membranes and a useful marker for the outline of blood vessels (see Fig. 4).

Pathobiology

The prevailing concept is that dysfunctional endothelial cells play the key pathobiologic role in PH [20]. However, the pathogenesis of intimal vascular lesions remains mostly undetermined. These lesions may result from injuries to the endothelium, followed by activation of smooth muscle cell migration, extracellular matrix deposition, and endothelial cell proliferation. These lesions may occur from organization of microthrombi. In animal models, only the association of the alkaloid monocrotaline (MCT) and high shear stress caused by shunting between the systemic and pulmonary circulations lead to marked intima thickening by smooth muscle cells and severe PH in rats [21]. The intimal cells express smooth muscle cell markers and fibronectin [19].

The authors have proposed that plexiform lesions represent a process of misguided angiogenesis based on the findings of expression of vascular endothelial growth factor (VEGF), its receptors 1 (flt) and 2 (kdr), and hypoxia inducible factor (HIF)-1α and -β [22]. The finding of monoclonality of endothelial cells in plexiform lesions in IPAH, but not in similar lesions in PH associated with congenital heart malformation, suggests that these lesions might arise from mutations in tumor suppressor genes [23]. Somatic loss of expression of TGF-β receptor 2 and the proapoptotic Bax, potentially caused by microsatellite instability, is also documented in IPAH plexiform lesions [24]. Heterozygous germline mutations of bone morphogenetic protein receptor 2 (BMPR2) (a component of the TGF-β family) is found to underlie up to 60% of cases of familial IPAH [25,26]. BMPR2 expression is documented in plexiform lesions [12] and remodeled pulmonary arteries in IPAH lungs, predominantly in endothelial cells. However, studies show that the cells in the central core of plexiform lesions lack the expression of TGF-β receptor 2 and TGF-β receptor 1 and their signaling Smads, Smad2, Smad1 (which shares common epitopes with Smad5 and Smad8), Smad3, and Smad4, including the phosphorylated Smad(1, 5, 8) and Smad2. The absence of expression of these phosphorylated Smads is the best indication that these cells have no TGF-β (by way of Smad 2 or Smads 1/5/8) or bone morphogenetic protein (BMP) (by way of Smads 1/5/8) signaling [27]. Loss of cytostatic signaling from TGF-β would allow the plexiform cells to abnormally proliferate. Notwithstanding the evidence of preserved BMPR expression and signaling in IPAH endothelial cells, recent studies indicate that BMP signaling protects against endothelial cell apoptosis in vitro [28]. The loss of this protection from germline mutations in BMPR2 would thus favor enhanced susceptibility to apoptosis of lung endothelial cells.

The potential role for early endothelial cell apoptosis in the pathogenesis of uncontrolled proliferation of pulmonary endothelial cells was first documented in the rat model of severe PH caused by the combination of VEGF receptor blockade with SU5416 and chronic hypoxia [29]. The role of endothelial cell apoptosis in the pathogenesis of PH was also extended to the monocrotaline model [30]. Initial endothelial cell apoptosis might favor the emergence of apoptosis-resistant endothelial cells, with potential for uncontrolled proliferation [29,31].

express moderate-to-intense immunohistochemical expression of MMP-2, whereas myofibroblasts display low levels of this extracellular protease [63]. Membrane type-1 MMP was also expressed in endothelial and myofibroblastic cells of concentric and plexiform lesions. These results and those in the monocrotaline model suggest that the inhibition of elastases or MMPs might be beneficial in IPAH, as shown in the monocrotaline model of PH [64], potentially leading to the apoptosis of smooth muscle cells.

It is becoming clear that the ultimate fate of vascular smooth muscle cells in PH is determined by their resistance to apoptosis. In fact, apoptosis resistance might play a central role in both the endothelial- and smooth muscle cell–based pulmonary vascular lesions [65], because IPAH lungs have a lower number of apoptotic cells than normal or emphysematous lungs [66]. As growth signals originated by PDGF, TGF-β, EGF, serotonin, and extracellular matrix proteins are interrupted in animal models of PH, pulmonary arteries undergo de-remodeling associated with apoptosis of pulmonary artery smooth muscle cells [64]. Targeting apoptosis of the hypertrophic smooth muscle cells might represent a more viable approach to treatment.

Recent studies of K^+ channel activity have provided a novel insight into the lack of proapoptotic signals in IPAH smooth muscle cells. An exciting and complementary paradigm based on the interplay between K^+ channels and apoptosis in pulmonary artery smooth muscle cells has emerged based on the demonstration that activation of K^+ channels causes cytochrome C release from the mitochondria and water efflux from the dying cells [67]. Conversely, inhibition of K^+ channels causes cell depolarization, enhances contractility, and decreases apoptosis of pulmonary artery smooth muscle cells. One potential mechanism linking this paradigm to BMPR2 mutations is the finding that BMPR2 activation up-regulates K^+ channels [68] and causes apoptosis of normal pulmonary artery smooth muscle cells, but not of cells from patients who have IPAH [69]. McMurtry and colleagues [34] recently provided additional evidence that mechanisms akin to cancer operate in pulmonary vascular remodeling. Survivin protects cancer cells against apoptosis by inhibiting caspase activation and apoptosis-inducing factor [70]. Not only do pulmonary artery smooth muscle cells in IPAH lungs express higher levels of the antiapoptotic survivin, but monocrotaline-induced

pulmonary vascular remodeling requires survivin expression. Transduction of a functionally deficient survivin in monocrotaline-treated lungs prevents pulmonary vascular remodeling and, when administered after monocrotaline treatment, enhances apoptosis of pulmonary artery smooth muscle cells and reduces pulmonary artery pressures. This mutant survivin increases levels of K^+ channel activity and leads to depolarization of mitochondria with enhanced cytochrome C release.

Adventitial remodeling

Pathology

The adventitia is mostly composed of fibroblasts. Growing evidence shows that, rather than being just a structural support to pulmonary vessels, the adventitia may also play a role in regulating pulmonary vascular function from the "outside-in" [71]. The normal adventitia represents approximately 15% of the external diameter of pulmonary arteries larger than 50 μm in diameter. In IPAH arteries, the adventitial thickness increases to 28% of artery diameter, predominantly because of collagen deposition [15]. Experts have not noted the presence of a vasa vasorum in the adventitia of medium-sized pulmonary arteries in PH. Whether the adventitia is thickened or presents with a heterogeneous stromal cell population in other forms of PH remains unclear. The diagnostic significance of the extent of adventitial thickening or its role in the differentiation between mild-to-moderate and severe PH is equally unknown. The adventitia contains a perivascular cuff of inflammatory cells, which might modulate the growth of, or transdifferentiate themselves into, vascular structural cells in the pulmonary vascular wall.

Pathobiology

The adventitial fibroblasts react promptly to vascular stresses, notably those caused by hypoxia, high-perfusion flow models, and, to a lesser extent, the alkaloid monocrotaline treatment [71]. Fibroblasts undergo a marked increase in cell proliferation, reaching an 11-fold increase in labeling index in hilar vessels at day 3 of chronic hypoxia exposure [43]. In the monocrotaline model, proliferation rate of adventitial fibroblasts reaches a fivefold increase at day 21 [44]. These findings underscore the powerful abilities of adventitial fibroblasts to undergo proliferation, which is one of the most characteristic properties of these cells. Moreover, adventitial fibroblasts can (1) differentiate into smooth muscle cells and migrate into the remodeled media; (2) trigger smooth muscle cell proliferation by secreting growth factors; (3) allow for the recruitment of inflammatory and bone marrow progenitor cells; or (4) create a vasculogenic and angiogenic niche for the expansion of newly formed vessels (vasa vasorum). Adventitial fibroblasts might represent heterogeneous clusters of cells, such as those found in the medial smooth muscle cells [71]. This biologic heterogeneity is readily apparent in the neonatal bovine model of hypoxic PH. A potentially important finding is the contribution of circulating fibrocytes (precursor cells sharing the expression of the fibroblast marker α1-collagen and peripheral leukocyte markers CD45, CD34, CD11b, and CD14) to experimental hypoxic PH [71]. Adventitial fibroblasts sense alterations in their redox status, with the ensuing activation of cell growth, cytokine release, and generation of oxidants through activation of nicotinamide adenine dinucleotide phosphate oxidase [71]. The redox regulation of adventitial cell function is supported by the identification of markers of oxidative stress in remodeled pulmonary arteries of IPAH lungs [72].

Venous pathology

Pathology

The pulmonary veins are primarily involved in the pathogenesis of postcapillary PH, such as that caused by veno-occlusive disease, capillary hemangiomatosis, mitral valve and other forms of left heart dysfunction, and extrinsic main pulmonary vein obstructions. Veno-occlusive disease and pulmonary capillary hemangiomatosis are rare causes of idiopathic PH. Veno-occlusive disease is characterized by variable luminal obstruction by intraluminal bands or eccentrically placed fibrous tissue, which is firmly attached to the intima, potentially representing organized thrombi. Interlobular septal veins become muscularized, and marked capillary distention occurs in periseptal alveoli, leading to a pattern suggestive of interstitial lung disease (Fig. 5). Pulmonary

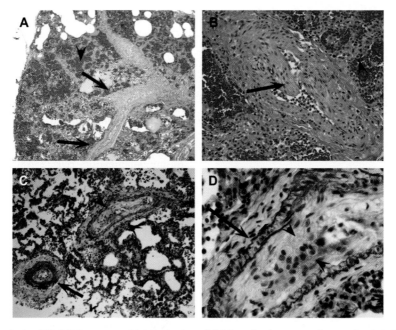

Fig. 5. Veno-occlusive PH. (*A*) Low-power histologic view of thickened pulmonary veins running into the lung parenchyma from the pleural surface (left edge) (*arrows*). Note marked vein wall thickening and decreased lumen. Adjacent alveoli are filled with blood and show septal thickening with engorged capillaries (*arrowhead*). (*B*) Marked vein thickening with intimal projection probably representing organized thrombus (*arrow*). Alveolar hemorrhage and septal thickening are highlighted with arrowhead. (*C*, *D*) Movat stained pulmonary vein showing arterialization pattern with internal and external elastic layers (*arrow*). The vein shows marked intima thickening with organized thrombus (*arrowheads*).

capillary hemangiomatosis is characterized by a neoplastic-like proliferation of endothelial cells, often forming capillaries, and infiltrating alveolar septa and venous and arterial pulmonary arteries.

Left heart failure or mitral valve dysfunction is often severe and one of the most frequent causes of PH. Lung vascular pathology is of limited help in diagnosing PH and in studies of its pathogenesis, because most patients who have left heart failure show chronic passive congestion with hemosiderin-laden macrophages. However, this finding is common to patients who have PH and those who do not have the disease. Pulmonary arteries show mild medial thickening.

Pulmonary arteries also undergo remodeling in venous PH, which might reflect the effect of the progressive buildup of pressures in the pulmonary arterial side of the pulmonary circulation. Pulmonary arteries undergo a smooth muscle cell–based remodeling with intima (eccentric lesions) and medial thickening. The extent and pattern of arterial remodeling is similar to that seen in arterial PH. Therefore, careful examination of pulmonary veins in any potential case of PH is warranted, because pulmonary veins show intimal thickening in precapillary PH [15].

Pathobiology

Little is known about the functional alterations of endothelial, smooth muscle, and adventitial fibroblasts in venous PH. Pulmonary veins are difficult to identify in lung sections because they are located in the midst of the alveolated tissue. Only vein segments present in interlobular septa (ie, invaginations of pleural connective tissue containing veins and lymphatics) can be more easily recognized. The development of endothelial cell markers unique to pulmonary veins would aid in the proper assessment of the contribution of endothelial cell dysfunction in venous PH. The same limitations apply to venous smooth muscle cells and fibroblasts.

Inflammation, circulating progenitor cells, and viral agents

Pathology

Perivascular cuffing of remodeled pulmonary arteries is present in IPAH lungs and severe PH associated with underlying conditions, such as HIV infection and CREST (see Fig. 5) [16,73]. B cells, T cells, and macrophages infiltrate the vessel wall and are present within intimal lesions (Fig. 6)

[16]. Both CD4 and CD8 cells are present, and many of these express the memory T-cell marker CD45RO, which might also indicate cell activation (see Fig. 6). Perivascular inflammation is more frequently seen in severe PH than in mild-to-moderate and normal lungs, but whether this finding pertains to autopsied lung specimens or occurs during the progression of the disease is unclear.

Some of the so-called inflammatory cells might represent circulating blood progenitor cells. No detailed investigation into the lung homing of circulating blood progenitor cells has been performed in PH. The lone evidence is provided by studies that reported AC133+ and CD45+ cells infiltrating the remodeled intima of patients who had COPD [74].

Pathobiology

Although perivascular inflammation has limited value in the pathologic workup of PH cases, it is one of the most promising areas of investigation in the disease. Inflammatory cells may interact with viral factors, which have emerged as potential etiologic and pathogenetic agents in PH.

Compelling evidence shows global immunologic alterations in patients who have IPAH [75,76] and that PH occurs in the setting of profound immune deregulation underlying HIV infection and collagen vascular diseases. The recognition of an inflammatory component in PH [16,73] supports the investigation into the expression of cytokines that might potentially drive perivascular inflammation and thus contribute to the disease. Remodeled pulmonary arteries express interleukin (IL)-1, IL-6, and PDGF in infiltrating inflammatory cells [77,78]; the chemokine RANTES (*regulated on activation, normal T-cell expressed and secreted*), which is an important chemoattractant for monocytes and T cells [79]; and the macrophage inflammatory protein-1α (MIP-1α) [75]. Lungs of patients who have IPAH show increased expression of fractalkine, a chemokine involved in T-cell trafficking and monocyte recruitment, and their circulating CD4 and CD8 T-cells have higher levels of the fractalkine receptor CX3CR1 than those of controls or patients who have thromboembolic PH [80].

Inflammatory cells infiltrating remodeled pulmonary arteries may include subpopulations of vascular precursor or early-progenitor cells, also potential contributors to pulmonary vascular remodeling in PH. Pulmonary arteries in PH caused by chronic hypoxia contain an infiltrating

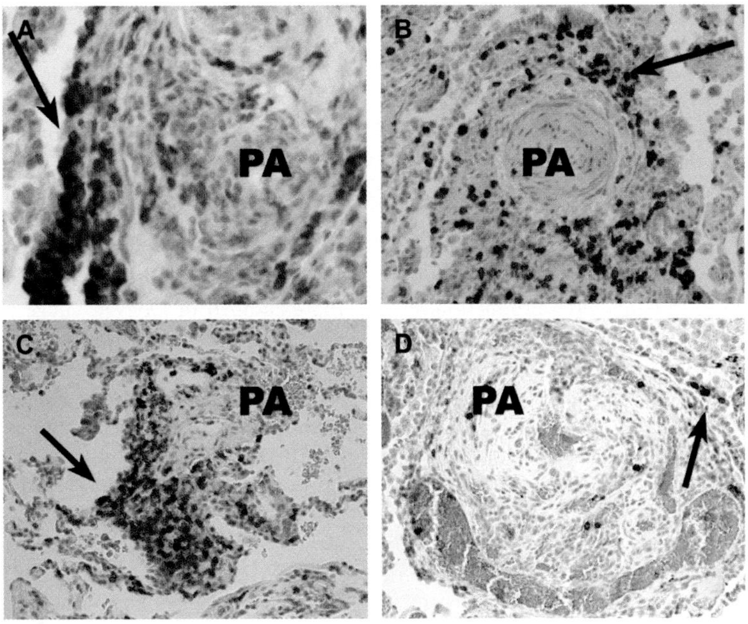

Fig. 6. Inflammatory cell infiltrate in severe PH. (*A*) Lymphomonuclear cells positive for CD45RO (*arrow*), surrounding a plexiform lesion (PA). (*B*) Clustering of CD4 lymphocytes around a pulmonary artery (PA) with concentric thickening (*arrow*). (*C*) Clustering of CD8 lymphocytes around a remodeled pulmonary artery (PA) (*arrow*). (*D*) Few cells stain positively for CD45RA marker (indicative of naïve T cells).

subpopulation of fibrocytes, identified by the expression mononuclear cell markers CD45, CD11b, CD14, and the fibroblast marker α1-procollagen. Approximately 15% and 20% of these cells also undergo proliferation and express smooth muscle α-actin, respectively [81]. These studies also document that depletion of circulating monocytic cells alleviates pulmonary vascular remodeling caused by chronic hypoxia. Endothelial cell precursors may play a beneficial role in PH because their administration to monocrotaline-treated rats has shown dramatic healing effects in remodeled pulmonary arteries, notably when transfected with the endothelial nitric oxide synthase gene [82]. The potential for either deleterious or beneficial effects from manipulations that increase the progenitor cell pool underscores the need for careful and detailed studies into the human disease before embarking on clinical trials.

Viral infection may disrupt normal immunoregulatory and homeostatic cellular pathways, which result in endothelial or smooth muscle cell injury and activate inflammation. Most pathways involved in virus pathogenesis converge on either pro-survival or pro-angiogenic signals, the same signals associated with severe PH.

The important role of inflammation is further highlighted in cases of PH where a viral origin can be identified. For HIV-related PH, the first clinical report of an association between infection and the development of lesions appeared in 1987 [83], followed by other reports [84–86], but with no evidence of the virus in PH vascular lesions. Because PH is frequently diagnosed when it is in advanced stages, its incidence in patients infected with HIV is likely underestimated, although a recent report shows a high prevalence of PH in children infected with HIV [87]. BMPR2 mutations are not required for severe PH to occur in patients infected with HIV, although the vascular lesions in the lungs of these patients [85] are identical to those of patients who have familial PH and sporadic IPAH with BMPR2 mutations.

Some studies showed no correlation between viral load and right heart changes [88,89]. However, a case report [90] and recent unpublished observation showed that viral load control with highly active antiretroviral therapy (HARRT) can be associated with an improved clinical outcome (M. Humbert, personal communication, 2005). Furthermore, bosentan, an endothelin receptor antagonist, has been successful in some patients who have HIV and PH [91], suggesting that shear stress contributes to the disease independent of the viral load.

In the lung, HIV-1 primarily infects macrophages, providing not only a potential reservoir for the transmission of the virus to circulating T cells but also a source for localized viral proteins, such as Nef, Tat, and gp120, all of which may have direct effects on innocent bystander cells. The chronic exposure to viral products in the lung, a deficiency in regulatory T cells, and an altered production of chemokines and cytokines, may all contribute to pulmonary vascular dysfunction, with endothelial cells being particularly sensitive targets.

The HIV Nef (representing *negative factor*) protein is found in plexiform lesions of macaques infected with a chimeric virus containing the simian immunodeficiency virus (SIV) backbone with the HIV Nef (in place of SIV Nef) [92]. Nef is also present in endothelial cells of patients infected with HIV who have PH (Fig. 7) [92]. Recent studies suggest that the viral protein may exert direct effects on cells not necessarily permissive for viral replication. Foci of mononuclear cells and ectopic lymphoid tissues characteristically found in regions adjacent to the lesions may be sources of this viral protein (see Fig. 5).

The Nef protein seems to be dispensable for viral replication in vitro, but is a critical virulence factor for pathogenesis and maintaining high viral loads in vivo [93,94]. Nef is an *N*-terminus-myristoylated protein with a relative molecular mass of 27 kd associated with cellular membranes and the cytoskeleton [95]. Myristoylation is essential for almost all functions ascribed to Nef, including membrane localization within lipid raft microdomains. The localization and adaptor functions recruit signaling proteins to discrete regions in the membrane and affect T-cell signaling pathways [96]. Proteins associated with a survival and proangiogenic phenotype in severe PH, such as PI-3 kinase, MAP kinases, and a p21 kinase-2, are all recruited to the rafts by Nef [97–100]. In human monocyte–derived macrophages (MDMs), Nef activates the STAT1 pathway and the secretion of MIP-1, IL-1-α, IL-6, and TNF-α [101]. Extracellular Nef found in patients who have HIV (approximately 10 ng/mL) enters the vascular endothelium in vivo by way of CXCR4 [102]. Finally, Nef can be proapoptotic or pro-survival, depending on the context of expression and particular cell type [103]. Thus, localization of Nef to the lipid rafts may be sufficient to trigger the changes associated with the endothelial cell–expansion characteristic of plexiform lesions. On the other hand, a second hit, such as infection with other viruses (eg, gammaherpesviruses such as human herpesvirus 8 [HHV8]), or a genetic susceptibility also may be necessary.

HHV8 is a gammaherpesvirus, also known as Kaposi's sarcoma–associated herpesvirus [104,105]. Evidence of HHV8 is found in a large percentage of plexiform lesions of patients who have PH examined in Denver, suggesting for the first time that this virus was a contributing factor [106]. Several proangiogenic or oncogenic genes are present in its genome, including a viral IL-8 and a viral IL-6, both shown to play a role in IPAH. In addition, the genome encodes a seven-transmembrane–spanning G protein–coupled receptor (GPCR) with extensive sequence similarity to cellular chemokine receptors [107]. When expressed in NIH 3T3 fibroblasts, this gene increases their ability to grow in soft agar and to induce tumor formation in nude mice [108]. GPCR increases secretion of VEGF and activation of the ERK1/2 (p44/42) MAP kinase signaling pathway [109]. Endothelial cells that express this gene become immortalized with constitutive activation of the VEGF-receptor 2 (KDR) [110]. In addition, this gene can cause Kaposi's sarcoma–like lesions in nude mice [108], and overexpression within hematopoietic cells results in angioproliferative lesions resembling those found in Kaposi's sarcoma [111]. These viral factors have the potential to alter cellular phenotype in the absence of viral replication.

Nevertheless, despite the recognized angioproliferative potential of HHV8 and its initial association with plexiform lesions, several studies have not reproduced these results [112]. Studies of patients from a San Francisco clinic and Japanese and German cohorts show no evidence of latent virus in the lesions or serum antibodies against viral antigens [113–116]. The divergent findings among groups may be caused by the methodology used to detect the virus, or regional (genetic and environmental) differences in the study population. Latency-associated transcripts may be undetectable if the virus is undergoing a lytic replication cycle. In addition, serologic tests for viral antibodies are notoriously difficult and often difficult to interpret. Therefore, further studies are necessary to address these questions.

PH represents one of the extrahepatic complications of hepatitis C virus infection, with

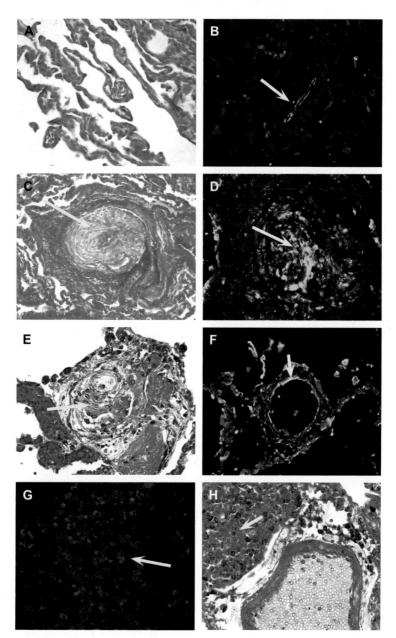

Fig. 7. HIV-1 Nef localization in HIV-1–associated PH. (*A*) Normal precapillary vessels, highlighted with methyl green. (*B*) Localization of factor VIII–related antigen stained with Alexa Fluor 488, shown in green, and Nef stained with Vector Red. Note lack of expression of Nef in normal pulmonary arteries, resulting in a green signal in the endothelial cells (*arrow*). (*C*) Markedly remodeled pulmonary artery with a concentric/plexiform lesion, highlighted with methyl green (*arrow*). (*D*) Colocalization of factor VIII–related antigen (*green*) with Nef (*red*), resulting in a yellow signal (*arrow*). (*E*) Plexiform lesion in HIV--associated PH, highlighted with methyl green (*arrow*). (*F*) Co-localization of factor VIII–related antigen (*green*) with Nef (*red*), resulting in a yellow signal (*arrow*) in endothelial cells of pulmonary arteries with mild remodeling (*arrow*). (*G, H*) Lymph node of an SIV-infected monkey, showing extensive expression of Nef (red in G and brown in H, *arrows*) in a hilar lymph node. (*Reproduced from* Marecki JC, Cool CD, Parr JE, et al. HIV-1 Nef is associated with complex pulmonary vascular lesions in SHIV-nef-infected macaques. Am J Respir Crit Care Med 2006;174:437–45; with permission.)

a prevalence of 1% to 5% [117]. In most patients, portal hypertension precedes PH [117,118]. The pathogenesis is also poorly understood, but the histologic hallmarks are similar to IPAH. Whether these lesions are secondary to increased inflammatory cytokine production, direct viral replication, or presence of viral products in the lung remains to be determined. As in HIV-mediated PH, an associated immune dysregulation may trigger uncontrolled intrapulmonary angiogenesis.

Some case reports of patients who had PH showed lung endothelial cells infected with other viruses, such as herpes simplex type 2 or cytomegalovirus. The fact that both viruses belong to the viral family Herpesviridae suggests that they may share some of the angioproliferative potential of HHV8. Nevertheless, because both patients were HIV-positive, the contribution of each virus to the angioproliferation is difficult to dissect.

Summary

The secondary role taken by the pathology in the present clinical management of PH reflects to some extent the limitations of the current understanding of the disease. Ample room exists for the diagnostic translation of the pathobiologic studies, with the goal of improving the diagnostic and prognostic power of the pathologic assessment of pulmonary vascular remodeling. This article seeks to show the complementarities of the pathology and pathobiology of PH. The authors forecast that the pathogenetic insights will allow experts to further reclassify the disease as angioproliferative [119] or myofibroblastic (as in idiopathic pulmonary fibrosis), neoplastic-like, or a reaction to injury, with clear implications to biomarker discovery, disease-tailored therapies, genetic association studies, and other areas of investigation. Based solely on the advances in the past 10 years, the potential exists to refine the diagnostic tools using genomics of peripheral blood cells of patients who have PH [120] and also to breakdown the apparently unifying pathology of severe PH using genomics applied to lung tissue [121]. As illustrated in the figures, a lung with severe PH shows a range of ongoing vascular lesions, with distinct severities and cellular compositions. The authors hope that this article will be rewritten in the future with a deeper insight into the role of specific pulmonary vascular lesions, ultimately aiding novel treatments targeting PH.

References

[1] Tuder RM, Cool CD, Yeager ME, et al. The pathobiology of pulmonary hypertension: endothelium. Clin Chest Med 2001;22(3):405–18.

[2] Strange C, Highland KB. Pulmonary hypertension in interstitial lung disease. Curr Opin Pulm Med 2005;11(5):452–5.

[3] Kessler R, Faller M, Weitzenblum E, et al. "Natural history" of pulmonary hypertension in a series of 131 patients with chronic obstructive lung disease. Am J Respir Crit Care Med 2001;164(2): 219–24.

[4] Haworth SG, Rabinovitch M, Meyrick B, et al. Primary pulmonary hypertension: executive summary from the World Symposium—Primary Pulmonary Hypertension. Rich S, editor. World Health Organization; 1998. p. 2–5.

[5] Pietra GG, Capron F, Stewart S, et al. Pathologic assessment of vasculopathies in pulmonary hypertension. J Am Coll Cardiol 2004;43(12 Suppl S): 25S–32S.

[6] Tuder RM, Zaiman AL. Pathology of pulmonary vascular disease. In: Peacock A, Rubin LJ, editors. Pulmonary circulation. 2nd edition. London: Arnold; 2003.

[7] Wagenvoort CA, Wagenvoort N. Normal circulation of the lungs. In: Wagenvoort CA, Wagenvoort N, editors. Pathology of pulmonary hypertension. 1st edition. New York: John Wiley & Sons; 1977. p. 1–8.

[8] Zaiman A, Fijalkowska I, Hassoun PM, et al. One hundred years of research in the pathogenesis of pulmonary hypertension. Am J Respir Cell Mol Biol 2005;33(5):425–31.

[9] Cool CD, Kennedy D, Voelkel NF, et al. Pathogenesis and evolution of plexiform lesions in pulmonary hypertension associated with scleroderma and human immunodeficiency virus infection. Hum Pathol 1997;28(4):434–42.

[10] Santos S, Peinado VI, Ramirez J, et al. Characterization of pulmonary vascular remodelling in smokers and patients with mild COPD. Eur Respir J 2002;19(4):632–8.

[11] Cool CD, Stewart JS, Werahera P, et al. Three-dimensional reconstruction of pulmonary arteries in plexiform pulmonary hypertension using cell specific markers: evidence for a dynamic and heterogeneous process of pulmonary endothelial cell growth. Am J Pathol 1999;155(2):411–9.

[12] Atkinson C, Stewart S, Upton PD, et al. Primary pulmonary hypertension is associated with reduced pulmonary vascular expression of type II bone morphogenetic protein receptor. Circulation 2002; 105(14):1672–8.

[13] Yamashita J, Itoh H, Hirashima M, et al. Flk1-positive cells derived from embryonic stem cells serve as vascular progenitors. Nature 2000; 408(6808):92–6.

[14] Frid MG, Kale VA, Stenmark KR. Mature vascular endothelium can give rise to smooth muscle cells via endothelial-mesenchymal transdifferentiation—in vitro analysis. Circ Res 2002;90(11):1189–96.

[15] Chazova I, Loyd JE, Newman JH, et al. Pulmonary artery adventitial changes and venous involvement in primary pulmonary hypertension. Am J Pathol 1995;146(2):389–97.

[16] Tuder RM, Groves BM, Badesch DB, et al. Exuberant endothelial cell growth and elements of inflammation are present in plexiform lesions of pulmonary hypertension. Am J Pathol 1994;144(2):275–85.

[17] Heath D, Smith P, Gosney J. Ultrastructure of early plexogenic pulmonary arteriopathy. Histopathology 1988;12(1):41–52.

[18] Voelkel NF, Tuder RM, Cool CD, et al. Severe chronic pulmonary hypertension and the pressure-overloaded right ventricle. In: Banner NR, Polak JM, Yacoub M, editors. Lung Transplantation. 1st edition. Cambridge: Cambridge University Press; 2003. p. 29–38.

[19] Mitani Y, Ueda M, Komatsu R, et al. Vascular smooth muscle cell phenotypes in primary pulmonary hypertension. Eur Respir J 2001;17(2):316–20.

[20] Budhiraja R, Tuder RM, Hassoun PM. Endothelial dysfunction in pulmonary hypertension. Circulation 2004;109(2):159–65.

[21] Tanaka Y, Schuster DP, Davis EC, et al. Role of vascular injury and hemodynamics in rat pulmonary artery remodeling. J Clin Invest 1996;98(2):434–42.

[22] Tuder RM, Chacon M, Alger LA, et al. Expression of angiogenesis-related molecules in plexiform lesions in severe pulmonary hypertension: evidence for a process of disordered angiogenesis. J Pathol 2001;195(3):367–74.

[23] Lee SD, Shroyer KR, Markham NE, et al. Monoclonal endothelial cell proliferation is present in primary but not secondary pulmonary hypertension. J Clin Invest 1998;101(5):927–34.

[24] Yeager ME, Halley GR, Golpon HA, et al. Microsatellite instability of endothelial cell growth and apoptosis genes within plexiform lesions in primary pulmonary hypertension. Circ Res 2001;88(1):e8–11.

[25] The International PPH Consortium. Lane KB, Machado RD, Pauciulo MW, et al. Heterozygous germline mutations in BMPR2 encoding a TGF-B receptor cause familiar pulmonary hypertension. Nat Genet 2000;26(1);81–4.

[26] Deng Z, Morse JH, Slager SL, et al. Familial primary pulmonary hypertension (gene PPH1) is caused by mutations in the bone morphogenetic protein receptor-II gene. Am J Hum Genet 2000;67(3):737–44.

[27] Richter A, Yeager ME, Zaiman A, et al. Impaired transforming growth factor-beta signaling in idiopathic pulmonary arterial hypertension. Am J Respir Crit Care Med 2004;170(12):1340–8.

[28] Teichert-Kuliszewska K, Kutryk MJ, Kuliszewski MA, et al. Bone morphogenetic protein receptor-2 signaling promotes pulmonary arterial endothelial cell survival: implications for loss-of-function mutations in the pathogenesis of pulmonary hypertension. Circ Res 2006;98(2):209–17.

[29] Taraseviciene-Stewart L, Kasahara Y, Alger L, et al. Inhibition of the VEGF receptor 2 combined with chronic hypoxia causes cell death-dependent pulmonary endothelial cell proliferation and severe pulmonary hypertension. FASEB J 2001;15(2):427–38.

[30] Campbell AIM, Zhao YD, Sandhu R, et al. Cell-based gene transfer of vascular endothelial growth factor attenuates monocrotaline-induced pulmonary hypertension. Circulation 2001;104(18):2242–8.

[31] Sakao S, Taraseviciene-Stewart L, Lee JD, et al. Initial apoptosis is followed by increased proliferation of apoptosis-resistant endothelial cells. FASEB J 2005;19(9):1178–80.

[32] Giaid A, Yanagisawa M, Langleben D, et al. Expression of endothelin-1 in the lungs of patients with pulmonary hypertension. N Engl J Med 1993;328(24):1732–9.

[33] Bonnet S, Michelakis ED, Porter CJ, et al. An abnormal mitochondrial-hypoxia inducible factor-1 alpha-Kv channel pathway disrupts oxygen sensing and triggers pulmonary arterial hypertension in fawn hooded rats—similarities to human pulmonary arterial hypertension. Circulation 2006;113(22):2630–41.

[34] McMurtry MS, Archer SL, Altieri DC, et al. Gene therapy targeting survivin selectively induces pulmonary vascular apoptosis and reverses pulmonary arterial hypertension. J Clin Invest 2005;115(6):1479–91.

[35] Giaid A, Saleh D. Reduced expression of endothelial nitric oxide synthase in the lungs of patients with pulmonary hypertension. N Engl J Med 1995;333(4):214–21.

[36] Tuder RM, Cool CD, Geraci MW, et al. Prostacyclin synthase expression is decreased in lungs from patients with severe pulmonary hypertension. Am J Respir Crit Care Med 1999;159(6):1925–32.

[37] Achcar RO, Demura Y, Rai PR, et al. Loss of caveolin and heme oxygenase expression in severe pulmonary hypertension. Chest 2006;129(3):696–705.

[38] Voelkel NF, Cool CD, Lee SD, et al. Primary pulmonary hypertension between inflammation and cancer. Chest 1999;114(Suppl 3):225S–30S.

[39] Yamaki S, Wagenvoort CA. Comparison of primary plexogenic arteriopathy in adults and children. A morphometric study in 40 patients. Br Heart J 1985;54(4):428–34.

[40] Yi ES, Kim H, Ahn H, et al. Distribution of obstructive intimal lesions and their cellular phenotypes in chronic pulmonary hypertension. A morphometric and immunohistochemical study. Am J Respir Crit Care Med 2000;162(4):1577–86.

[41] Palevsky HI, Schloo BL, Pietra GG, et al. Primary pulmonary hypertension. Vascular structure, morphometry, and responsiveness to vasodilator agents. Circulation 1989;80(5):1207–21.

[42] Balk AG, Dingemans KP, Wagenvoort CA. The ultrastructure of the various forms of pulmonary arterial intimal fibrosis. Virchows Arch A Pathol Anat Histol 1979;382(2):139–50.

[43] Meyrick B, Reid L. Hypoxia and incorporation of 3H-thymidine by cells of the rat pulmonary arteries and alveolar wall. Am J Pathol 1979; 96(1):51–70.

[44] Meyrick BO, Reid LM. Crotalaria-induced pulmonary hypertension. Uptake of 3H-thymidine by the cells of the pulmonary circulation and alveolar walls. Am J Pathol 1982;106(1):84–94.

[45] Reid L, Anderson G, Simon G. Comparison of primary and thromboembolic pulmonary hypertension. Thorax 1972;27(2):263–4.

[46] Tuder RM, Zaiman AL. Prostacyclin analogs as the brakes for pulmonary artery smooth muscle cell proliferation. Is it sufficient to treat severe pulmonary hypertension? Am J Respir Cell Mol Biol 2002;26(2):171–4.

[47] Frid MG, Aldashev AA, Dempsey EC, et al. Smooth muscle cells isolated from discrete compartments of the mature vascular media exhibit unique phenotypes and distinct growth capabilities. Circ Res 1997;81(6):940–52.

[48] Morrell NW, Yang X, Upton PD, et al. Altered growth responses of pulmonary artery smooth muscle cells from patients with primary pulmonary hypertension to transforming growth factor-beta(1) and bone morphogenetic proteins. Circulation 2001;104(7):790–5.

[49] Yang X, Long L, Southwood M, et al. Dysfunctional Smad signaling contributes to abnormal smooth muscle cell proliferation in familial pulmonary arterial hypertension. Circ Res 2005;96(10): 1053–63.

[50] Song YL, Jones JE, Beppu H, et al. Increased susceptibility to pulmonary hypertension in heterozygous BMPR2-mutant mice. Circulation 2005;112(4): 553–62.

[51] Launay JM, Herve P, Peoc'h K, et al. Function of the serotonin 5-hydroxytryptamine 2B receptor in pulmonary hypertension. Nat Med 2002;8(10): 1129–35.

[52] Eddahibi S, Humbert M, Fadel E, et al. Serotonin transporter overexpression is responsible for pulmonary artery smooth muscle hyperplasia in primary pulmonary hypertension. J Clin Invest 2001; 108(8):1141–50.

[53] Eddahibi S, Hanoun N, Lanfumey L, et al. Attenuated hypoxic pulmonary hypertension in mice lacking the 5- hydroxytryptamine transporter gene. J Clin Invest 2000;105(11):1555–62.

[54] Botney MD, Bahadori L, Gold LI. Vascular remodeling in primary pulmonary hypertension. Potential role for transforming growth factor-beta. Am J Pathol 1994;144(2):286–95.

[55] Schermuly RT, Dony E, Ghofrani HA, et al. Reversal of experimental pulmonary hypertension by PDGF inhibition. J Clin Invest 2005;115(10): 2811–21.

[56] Ghofrani HA, Seeger W, Grimminger F. Imatinib for the treatment of pulmonary arterial hypertension. N Engl J Med 2005;353(13):1412–3.

[57] Jones PL, Cowan KN, Rabinovitch M. Tenascin-C, proliferation and subendothelial fibronectin in progressive pulmonary vascular disease. Am J Pathol 1997;150(4):1349–60.

[58] Rabinovitch M. EVE and beyond, retro and prospective insights. Am J Physiol 1999;277(1 Pt 1): L5–12.

[59] Cowan KN, Jones PL, Rabinovitch M. Elastase and matrix metalloproteinase inhibitors induce regression, and tenascin-C antisense prevents progression, of vascular disease. J Clin Invest 2000; 105(1):21–34.

[60] Merklinger SL, Jones PL, Martinez EC, et al. Epidermal growth factor receptor blockade mediates smooth muscle cell apoptosis and improves survival in rats with pulmonary hypertension. Circulation 2005;112(3):423–31.

[61] Vieillard-Baron A, Frisdal E, Eddahibi S, et al. Inhibition of matrix metalloproteinases by lung TIMP-1 gene transfer or doxycycline aggravates pulmonary hypertension in rats. Circ Res 2000; 87(5):418–25.

[62] Lepetit H, Eddahibi S, Fadel E, et al. Smooth muscle cell matrix metalloproteinases in idiopathic pulmonary arterial hypertension. Eur Respir J 2005;25(5):834–42.

[63] Matsui K, Takano Y, Yu ZX, et al. Immunohistochemical study of endothelin-1 and matrix metalloproteinases in plexogenic pulmonary arteriopathy. Pathol Res Pract 2002;198(6):403–12.

[64] Cowan KN, Heilbut A, Humpl T, et al. Complete reversal of fatal pulmonary hypertension in rats by a serine elastase inhibitor. Nat Med 2000;6(6): 698–702.

[65] Tuder RM, Yeager ME, Geraci M, et al. Severe pulmonary hypertension after the discovery of the familial primary pulmonary hypertension gene. Eur Respir J 2001;17(6):1065–9.

[66] Kasahara Y, Tuder RM, Cool CD, et al. Endothelial cell death and decreased expression of vascular endothelial growth factor and vascular endothelial growth factor receptor 2 in emphysema. Am J Respir Crit Care Med 2001;163(3):737–44.

[67] Remillard CV, Yuan JXJ. Activation of K+ channels: an essential pathway in programmed cell death. Am J Physiol Lung Cell Mol Physiol 2004;286(1):L49–67.

[68] Fantozzi I, Platoshyn O, Wong AH, et al. Bone morphogenetic protein-2 upregulates expression and function of voltage-gated K+ channels in human pulmonary artery smooth muscle cells. Am J Physiol Lung Cell Mol Physiol 2006;291(5):L993–1004.

[69] Dawson CA. Hypoxic pulmonary vasoconstriction: heterogeneity. In: Yuan JX, editor. Hypoxic pulmonary vasoconstriction: cellular and molecular mechanisms. Norwell (MA): Kluwer Academic Publishers; 2002. p. 15–32.

[70] Altieri DC. Validating survivin as a cancer therapeutic target. Nat Rev Cancer 2003;3(1):46–54.

[71] Stenmark KR, Davie N, Frid M, et al. Role of the adventitia in pulmonary vascular remodeling. Physiology (Bethesda) 2006;21(2):134–45.

[72] Bowers R, Cool C, Murphy RC, et al. Oxidative stress in severe pulmonary hypertension. Am J Respir Crit Care Med 2004;169(6):764–9.

[73] Caslin AW, Heath D, Madden B, et al. The histopathology of 36 cases of plexogenic pulmonary arteriopathy. Histopathology 1990;16(1):9–19.

[74] Peinado VI, Ramirez J, Roca J, et al. Identification of vascular progenitor cells in pulmonary arteries of patients with chronic obstructive pulmonary disease. Am J Respir Cell Mol Biol 2006;34(3):257–63.

[75] Dorfmuller P, Perros F, Balabanian K, et al. Inflammation in pulmonary arterial hypertension. Eur Respir J 2003;22(2):358–63.

[76] Nicolls MR, Taraseviciene-Stewart L, Rai PR, et al. Autoimmunity and pulmonary hypertension: a perspective. Eur Respir J 2005;26(6):1110–8.

[77] Humbert M, Monti G, Brenot F, et al. Increased interleukin-1 and interleukin-6 serum concentrations in severe primary pulmonary hypertension. Am J Respir Crit Care Med 1995;151(5):1628–31.

[78] Humbert M, Monti G, Fartoukh M, et al. Platelet-derived growth factor expression in primary pulmonary hypertension: comparison of HIV seropositive and HIV seronegative patients. Eur Respir J 1998;11(3):554–9.

[79] Dorfmuller P, Zarka V, Durand-Gasselin I, et al. Chemokine RANTES in severe pulmonary arterial hypertension. Am J Respir Crit Care Med 2002; 165(4):534–9.

[80] Balabanian K, Foussat A, Dorfmuller P, et al. CX3C chemokine fractalkine in pulmonary arterial hypertension. Am J Respir Crit Care Med 2002; 165(10):1419–25.

[81] Frid MG, Brunetti JA, Burke DL, et al. Hypoxia-induced pulmonary vascular remodeling requires recruitment of circulating mesenchymal precursors of a monocyte/macrophage lineage. Am J Pathol 2006;168(2):659–69.

[82] Zhao YDD, Courtman DW, Deng YP, et al. Rescue of monocrotaline-induced pulmonary arterial hypertension using bone marrow-derived endothelial-like progenitor cells—efficacy of combined cell and eNOS gene therapy in established disease. Circ Res 2005;96(4):442–50.

[83] Kim KK, Factor SM. Membranoproliferative glomerulonephritis and plexogenic pulmonary arteriopathy in a homosexual man with acquired immunodeficiency syndrome. Hum Pathol 1987; 18(12):1293–6.

[84] Kanmogne GD, Kennedy RC, Grammas P. Is HIV involved in the pathogenesis of non-infectious pulmonary complications in infected patients? Curr HIV Res 2003;1(4):385–93.

[85] Mette SA, Palevsky HI, Pietra GG, et al. Primary pulmonary hypertension in association with human immunodeficiency virus infection. A possible viral etiology for some forms of hypertensive pulmonary arteriopathy. Am Rev Respir Dis 1992;145(5): 1196–200.

[86] Pellicelli AM, Barbaro G, Palmieri F, et al. Primary pulmonary hypertension in HIV patients: a systematic review. Angiology 2001;52(1):31–41.

[87] Pongprot Y, Sittiwangkul R, Silvilairat S, et al. Cardiac manifestations in HIV-infected Thai children. Ann Trop Paediatr 2004;24(2):153–9.

[88] Recusani F, Di M, Gambarin F, et al. Clinical and therapeutical follow-up of HIV-associated pulmonary hypertension: prospective study of 10 patients. AIDS 2003;17(Suppl 1):S88–95.

[89] Barbaro G, Lucchini A, Pellicelli AM, et al. Highly active antiretroviral therapy compared with HAART and bosentan in combination in patients with HIV-associated pulmonary hypertension. Heart 2006;92(8):1164–6.

[90] Speich R, Jenni R, Opravil M, et al. Regression of HIV-associated pulmonary arterial hypertension and long-term survival during antiretroviral therapy. Swiss Med Wkly 2001;131(45–46):663–5.

[91] Sitbon O, Gressin V, Speich R, et al. Bosentan for the treatment of human immunodeficiency virus-associated pulmonary arterial hypertension. Am J Respir Crit Care Med 2001;170(11):1212–7.

[92] Marecki JC, Cool CD, Parr JE, et al. HIV-1 Nef is associated with complex pulmonary vascular lesions in SHIV-nef-infected Macaques. Am J Respir Crit Care Med 2006;174(4):437–45.

[93] Kirchhoff F, Greenough TC, Brettler DB, et al. Brief report: absence of intact nef sequences in a long-term survivor with nonprogressive HIV-1 infection. N Engl J Med 1995;332(4):228–32.

[94] Kestler HW, Ringler DJ, Mori K, et al. Importance of the nef gene for maintenance of high virus loads and for development of AIDS. Cell 1991;65(4): 651–62.

[95] Harris M. The role of myristoylation in the interactions between human immunodeficiency virus type I Nef and cellular proteins. Biochem Soc Trans 1995;23(3):557–61.

[96] Wang JK, Kiyokawa E, Verdin E, et al. The Nef protein of HIV-1 associates with rafts and primes T cells for activation. Proc Natl Acad Sci U S A 2000;97(1):394–9.

[97] Graziani A, Galimi F, Medico E, et al. The HIV-1 nef protein interferes with phosphatidylinositol 3-kinase activation 1. J Biol Chem 1996;271(12): 6590–3.

[98] Linnemann T, Zheng YH, Mandic R, et al. Interaction between Nef and phosphatidylinositol-3-kinase leads to activation of p21-activated kinase and increased production of HIV. Virology 1915; 294(2):246–55.

[99] He JC, Husain M, Sunamoto M, et al. Nef stimulates proliferation of glomerular podocytes through activation of Src-dependent Stat3 and MAPK1,2 pathways. J Clin Invest 2004;114(5):643–51.

[100] Krautkramer E, Giese SI, Gasteier JE, et al. Human immunodeficiency virus type 1 Nef activates p21-activated kinase via recruitment into lipid rafts. J Virol 2004;78(8):4085–97.

[101] Olivetta E, Percario Z, Fiorucci G, et al. HIV-1 Nef induces the release of inflammatory factors from human monocyte/macrophages: involvement of Nef endocytotic signals and NF-kappa B activation. J Immunol 1915;170(4):1716–27.

[102] James CO, Huang MB, Khan M, et al. Extracellular Nef protein targets CD4+ T cells for apoptosis by interacting with CXCR4 surface receptors. J Virol 2004;78(6):3099–109.

[103] Choi HJ, Smithgall TE. HIV-1 Nef promotes survival of TF-1 macrophages by inducing Bcl-XL expression in an extracellular signal-regulated kinase-dependent manner. J Biol Chem 2003; 279(49):51688–96.

[104] Damania B, Desrosiers RC. Simian homologues of human herpesvirus 8. Philos Trans R Soc Lond B Biol Sci 1929;356(1408):535–43.

[105] Desrosiers RC, Sasseville VG, Czajak SC, et al. A herpesvirus of rhesus monkeys related to the human Kaposi's sarcoma-associated herpesvirus. J Virol 1997;71(12):9764–9.

[106] Cool CD, Rai MD, Yeager ME, et al. Expression of human herpesvirus 8 in primary pulmonary hypertension. N Engl J Med 2003;349(12):1113–22.

[107] Boshoff C, Endo Y, Collins PD, et al. Angiogenic and HIV-inhibitory functions of KSHV-encoded chemokines. Science 1997;278(5336):290–4.

[108] Guo HG, Sadowska M, Reid W, et al. Kaposi's sarcoma-like tumors in a human herpesvirus 8 ORF74 transgenic mouse. J Virol 2003;77(4): 2631–9.

[109] Estep RD, Axthelm MK, Wong SW. A G protein-coupled receptor encoded by rhesus rhadinovirus is similar to ORF74 of Kaposi's sarcoma-associated herpesvirus. J Virol 2003;77(3):1738–46.

[110] Bais C, Van Geelen A, Eroles P, et al. Kaposi's sarcoma associated herpesvirus G protein-coupled receptor immortalizes human endothelial cells by activation of the VEGF receptor-2/KDR. Cancer Cells 2003;3(2):131–43.

[111] Yang TY, Chen SC, Leach MW, et al. Transgenic expression of the chemokine receptor encoded by human herpesvirus 8 induces an angioproliferative disease resembling Kaposi's sarcoma. J Exp Med 2000;191(3):445–54.

[112] Galambos C, Montgomery J, Jenkins FJ. No role for kaposi sarcoma-associated herpesvirus in pediatric idiopathic pulmonary hypertension. Pediatr Pulmonol 2006;41(2):122–5.

[113] Laney AS, De M, Peters JS, et al. Kaposi sarcoma-associated herpesvirus and primary and secondary pulmonary hypertension. Chest 2005; 127(3):762–7.

[114] Katano H, Ito K, Shibuya K, et al. Lack of human herpesvirus 8 infection in lungs of Japanese patients with primary pulmonary hypertension. J Infect Dis 2001;191(5):743–5.

[115] Nicastri E, Vizza CD, Carletti F, et al. Human herpesvirus 8 and pulmonary hypertension. Emerg Infect Dis 2005;11(9):1480–2.

[116] Henke-Gendo C, Mengel M, Hoeper MM, et al. Absence of Kaposi's sarcoma-associated herpesvirus in patients with pulmonary arterial hypertension. Am J Respir Crit Care Med 1915;172(12): 1581–5.

[117] Moorman J, Saad M, Kosseifi S, et al. Hepatitis C virus and the lung: implications for therapy. Chest 2005;128(4):2882–92.

[118] Robalino BD, Moodie DS. Association between primary pulmonary hypertension and portal hypertension: analysis of its pathophysiology and clinical, laboratory and hemodynamic manifestations. J Am Coll Cardiol 1991;17(2):492–8.

[119] Voelkel NF, Tuder RM. Severe pulmonary hypertensive diseases: a perspective. Eur Respir J 1999; 14(6):1246–50.

[120] Bull TM, Coldren CD, Moore M, et al. Gene microarray analysis of peripheral blood cells in pulmonary arterial hypertension. Am J Respir Crit Care Med 2004;170(8):911–9.

[121] Geraci MW, Gao B, Hoshikawa Y, et al. Genomic approaches to research in pulmonary hypertension. Respir Res 2001;2(4):210–5.

ELSEVIER
SAUNDERS

Clin Chest Med 28 (2007) 43–57

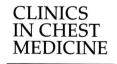

CLINICS
IN CHEST
MEDICINE

Genetics and Mediators in Pulmonary Arterial Hypertension

Eric D. Austin, MD[a],*, James E. Loyd, MD[b]

[a]*Division of Pediatric Pulmonary Medicine, Department of Pediatrics,
Vanderbilt University Medical Center, T-1217 Medical Center North, Nashville, TN 37232-2650, USA*
[b]*Division of Allergy, Pulmonary, and Critical Care Medicine, Department of Medicine,
Vanderbilt University Medical Center, T-1217 Medical Center North, Nashville, TN 37232-2650, USA*

Background and synopsis of history

Idiopathic pulmonary arterial hypertension (IPAH), formerly known as primary pulmonary hypertension (PPH), was first described by Dresdale and colleagues [1] in 1951. This report was soon followed by a second publication in 1954, in which the same author described the occurrence of pulmonary hypertension among several members of the same family, comprising the first report of familial PPH, now known as familial pulmonary arterial hypertension (FPAH) [2].

After this initial description, slow progress in understanding the genetics of FPAH was made during the next 30 years, with individual reports describing 13 different families reported in the United States. In 1984, a follow-up analysis of these 13 families, including interval description of 8 new cases in 9 of the families and an additional 14th family, were reviewed. The additional family contained the largest number of affected family members described to that time, with six deaths caused by PPH during two generations [3]. That publication described inheritance patterns, including vertical transmission and father-to-son transmission, which suggested autosomal dominant pattern of inheritance indicative of a single gene defect. This report also caused experts to speculate that cases of PPH that seemed to occur in isolation may, in fact, have a familial basis, although this was difficult to recognize partly because of skip generations that resulted from incomplete penetrance [4].

The National Institutes of Health (NIH) PPH prospective registry [5] in the mid-1980s provided the benchmark for the clinical definition of IPAH, and facilitated interaction of participating investigators to collect and organize sufficient numbers of FPAH families to provide robust statistical power for a genome-wide search for FPAH loci. Two separate teams of investigators independently established linkage of a locus for the gene, named *PPH1*, for familial PPH to chromosome 2q31–32 in 1997 [6,7]. A few years later, both teams also showed that mutations in the gene encoding bone morphogenetic protein receptor type 2 (*BMPR2*), a receptor that is a member of the transforming growth factor beta (TGF-β) superfamily [8,9], was responsible for FPAH.

Epidemiology of pulmonary arterial hypertension

The frequency of PPH, which encompasses IPAH and FPAH, is estimated to be one to two cases per year per 1 million in the general population, with a female-to-male prevalence of 2:1 but with similar disease severity and outcome [10,11]. Even after 2 decades, the best available clinical information on the natural history of IPAH derives from the prospective NIH study of patients who had PPH and were followed up in the United States from 1981 to 1985. This report remains the benchmark because it

This work was supported by NIH NHLBI PO1 HL72058 and The Vanderbilt GCRC grant M01 RR 00095 NCRR/NIH.

* Corresponding author.

E-mail address: eric.austin@vanderbilt.edu (E.D. Austin).

meticulously described and followed up 187 patients who had PPH at 32 centers in the United States, and was conducted before effective therapies were developed. The ethnic background of patients was comparable to that of the U.S. population. The registry confirmed that PPH can develop at any age, with a mean age at diagnosis of 36 years. In general, women tended to present in the third decade of life and men in the fourth. The median survival after diagnosis was 2.8 years. The mean time from symptom onset to diagnosis was 2 years for the entire cohort, but this interval was shorter for patients who had a family history of PPH. In terms of familial prevalence, the NIH registry reported prevalence of 6% based on the finding that 12 of the 187 patients reported one or more immediate family member affected with PAH. These 12 FPAH patients did not differ from the 175 other patients in hemodynamic data or symptoms [5,12].

Similar findings were confirmed and extended in a national prospective registry of patients who have PAH that was established in France in 2000 and which recently reported 674 enrolled PAH cases. Investigators reported a PAH prevalence of 15 cases per 1 million adult French inhabitants. They identified a female-to-male ratio of 1.9:1, consistent with the NIH registry data. The distribution of PAH causes in the 674 cases showed 39.2% from IPAH, 3.9% from FPAH, 15.3% associated with connective tissue diseases (systemic sclerosis was leading cause), 11.3% related to congenital heart diseases, 10.4% related to portal hypertension, 9.5% associated with anorexigen use, 6.2% related to HIV, and 4.3% related to other causes. The design of this registry did not include children [13].

Genetics and the diagnosis of familial pulmonary arterial hypertension

IPAH and FPAH share the same clinical features, histopathology, and clinical course. The true incidence of FPAH is unknown and is difficult to completely elucidate [14]. Some investigators speculate that as knowledge of the complex genetics of PAH increases and mutation detection improves, the percentage of patients whose disease is identified as familial will continue to climb. Establishing the role of familial transmission is often difficult for several reasons. First, despite increasing awareness of the disease entity, misdiagnosis of pulmonary hypertension continues to occur. Second, despite the autosomal dominant

nature of the genetic defects in the *BMPR2* gene, the penetrance of disease expression is low and varies among families. As a result, generations of individuals carrying mutation may not develop clinical expression of FPAH. Estimates indicate that only approximately 20% of individuals with a known genetic mutation in *BMPR2* will develop PAH during their entire life, and that phenotypic expression may occur at any age. Finally, the high mobility of our society may hinder complete knowledge of family genealogic history, which can impair recognition of families not otherwise known to be related [15].

Only gender has been shown to influence clinical expression of the *BMPR2* mutation, demonstrated by the 2:1 female predominance. This finding implicates the role of gender in facilitating a predisposition to disease, suggesting some hormonal influence or X chromosome association for clinical expression [16]. Neither suggestion has been confirmed, but an abnormal gender ratio among progeny of obligate gene carriers has been described. Increased ratio of female live births suggests possible selective wastage of male fetuses or an abnormal primary sex ratio [17]. The fact that more women are affected may be caused by the loss of male fetuses from an unrecognized defect in embryologic development.

Data from national prospective registries in the United States and France described a 6% and 3.9% prevalence, respectively, of FPAH among patients who have PAH [5,13]. Discovery of the molecular basis of FPAH and IPAH has advanced investigations into the true impact of genetics on the diagnosis of PAH. The family reported to be most heavily affected with FPAH was described in an investigation that connected five previously independent Tennessee families, including 18 affected members, 12 of whom were erroneously believed to have IPAH. These five family branches, not formerly known to the investigators to be related, shared the same *BMPR2* missense mutation and a common ancestry [18]. Currently, 23 patients (20 women, and 3 men) who have FPAH have been identified in the extended kindred (Fig. 1), including a new family branch discovered in 2006.

FPAH seems to show no predilection for geographic location; it has been reported around the globe. FPAH predominantly affects Caucasians in the United States, but ethnic or racial distribution has not been investigated in depth [15]. The registry at Vanderbilt University currently contains 100 families that have two or more affected members.

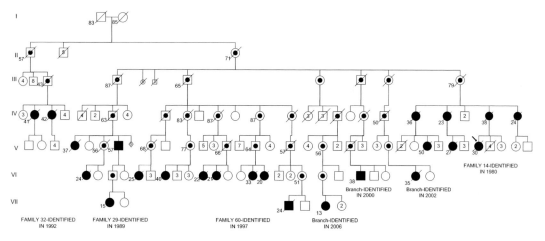

Fig. 1. Pedigree of an extended kindred with familial pulmonary arterial hypertension (FPAH). This pedigree now links six families that were previously labeled as independent, and 23 total patients who had FPAH. Solid symbols represent individuals who have disease; circles represent women, squares represent men. Line through symbol represents death. Dot inside symbol represents obligate carrier of the *BMPR2* mutation. Numbers below symbols represent age at death or current living age. Numbers inside symbols represent numbers of unaffected siblings of each gender. *S* inside symbol represents stillbirth. Diamond symbol represents sex unknown.

Of the 3750 total individuals followed up, 352 subjects meet criteria for PAH.

Reduced penetrance

Initial pedigree studies of families with PAH showed phenotypic expression in fewer individuals than expected. In fact, individuals known to be at risk for disease through pedigree analysis did not express PAH consistently [3]. From genetic analysis, mutant *BMPR2* alleles are known to display reduced penetrance among PAH kindreds, indicating that heterozygous mutation of the gene is required, but not sufficient, to precipitate clinical expression of disease [10]. The mechanisms of reduced penetrance are unknown, and are the subject of intense investigation because of the possible role of genetic or environmental modifiers of disease expression [19].

The registry at Vanderbilt continues to display reduced penetrance. In fact, of the 3750 total subjects followed up, approximately 2250 are within family bloodlines, but only 15.6% of subjects were diagnosed with PAH. Furthermore, pedigree analysis of the six most heavily affected families shows that 24.2% of first-degree relatives of patients who have PAH were also diagnosed with this disease (Eric D. Austin, MD; Lisa Wheeler; James E. Loyd, MD, unpublished data, 2006). These heavily affected families provide a valuable opportunity for genetic and environmental evaluation of disease modifiers, which is underway.

Genetic anticipation

Several reports have shown earlier age of FPAH onset in subsequent generations. This early onset is one manifestation of genetic anticipation that was observed in some of the earliest reports of individual families in the 1960s, and was again substantiated in a summary analysis of multiple families in 1984 [3]. The age at death in each successive generation decreased serially by approximately a decade. For example, age of death in successive generations statistically decreased from a mean of 45.6 years to 36.3 years to 24.2 years. Historically, genetic anticipation was attributed to ascertainment and other possible bias. In a method designed to overcome artefactual bias, 60 pairs, including an affected parent and child, were analyzed with the finding that age at death was significantly less (15 years younger) for the affected child than for the parent, confirming a biologic basis for genetic anticipation as best possible [20].

The molecular mechanism of genetic anticipation in FPAH remains unknown, despite the recent advances in knowledge about central pathogenesis. Many other disease examples of genetic anticipation exist and may lend clues. Several neurologic diseases, including fragile X syndrome, myotonic dystrophy, and Huntington's disease, exhibit genetic anticipation in association with trinucleotide repeat expansion (TRE). In these diseases, TRE has been confirmed as the molecular basis for not only genetic anticipation but also incomplete penetrance and variable age of onset [21,22]. All three phenomena are also similarly observed in FPAH. TRE has not been identified in the primary gene defects in *BMPR2*, but efforts continue to identify relevant regions containing expanded repeats. Meanwhile, speculation continues that TRE might be present in a modifier gene (not yet identified) that facilitates disease expression. Alternatively, another molecular mechanism, not yet recognized, may cause genetic anticipation.

Mutations in *BMPR2* cause familial pulmonary arterial hypertension

The discovery of the genetic basis of FPAH was made possible by the collaborative development of family cohorts with banked DNA, and facilitated by advances in molecular genetics and availability of information from the human genome project [23]. As families were identified with PPH, DNA was collected and stored, so that by the mid-1990s the statistical power was sufficient to locate the genetic cause of PAH. Two separate groups used microsatellite markers and linkage analysis to focus the search to chromosome 2q33. Using DNA collected from 19 affected and 58 unaffected family members of six families with PPH that had pedigrees suggestive of an autosomal dominance pattern of gene transmission, Nichols and colleagues [6] used a microsatellite marker search to establish linkage to a 30 million base pair region on chromosome 2q33. Similarly, Morse and colleagues [24] independently identified the locus of a familial PPH gene to chromosome 2q31–32.

Because the segment on chromosome 2 was longer than could readily be sequenced in that era, the investigators used a positional candidate gene approach, targeting and testing several genes in this region with known gene products of potential relevance [15]. Because it is a member of the TGF-β superfamily of receptors, *BMPR2* was selected for evaluation. In 2000, two separate teams of investigators characterized multiple heterozygous mutations in this large gene, which resides on chromosome 2q33 and has 13 exons, as the cause of disease in several affected kindreds [8,9].

Prevalence of *BMPR2* mutations in familial pulmonary arterial hypertension

Since the discovery of *BMPR2* mutations in several families with FPAH in 2000, investigators have worked to identify mutations in other families and in those with apparently "sporadic" PAH (IPAH). Molecular testing for *BMPR2* abnormalities has shown mutations among many different ethnic groups [25–27]. By 2005, approximately 65% of known FPAH families had *BMPR2* mutations identifiable through gene sequencing. A summary report described 144 distinct mutations among 210 subjects, and most of these coded frameshift, nonsense, or splice site donor/acceptance site mutations [28]. By expanding the mutation screening methods in 2005, Cogan and colleagues [29] showed that 48% of the 21 mutations discovered in 30 unrelated affected families were deletions or duplications of exons. These investigators used Multiplex Ligation-dependent Probe Amplification (MLPA) analysis of genomic DNA, confirmed with real-time polymerase chain reaction. They concluded that these techniques improved the identification of genetic abnormalities in *BMPR2* in FPAH, showing that 70% or more of families have identifiable *BMPR2* mutations. A different group also recently reported using MLPA analysis of genomic DNA, with mutations discovered in 28% of families previously reported to lack *BMPR2* mutations [30]. These reports further support the primary role of *BMPR2* in the central pathogenesis of disease in FPAH. In the Vanderbilt cohort, DNA specimens are available from at least one affected patient in 55 families, and using current methods *BMPR2* mutations are found to be present in 46 families, but not in 9. Fig. 2 displays the distribution of most reported recurrent mutations in the *BMPR2* gene, including their domain location.

BMPR2 mutations in sporadic or idiopathic PAH

Although further analysis of larger IPAH cohorts is needed, it is already clear that a significant proportion of patients who have IPAH harbor mutations in the *BMPR2* gene. These mutations may occur in the setting of low-penetrance germline mutations, in which other family members transmit the mutation without disease expression, or the mutations may develop de novo [31]. This fact is not surprising, given that low penetrance and genetic anticipation are hallmarks of FPAH. Although the rate of *BMPR2* mutation in the

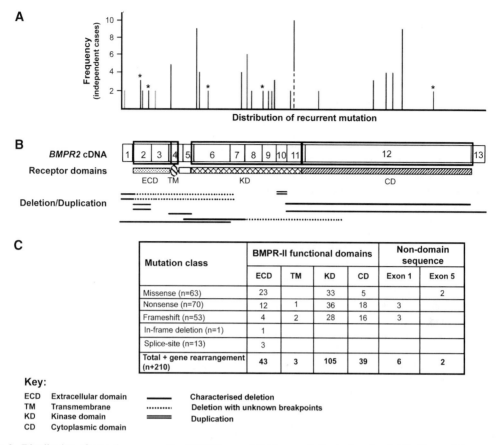

Fig. 2. Distribution of mutations across the *BMPR2* gene. (*A*) Line graph illustrating the distribution and frequency of recurrent mutations. The *x*-axis represents the position of mutations relative to the *BMPR2* cDNA below, and the *y*-axis defines the number of unrelated probands observed to harbor each mutation. The contiguous black and dotted line identifies the two amino acid substitutions recurrent at position 491. (*B*) Proportional representation of the *BMPR2* cDNA, with exons 1–13 indicated. The boxed regions delineate the extracellular (ECD), transmembrane (TM), kinase (KD), and cytoplasmic (CD) domains of the receptor depicted below. Large gene rearrangements (deletions and duplications) identified in PAH cases are arrayed below the cDNA. (*C*) Table summarizing the total number of PAH-causing mutations observed in each functional domain and nondomain encoding sequence. (*From* Machado RD, Aldred MA, James V, et al. Mutations of the TGF-β type II receptor *BMPR2* in pulmonary arterial hypertension. Human Mutation 2006; 27(2):121–32; with permission).

general population is not known, it seems to be extremely low given that no mutations have been detected among a few hundred control samples [15].

Reports of mutation prevalence in patients who have IPAH are limited, and these depend partly on which detection techniques were used, because these techniques continue to improve. The true prevalence is currently unknown, with reports ranging from 11% to 40% [14,26,27]. As with FPAH, more mutations were detected when newer molecular techniques were applied to IPAH cohorts. Aldred and colleagues [30] noted that 6 of 106 (5.7%) patients who had IPAH previously labeled *BMPR2* mutation–negative had detectable gene rearrangements. Parental evaluation in three of these patients showed that two of the mutations were de novo, whereas one was inherited from an unaffected mother.

BMPR2 and the expression of disease

Haploinsufficiency describes the condition in which heterozygosity for a gene mutation leads to insufficient protein product, with decreased protein function leading to phenotypic expression of disease. In 2001, Machado and colleagues [25] examined the role of *BMPR2* mutation in terms of genotype–phenotype relationships, proposing that a model of haploinsufficiency explains the development of pulmonary hypertension from a molecular perspective. They suggested that 60% of the reported pathogenic mutations should result in premature truncation codons of the *BMPR2* transcript, which would lead to nonsense-mediated decay. Recent studies have supported this by showing deletions within exons 2–13, which would confer nonfunctional peptide [29,30]. These studies suggest that haploinsufficiency contributes to the molecular mechanisms underlying PAH through reduction in the available level of *BMPR2* protein, at least in some cases.

Investigation of downstream molecular effects of the *BMPR2* signaling pathway have also shown that specific disease-causing mutations in the ligand-binding and kinase domains of *BMPR2* seem to exert dominant negative effects on BMP signaling. Therefore, disruption of BMP signaling may lead to absence of critical mechanisms in the antiproliferative and differentiation mechanisms in the pulmonary vasculature [28]. In fact, functional studies have shown dominant negative effects on BMP signaling in vitro in the setting of point mutations or truncations in the kinase domain of *BMPR2* [32].

Multiple "hits": Is one abnormal *BMPR2* allele sufficient to cause pulmonary arterial hypertension?

The observation of reduced penetrance implies that mutation of the *BMPR2* gene is required but is not sufficient alone for phenotypic expression. This fact suggests that other genetic or environmental modifiers likely mediate the clinical expression of disease [10]. Given this information, individuals who carry the *BMPR2* mutation and others may express disease in the setting of a "multiple hit" model, analogous to models of sequential mutations in the genesis of neoplasia.

Plexiform lesions are a characteristic histopathologic microvascular abnormality found in the lungs of many patients who have PAH [33]. Some investigators have suggested that they represent a neoplastic-like proliferative process, with resultant endothelial and smooth muscle cell proliferation and diminished apoptosis. In support of this, evidence of monoclonal proliferation of local endothelial cells and the migration and local proliferation of smooth muscle cells exists [34]. Furthermore, investigations suggest a role for *BMPR2* signaling in these events [35]. In contrast, the plexiform lesions in patients who have secondary pulmonary hypertension contain endothelial cells that are polyclonal [36]. In addition, experts have suggested that circulating endothelial precursor cells that migrate to the pulmonary vasculature may participate in the pathogenesis of PAH [37].

Immunohistochemical staining of lung tissue from patients who have FPAH shows nearly complete absence of *BMPR2* protein in those who demonstrate heterozygosity through genetic testing [38]. This finding is somewhat unexpected, because at least some protein production is anticipated in the setting of one wild-type and one germline mutated allele. To examine this, Machado and colleagues [19] investigated whether inactivation of the remaining wild-type *BMPR2* allele through somatic mutation prompts disease expression, similar to the loss of a second tumor suppressor gene in cancer development. However, results suggested that microsatellite instability with somatic loss of function in the remaining wild-type *BMPR2* allele did not contribute to disease development. This area needs more investigation to evaluate whether de novo mutations or common polymorphisms in other genes function as multiple genetic "hits" that interact with the heterozygous *BMPR2* mutation to create a molecular environment suitable to trigger phenotypic expression of disease [39].

BMPR2 signaling pathway

Expressed ubiquitously, *BMPR2* is a receptor for a family of cytokines known as *bone morphogenetic proteins* (BMPs). BMPs are members of the TGF-β superfamily of proteins. The TGF-β family of proteins and their receptors are highly conserved throughout nature. Originally identified for their role in ectopic bone and cartilage formation, BMPs play a crucial role in regulating mammalian development, such as embryonic lung morphogenesis [40]. Although genetic studies strongly implicate the TGF-β superfamily in the regulation of pulmonary vascular cell growth and differentiation, investigations have not shown the precise molecular mechanisms involved. Nonetheless, progress has been made in evaluating their contribution to lung vascular development.

The BMP signaling pathway involves hetero-dimerization of the serine/threonine transmem-brane kinases, *BMPR1* and *BMPR2*. Four functional domains comprise *BMPR2*: ligand binding, kinase, transmembrane, and cytoplasmic domains. Activation of the *BMPR2/BMPR1* receptor complex leads to phosphorylation of a se-ries of cytoplasmic mediators, which include the Smad family. Specifically, Smad proteins 1, 5, and 8 are phosphorylated, and subsequently com-plex with Smad 4 for translocation into the nu-cleus to regulate target gene transcription. The Smad signaling pathway seems to participate in the inhibition of cell growth and induction of ap-optosis [41]. Perhaps mutations in *BMPR2* elimi-nate a critical growth regulatory function in pulmonary vascular cells. Why other types of vas-culature in the body are spared remains a mystery.

In addition to Smad pathway activation, other substrates are affected by *BMPR2/BMPR1* recep-tor activation, including mitogen-activated protein kinases (MAPKs), NH_2-terminal kinase, and others [42]. Recent studies have implicated not only Smad signaling but also unopposed MAPK function in association with *BMPR2* mutations. Yang and colleagues [32] showed that kinase do-main mutations of *BMPR2* found in PAH patients result in down-regulation of Smad signaling in pul-monary artery smooth muscle cells (PASMCs), with resultant loss of antiproliferative effect. The resulting imbalance between Smad and MAPK function may lead to proproliferative and antia-poptotic effects that promote the development of PAH.

BMPR2 mutations in other disease states

The discovery of mutations in *BMPR2* in pa-tients who have FPAH and IPAH has prompted searches for this abnormality in other patients who have pulmonary hypertension. Mutations in this gene generally have not been found consis-tently, further supporting the relationship between these two disease entities, which may in fact exist together along a continuum.

Patients have been evaluated who have pul-monary veno-occlusive disease (PVOD), a rare form of pulmonary hypertension in which the vascular changes originate in the small pulmonary veins and venules. Runo and colleagues [43] docu-mented a novel mutation in exon 1 of the *BMPR2* gene, resulting in a truncated protein predicted to have no function, in a 36-year-old woman who

had biopsy-confirmed PVOD. Further investiga-tion showed that the proband's mother died of pulmonary hypertension, whereas laboratory evaluation confirmed an identical *BMPR2* muta-tion in the proband's healthy sister. Similarly, Al-dred and colleagues [30] discovered a genetic mutation in exon 2 of *BMPR2* in a patient who had PVOD. This patient had three first-degree rel-atives who died with the diagnosis of pulmonary hypertension. This mutation of *BMPR2* had pre-viously been described in a family that had FPAH with no evidence of PVOD. These results suggest that the molecular alterations associated with *BMPR2* mutations may exhibit phenotypic heterogeneity (ie, the ability of an allelic mutation at a single locus to produce more than one expres-sion of disease). Furthermore, PVOD and FPAH may represent different spectra of the same dis-ease, with phenotype influenced by genetic or en-vironmental modifiers [43].

Another cause of PAH is associated with drug exposure. Specifically, PAH has been reported in conjunction with exposure to appetite suppres-sants, such as fenfluramine and dexfenfluramine [44,45]. The exact mechanism of PAH promotion has not been elucidated, but these drugs may serve as an environmental mediator to facilitate disease expression, possibly in genetically susceptible indi-viduals. Individual factors of susceptibility are particularly plausible given the low numbers of PAH in those exposed to fenfluramine (approxi-mately 1 case per 10,000 people exposed) [46]. Humbert and colleagues [47] found distinct *BMPR2* mutations, each predicted to result in di-minished receptor function, in 9% of unrelated pa-tients who had PAH associated with fenfluramine exposure. They found no *BMPR2* mutations in 130 normal control subjects. When compared with other patients who had PAH associated with fenfluramine, patients who had *BMPR2* mu-tation expressed disease after a shorter interval of exposure to fenfluramine, which was also statisti-cally significant. This information, although in requiring further study, again emphasizes the im-portance of additional genetic and environmental factors required to produce disease expression.

Insufficient data exist for an exhaustive discus-sion of congenital heart disease and *BMPR2* mu-tations. A report by Roberts and colleagues [48] noted that 6% of 106 children and adults who had congenital heart disease possessed mutations of the *BMPR2* gene. They noted that this finding agreed with reports in mouse models of vasculo-genesis and cardiac anomalies, which implicate abnormalities of the TGF-β pathway. These findings clearly warrant further investigation.

The serotonin pathway and pulmonary arterial hypertension mediation

Although the modifier genes of PAH pathogenesis are currently unknown, investigations are underway to elucidate these pathways. The neurotransmitter serotonin (5-hydroxytryptamine [5-HT]) has been implicated. Common genetic variations (polymorphisms) in the serotonin pathway or polymorphisms in the serotonin transporter (*SERT*) gene may contribute, either independently or related to the presence of a *BMPR2* mutation. Serotonin has been shown to be a cellular mitogen, and stimulates PASMC proliferation through a signaling pathway mediated by *SERT* [49].

In 1995, Herve and colleagues [50] described increased plasma serotonin levels caused by abnormal platelet serotonin storage in 16 patients who had PPH. Subsequently, Eddahibi and colleagues [51,52] found increased growth of PASMCs in culture from patients who had PPH compared with controls when stimulated by serotonin or serum, and this proliferative response was augmented in the setting of hypoxia. The investigators attributed these mitogenic effects to increased expression of *SERT*. Furthermore, they proposed a clinical link to the molecular cause for *SERT* overexpression in the form of variations in the *SERT* gene promoter by comparing 89 people who had severe PPH and 84 control subjects. Homozygosity for a long promoter variant (L-allelic variant) was present in approximately 65% of patients (LL genotype individuals) who had PPH but only 27% of controls [52].

Continued work on the role of serotonin as a cellular mitogen has shown that internalization of 5-HT by *SERT* leads to downstream activation of the MAPK cascade, partly through the production of reactive oxygen species, which ultimately stimulates transcription of genes to drive cellular proliferation. PASMCs respond strongly to these stimulatory effects in vitro [53,54]. Therefore, up-regulation of the MAPK cascade as an effect of abnormal serotonin signaling has garnered attention as a potential antagonist to the growth inhibitory effects of BMP signaling pathways, and possibly confers susceptibility to PAH expression.

Genetic abnormalities may lead to an imbalance of these cellular processes that facilitates abnormal PASMC proliferation and the development of PAH. Seeking to confirm disease susceptibility alleles using a larger cohort, Machado and colleagues [55] recently examined the role of polymorphic variation within the *SERT* gene in the predisposition to and modification of PAH in 528 affected patients. This study evaluated 133 patients who had FPAH or IPAH and known *BMPR2* mutation, 259 patients who had IPAH, 136 patients who had PAH associated with other diseases or exposures, and 353 control subjects. Results showed no difference in frequency of *SERT* gene alleles among any groups, suggesting that the *SERT* mutations evaluated are not likely to contribute to phenotypic expression of PAH in patients carrying a *BMPR2* mutation and those who are not. Likewise, genetic variation of the *SERT* promoter gene locus did not correlate with differences in age of onset of disease, nor did this variation differ by gender, which is the only known risk factor for PAH development.

The authors' group also investigated the role of polymorphisms in the *SERT* gene, specifically the L allele, in a cohort of patients who had IPAH and FPAH. This cohort included 83 patients who had IPAH, 99 patients who had FPAH, 67 unaffected carriers of a known *BMPR2* mutation, and 125 controls [54]. Overall, results comparable to those found in the study by Machado and colleagues [55] were found, including no difference in *SERT* genotype distribution among groups. Again, a lack of difference between diseased patients who had FPAH and unaffected patients carrying a *BMPR2* mutation suggested that the polymorphisms studied do not affect disease penetrance. However, other polymorphisms within the *SERT* gene have not been investigated and could function as modifier genes. Lastly, although patients who had FPAH were diagnosed earlier than those who had IPAH, patients who had FPAH and were homozygous for the L allele (LL genotype) showed an even earlier age at diagnosis than patients who had FPAH and did not have this polymorphism. This finding may reflect unappreciated interactions between *BMPR2* mutations and polymorphisms in the *SERT* gene that affect disease expression [56].

Hereditary hemorrhagic telangiectasia (Osler-Weber-Rendu syndrome) and pulmonary arterial hypertension

Hereditary hemorrhagic telangiectasia (HHT), or Osler-Weber-Rendu syndrome, is a vascular dysplasia characterized by mucocutaneous telangiectasias that cause recurrent epistaxis, gastrointestinal bleeding, and arteriovenous malformations of the pulmonary, hepatic, and cerebral circulations. Defects in additional components of the TGF-β signaling superfamily receptor complex—activin receptor-like kinase 1 (*ALK1*) located on chromosome 12 and endoglin on chromosome 9—are pivotal in the pathogenesis of HHT [57,58]. Pulmonary hypertension is also known to occur in HHT, typically a secondary form related to a high cardiac output state. However, pulmonary hypertension that is clinically and histologically identical to FPAH and IPAH has recently been described in multiple unique kindreds with HTT associated with detectable mutations in *ALK1* [59,60]. Furthermore, a recent case report described an endoglin germline mutation in a patient who had HHT and PAH related to dexfenfluramine exposure [61]. Investigators also recently reported a child who had a mutation that resulted in abnormal splicing of the endoglin transcript that caused markedly reduced levels, suggesting haploinsufficiency leading to disease expression. This child initially presented at the age of 3 months with PAH and was later diagnosed with HHT at 8 years of age. The endoglin mutation was also detected in her asymptomatic father [62].

The finding of PAH in patients who have HHT and identifiable abnormalities of the TGF-β signaling pathway suggests that a common molecular pathway precipitates pulmonary vascular disease. A direct interaction between the gene products of the *BMPR2* gene and *ALK1* or endoglin genes has not been elucidated, and these receptors do not seem to share activating ligands [42,62]. However, each receptor mediates intracellular signaling through the Smad family of coactivators, suggesting interaction among these molecular receptors at some level [63]. TGF-β signaling pathway defects are likely to be diverse in type, interaction, and phenotypic expression, and require further study.

Additional mediators and mechanisms involved in pathogenesis

Many other mediators and mechanisms have been proposed to contribute to vasoconstriction and thrombosis and to pulmonary arterial obstruction caused by vascular proliferation and remodeling. Many of these topics are the focus of important ongoing studies but cannot be discussed in depth in this article. However, evaluation of these pathways at the molecular level may lead to important advances in earlier diagnosis, therapy, and outcomes [64].

Exuberant pulmonary vasoconstriction and inappropriate cell proliferation are strongly linked to endothelial cell dysfunction [65]. Endothelial cell dysfunction impairs local production of protective vasoactive compounds, such as prostacyclin and nitric oxide. Endothelial cell release of prostacyclin (prostaglandin-I_2), an endogenous vasodilator (through cyclic adenosine monophosphate [cAMP]-dependent pathways) and an inhibitor of platelet aggregation and suppressor of vascular smooth muscle cell proliferation, is diminished in patients who have PAH [66]. The pulmonary endothelial cells of these patients express far less prostacyclin synthase, leading to an imbalance in the local prostacyclin-to-thromboxane A2 ratio. Thromboxane A2 is a vasoconstrictor and a potent stimulant of platelet aggregation [67], which is particularly relevant considering the belief that platelet dysfunction and the development of thrombotic lesions are important processes in PAH, and the potential role of the serotonin pathway [65,68].

Reduced nitric oxide synthase expression in pulmonary endothelial cells results in diminished local production of nitric oxide, a potent pulmonary vasodilator and an inhibitor of pulmonary vascular smooth muscle proliferation [69,70]. Nitric oxide and atrial natriuretic peptide modulate pulmonary vascular resistance, and possibly remodeling, at least partly through manipulating intracellular cyclic guanosine monophosphate (cGMP)–mediated pulmonary vasodilatation [66,71]. Investigators continue to examine other mediators that affect the cGMP pathway, including vasoactive intestinal peptide. Vasoactive intestinal peptide is a neuropeptide that has potent systemic and pulmonary vasodilator effects and contributes to the inhibition of vascular smooth muscle cell proliferation and platelet aggregation. Vasoactive intestinal peptide, the effects of which are mediated through cGMP- and cAMP-dependent pathways, is deficient in the serum and lung tissue of patients who have IPAH compared with controls. Investigations to evaluate the response to vasoactive intestinal peptide as a therapeutic agent are underway [72].

Under pathologic conditions, endothelial cells increase production of compounds with vasoconstrictive, proliferative, and inflammatory properties, such as the peptides of the endothelin system [66]. Convincing evidence also exists for the role of endothelial cell–derived endothelin-1 in the pathogenesis of PAH, including the finding of increased endothelin-1 plasma levels and expression in patients who have pulmonary hypertension [69,73,74]. Endothelin-1 effects are mediated through two distinct endothelin receptor isoforms: endothelin receptors type A (ET$_A$) and B (ET$_B$). Activation of these receptors by endothelins results in variable, often competing, signals, including vasodilatory versus vasoconstrictive, proliferative versus antiproliferative, and inflammatory versus anti-inflammatory [65,75]. Investigations continue to examine the role of ET receptor blockade in the treatment of PAH.

Pathways that modulate vascular smooth muscle tone and proliferation often do so through PASMC membrane potential (*Em*) regulation [76]. Models of hypoxia show the critical role of various types of potassium channels, which are the primary regulators of *Em*. Hypoxic inhibition of potassium channels, and depressed potassium channel function for other reasons, ultimately trigger PASMC contraction and proliferation [77]. Pathways counteractive to hypoxic responses include cGMP signaling, which activates large-conductance calcium-activated potassium channels, causing vasodilatation [65]. In addition, potassium channel activity is important in activating apoptosis, and therefore defective channel function may facilitate cell proliferation [78]. Several studies have shown diminished potassium channel expression and function in patients who have PAH, implicating loss of function in the pathogenesis of this disease [65,77,79,80]. Most anorectic drugs, including dexfenfluramine, directly inhibit potassium channels [81,82].

The TGF-β superfamily, of which BMPs are a member, clearly has a critical role in a diverse array of cellular processes. Additional growth factors have been implicated in the pathogenesis of PAH, including vascular endothelial growth factor (VEGF) and platelet-derived growth factor (PDGF). The exact function of VEGF in the lung is unknown, but it is expressed at high levels and required for both lung development and structural maintenance, including endothelial cell survival. Studies of plexiform lesions in PAH showed elevated levels of VEGF expression, but current understanding of the complex interactions of this compound has not clarified whether its actions promote or inhibit apoptosis and remodeling in a beneficial manner in PAH [65,66]. A potent mitogen and pulmonary vascular smooth muscle cell chemoattractant, PDGF is postulated to contribute to pulmonary vasculature remodeling in various forms of pulmonary hypertension. It is also a stimulant for other mitogens, including endothelin-1 [83]. Elevated levels of PDGF have been seen in the lungs of individuals who have PAH, implicating this compound in disease pathogenesis [84,85]. Additional growth factors warrant continued examination as modulators of cellular proliferation in PAH, such as angiopietin-1, basic fibroblast growth factor, epidermal growth factor, and insulin-like growth factor-1, but are beyond the scope of this article [65].

The role of inflammation and autoimmunity in the pathogenesis of PAH is also a subject of ongoing investigation. It is well known that PAH develops more often in diseases known to be associated with immune disturbance, such as scleroderma, systemic lupus erythematosus, autoimmune thyroiditis, and HIV infection [86]. Histologic evaluation of plexiform lesions in various types of PAH shows perivascular inflammatory cell infiltrates, typically lymphocytic in nature [87,88]. Furthermore, elevated levels of autoantibodies such an antinuclear antibodies, and abnormally high levels of circulating proinflammatory cytokines such as IL-1 and IL-6, have been detected in some patients who have PAH [89]. Recently, Tamby and colleagues [90] identified the presence of antiendothelial cell antibodies in patients who had PAH, implicating a loss of tolerance with subsequent pulmonary vasculature attack. Meanwhile, other investigators have suggested that immune dysregulation related to dysfunctional regulatory T-cell activity underlies all of these inflammatory processes and facilitates the expression of PAH, but continued work is needed to elucidate these potential mechanisms [91].

Genetic implications for clinical evaluation and therapy

Although the potential is growing, scant information is available for evaluating the role of genotype in predicting therapeutic response in patients who have PAH. A small proportion of these have good long-term response to calcium channel blockers, but models for predicting who will respond on an acute and chronic basis are lacking [92,93]. Elliott and colleagues [94] retrospectively compared the results of vasoreactivity testing in patients who had PAH with the presence of known *BMPR2* gene changes that code for different amino acid products (nonsynonymous *BMPR2* sequence variations). They found that patients who had FPAH and IPAH with nonsynonymous *BMPR2* sequence variations were less likely to show vasoreactivity using standard testing. Their report highlights the potential to use information about known genetic variations in PAH to guide decisions about prognosis and treatment for individuals.

Screening and counseling

Siblings or children of patients who have FPAH, or of obligate heterozygotes for a *BMPR2* mutation, have an overall risk of 50% for inheriting the abnormal gene. Because the gene penetrance is approximately 20%, this yields an estimated risk of 10% for expressing disease [95]. Therefore, most relatives will be asymptomatic.

Current recommendations for asymptomatic family members of individuals who have FPAH advise echocardiographic screening at 3- to 5-year intervals [95]. Investigators in Germany proposed a screening process that uses estimation of systolic pulmonary artery pressure at rest and during exercise using echocardiography, based on studies of families of patients who have IPAH and FPAH. Using a systematic clinical assessment of pulmonary artery pressure at rest and during exercise in members of families with PAH, Grunig and colleagues [96] attempted to detect individuals who had abnormal pulmonary vascular response to supine bicycle exercise, and subsequently linked this response to inheritance of an abnormal genetic locus ultimately discovered to include the gene for *BMPR2*. In 2005, this group also reported an abnormal pulmonary artery pressure response to hypoxia during echocardiographic evaluation in individuals deemed at risk for developing PAH based on a known *BMPR2* mutation or a possible risk haplotype [97]. Although these efforts should be commended considering the profound need for earlier diagnosis of PAH, the use of stress echocardiography as a screening tool for PAH has not been widely accepted, and identifying a risk haplotype is challenging. Because both require more extensive evaluation and independent confirmation, they are not yet recommended for general use.

Genetic testing for mutations in the *BMPR2* gene are now available clinically, and therefore patients who have IPAH and FPAH and their families should be instructed about the availability of genetic testing and the potential risk for family members to develop PAH.

Genetic testing should only be provided after professional genetic counseling [15,95]. A negative test result can be helpful to members of a family with a known *BMPR2* mutation. If the test is negative, an individual FPAH family member's risk for disease declines from 1 in 10 to that of the population, which is approximately 1 in 1 million (100,000-fold risk reduction). Conversely, if an asymptomatic individual at risk is found to carry the known familial *BMPR2* mutation, risk increases only modestly to 1 in 5 (twofold risk increase) for expressing clinical disease throughout their lifetime.

Given the vast number of potential mutations in the large *BMPR2* gene, screening for a mutation is most efficient in an affected patient who has IPAH or FPAH, so that the specific mutation in their family can be identified if it is present. Clinical genetic testing of relatives of a patient who has PAH has no rationale unless a mutation is identified in the patient sample. The detection of a *BMPR2* mutation in a patient who has IPAH is often surprising and alarming, specifically because the familial basis was concealed by absence of knowledge about other cases in the family, and therefore it converts the concept of disease from one of a sporadic finding to that of a potentially familial disease. These family members are thus at increased risk and should be offered counseling about their risk and about testing for the known mutation.

Summary

Great strides in the evaluation and management of PAH have been made in relation to the genetics and pathogenic mechanisms of this devastating disease. The discovery that mutations in the *BMPR2* gene underlie most cases of FPAH and an important subset of IPAH cases has energized the field and prompted significant progress in understanding the molecular basis of PAH. Efforts continue to show the full genetic basis of FPAH and IPAH. Work is still needed to elucidate the causes of the variable penetrance of FPAH, including the identity and role of various modifiers of disease expression. These modifiers may also be the basis of genetic anticipation in FPAH. In addition, studies of genotype–phenotype interactions should include an exploration of the role of gender, which is the only known risk modifier.

Investigations should include evaluation of potential interactions between the *SERT* gene and members of the TGF-β signaling pathway, but also novel genes and proteins yet to be linked to PAH. The molecular mechanisms that converge to develop a milieu of cellular proliferation and vascular remodeling require aggressive investigation. Ultimately, a greater understanding of the genetic and molecular mechanisms of PAH should lead to earlier diagnosis, advanced pharmacogenetics, and, perhaps someday, disease prevention.

Acknowledgments

The authors thank the many patients and families who graciously contributed to this work, and Ms. Lisa Wheeler, whose service is invaluable as coordinator of the Vanderbilt Familial Primary Pulmonary Hypertension study.

References

[1] Dresdale DT, Schultz M, Michtom RJ. Primary pulmonary hypertension. I. Clinical and hemodynamic study. Am J Med 1951;11(6):686–705.

[2] Dresdale DT, Michtom RJ, Schultz M. Recent studies in primary pulmonary hypertension, including pharmacodynamic observations on pulmonary vascular resistance. Bull N Y Acad Med 1954; 30(3):195–207.

[3] Loyd JE, Primm RK, Newman JH. Familial primary pulmonary hypertension: clinical patterns. Am Rev Respir Dis 1984;129(1):194–7.

[4] Thomas AQ, Gaddipati R, Newman JH, et al. Genetics of primary pulmonary hypertension. Clin Chest Med 2001;22(3):477–91, ix.

[5] Rich S, Dantzker DR, Ayres SM, et al. Primary pulmonary hypertension. A national prospective study. Ann Intern Med 1987;107(2):216–23.

[6] Nichols WC, Koller DL, Slovis B, et al. Localization of the gene for familial primary pulmonary hypertension to chromosome 2q31-32. Nat Genet 1997; 15(3):277–80.

[7] Morse JH, Barst RJ. Detection of familial primary pulmonary hypertension by genetic testing. N Engl J Med 1997;337(3):202–3.

[8] Lane KB, Machado RD, Pauciulo MW, et al. Heterozygous germline mutations in BMPR2, encoding a TGF-beta receptor, cause familial primary pulmonary hypertension. The International PPH Consortium. Nat Genet 2000;26(1):81–4.

[9] Deng Z, Morse JH, Slager SL, et al. Familial primary pulmonary hypertension (gene PPH1) is caused by mutations in the bone morphogenetic protein receptor-II gene. Am J Hum Genet 2000;67(3): 737–44.

[10] Gaine SP, Rubin LJ. Primary pulmonary hypertension. Lancet 1998;352(9129):719–25.

[11] Runo JR, Loyd JE. Primary pulmonary hypertension. Lancet 2003;361(9368):1533–44.

[12] D'Alonzo GE, Barst RJ, Ayres AM, et al. Survival in patients with primary pulmonary hypertension. Results from a national prospective registry. Ann Intern Med 1991;115(5):343–9.

[13] Humbert M, Sitbon O, Chaouat A, et al. Pulmonary arterial hypertension in France: results from a national registry. Am J Respir Crit Care Med 2006; 173(9):1023–30.

[14] Thomson JR, Machado RD, Pauciulo MW, et al. Sporadic primary pulmonary hypertension is associated with germline mutations of the gene encoding BMPR-II, a receptor member of the TGF-beta family. J Med Genet 2000;37(10):741–5.

[15] Newman JH, Trembath RC, Morse JA, et al. Genetic basis of pulmonary arterial hypertension: current understanding and future directions. J Am Coll Cardiol 2004;43(12 Suppl S):33S–9S.

[16] Humbert M, Nunes H, Sitbon O, et al. Risk factors for pulmonary arterial hypertension. Clin Chest Med 2001;22(3):459–75.

[17] Kuhn KP, Byrne DW, Arbogast PG, et al. Outcome in 91 consecutive patients with pulmonary arterial hypertension receiving epoprostenol. Am J Respir Crit Care Med 2003;167(4):580–6.

[18] Newman JH, Wheeler L, Lane KB, et al. Mutation in the gene for bone morphogenetic protein receptor II as a cause of primary pulmonary hypertension in a large kindred. N Engl J Med 2001;345(5):319–24.

[19] Machado RD, James V, Southwood M, et al. Investigation of second genetic hits at the BMPR2 locus as a modulator of disease progression in familial pulmonary arterial hypertension. Circulation 2005; 111(5):607–13.

[20] Loyd JE, Butler MG, Foroud TM, et al. Genetic anticipation and abnormal gender ratio at birth in familial primary pulmonary hypertension. Am J Respir Crit Care Med 1995;152(1):93–7.

[21] Warren ST, Ashley CT Jr. Triplet repeat expansion mutations: the example of fragile X syndrome. Annu Rev Neurosci 1995;18:77–99.

[22] Ashley CT Jr, Warren ST. Trinucleotide repeat expansion and human disease. Annu Rev Genet 1995; 29:703–28.

[23] Newman JH. Pulmonary hypertension. Am J Respir Crit Care Med 2005;172(9):1072–7.

[24] Morse JH, Jones AC, Barst RJ, et al. Mapping of familial primary pulmonary hypertension locus (PPH1) to chromosome 2q31-q32. Circulation 1997; 95(12):2603–6.

[25] Machado RD, Pauciulo MW, Thomson JR, et al. BMPR2 haploinsufficiency as the inherited molecular mechanism for primary pulmonary hypertension. Am J Hum Genet 2001;68(1):92–102.

[26] Koehler R, Grunig E, Pauciulo MW, et al. Low frequency of BMPR2 mutations in a German cohort of

patients with sporadic idiopathic pulmonary arterial hypertension. J Med Genet 2004;41(12):e127.

[27] Morisaki H, Nakanishi N, Kyotani S, et al. BMPR2 mutations found in Japanese patients with familial and sporadic primary pulmonary hypertension. Hum Mutat 2004;23(6):632.

[28] Elliott CG. Genetics of pulmonary arterial hypertension: current and future implications. Semin Respir Crit Care Med 2005;26(4):365–71.

[29] Cogan JD, Pauciulo MW, Batchman AP, et al. High frequency of BMPR2 exonic deletions/duplications in familial pulmonary arterial hypertension. Am J Respir Crit Care Med 2006;174:590–8.

[30] Aldred MA, Vijayakrishnan J, James V, et al. BMPR2 gene rearrangements account for a significant proportion of mutations in familial and idiopathic pulmonary arterial hypertension. Hum Mutat 2006;27(2):212–3.

[31] Machado RD, Aldred MA, James V, et al. Mutations of the TGF-beta type II receptor BMPR2 in pulmonary arterial hypertension. Hum Mutat 2006;27(2):121–32.

[32] Yang X, Long L, Southwood M, et al. Dysfunctional Smad signaling contributes to abnormal smooth muscle cell proliferation in familial pulmonary arterial hypertension. Circ Res 2005;96(10):1053–63.

[33] Loyd JE, Atkinson JB, Pietra GG, et al. Heterogeneity of pathologic lesions in familial primary pulmonary hypertension. Am Rev Respir Dis 1988;138(4):952–7.

[34] Humbert M, Morrell NW, Archer SL, et al. Cellular and molecular pathobiology of pulmonary arterial hypertension. J Am Coll Cardiol 2004;43(12 Suppl S):13S–24S.

[35] Teichert-Kuliszewska K, Kutryk MJ, Kuliszewski MA, et al. Bone morphogenetic protein receptor-2 signaling promotes pulmonary arterial endothelial cell survival: implications for loss-of-function mutations in the pathogenesis of pulmonary hypertension. Circ Res 2006;98(2):209–17.

[36] Lee SD, Shroyer KR, Markham NE, et al. Monoclonal endothelial cell proliferation is present in primary but not secondary pulmonary hypertension. J Clin Invest 1998;101(5):927–34.

[37] Stewart DJ. Bone morphogenetic protein receptor-2 and pulmonary arterial hypertension: unraveling a riddle inside an enigma? Circ Res 2005;96(10):1033–5.

[38] Atkinson C, Stewart S, Upton PD, et al. Primary pulmonary hypertension is associated with reduced pulmonary vascular expression of type II bone morphogenetic protein receptor. Circulation 2002;105(14):1672–8.

[39] Yuan JX, Rubin LJ. Pathogenesis of pulmonary arterial hypertension: the need for multiple hits. Circulation 2005;111(5):534–8.

[40] De Caestecker M, Meyrick B. Bone morphogenetic proteins, genetics and the pathophysiology of primary pulmonary hypertension. Respir Res 2001;2(4):193–7.

[41] Derynck R, Zhang YE. Smad-dependent and Smad-independent pathways in TGF-beta family signaling. Nature 2003;425(6958):577–84.

[42] Shi Y, Massague J. Mechanisms of TGF-beta signaling from cell membrane to the nucleus. Cell 2003;113(6):685–700.

[43] Runo JR, Vnencak-Jones CL, Prince M, et al. Pulmonary veno-occlusive disease caused by an inherited mutation in bone morphogenetic protein receptor II. Am J Respir Crit Care Med 2003;167(6):889–94.

[44] Simonneau G, Galie N, Rubin LJ, et al. Clinical classification of pulmonary hypertension. J Am Coll Cardiol 2004;43(12 Suppl S):5S–12S.

[45] Abenhaim L, Moride Y, Brenot F, et al. Appetite-suppressant drugs and the risk of primary pulmonary hypertension. International Primary Pulmonary Hypertension Study Group. N Engl J Med 1996;335(9):609–16.

[46] Sztrymf B, Yaici A, Jais X, et al. Idiopathic pulmonary hypertension: what did we learn from genes? Sarcoidosis Vasc Diffuse Lung Dis 2005;22(Suppl 1):S91–S100.

[47] Humbert M, Deng Z, Simonneau G, et al. BMPR2 germline mutations in pulmonary hypertension associated with fenfluramine derivatives. Eur Respir J 2002;20(3):518–23.

[48] Roberts KE, McElroy JJ, Wong WP, et al. BMPR2 mutations in pulmonary arterial hypertension with congenital heart disease. Eur Respir J 2004;24(3):371–4.

[49] Lee SL, Wang WW, Moore BJ, et al. Dual effect of serotonin on growth of bovine pulmonary artery smooth muscle cells in culture. Circ Res 1991;68(5):1362–8.

[50] Herve P, Launay JM, Scrobohaci ML, et al. Increased plasma serotonin in primary pulmonary hypertension. Am J Med 1995;99(3):249–54.

[51] Eddahibi S, Hanoun N, Lanfumey L, et al. Attenuated hypoxic pulmonary hypertension in mice lacking the 5-hydroxytryptamine transporter gene. J Clin Invest 2000;105(11):1555–62.

[52] Eddahibi S, Humbert M, Fadel E, et al. Serotonin transporter overexpression is responsible for pulmonary artery smooth muscle hyperplasia in primary pulmonary hypertension. J Clin Invest 2001;108(8):1141–50.

[53] Liu Y, Suzuki YJ, Day RM, et al. Rho kinase-induced nuclear translocation of ERK1/ERK2 in smooth muscle cell mitogenesis caused by serotonin. Circ Res 2004;95(6):579–86.

[54] Lee SL, Wang WW, Finlay GA, et al. Serotonin stimulates mitogen-activated protein kinase activity through the formation of superoxide anion. Am J Physiol 1999;277(2 Pt 1):L282–91.

[55] Machado RD, Koehler R, Glissmeyer E, et al. Genetic association of the serotonin transporter in

pulmonary arterial hypertension. Am J Respir Crit Care Med 2006;173(7):793–7.

[56] Willers ED, Newman John H, Loyd James E, et al. Serotonin transporter polymorphisms in familial and idiopathic pulmonary arterial hypertension. Am J Respir Crit Care Med 2006;173(7):798–802.

[57] McAllister KA, Grogg KM, Johnson DW, et al. Endoglin, a TGF-beta binding protein of endothelial cells, is the gene for hereditary haemorrhagic telangiectasia type 1. Nat Genet 1994;8(4):345–51.

[58] Johnson DW, Berg JN, Baldwin MA, et al. Mutations in the activin receptor-like kinase 1 gene in hereditary haemorrhagic telangiectasia type 2. Nat Genet 1996;13(2):189–95.

[59] Trembath RC, Thomson JR, Machado RD, et al. Clinical and molecular genetic features of pulmonary hypertension in patients with hereditary hemorrhagic telangiectasia. N Engl J Med 2001;345(5): 325–34.

[60] Harrison RE, Flanagan JA, Sankelo M, et al. Molecular and functional analysis identifies ALK-1 as the predominant cause of pulmonary hypertension related to hereditary haemorrhagic telangiectasia. J Med Genet 2003;40(12):865–71.

[61] Chaouat A, Coulet F, Favre C, et al. Endoglin germline mutation in a patient with hereditary haemorrhagic telangiectasia and dexfenfluramine associated pulmonary arterial hypertension. Thorax 2004;59(5):446–8.

[62] Harrison RE, Berger R, Haworth SG, et al. Transforming growth factor-beta receptor mutations and pulmonary arterial hypertension in childhood. Circulation 2005;111(4):435–41.

[63] Fernandez LA, Sanz-Rodriguez F, Blanco FJ, et al. Hereditary hemorrhagic telangiectasia, a vascular dysplasia affecting the TGF-beta signaling pathway. Clin Med Res 2006;4(1):66–78.

[64] McLaughlin VV, McGoon MD. Pulmonary arterial hypertension. Circulation 2006;114(13):1417–31.

[65] Perros F, Dorfmuller P, Humbert M. Current insights on the pathogenesis of pulmonary arterial hypertension. Semin Respir Crit Care Med 2005;26(4): 355–64.

[66] Said SI. Mediators and modulators of pulmonary arterial hypertension. Am J Physiol Lung Cell Mol Physiol 2006;291:547–58.

[67] Christman BW, McPherson CD, Newman JH, et al. An imbalance between the excretion of thromboxane and prostacyclin metabolites in pulmonary hypertension. N Engl J Med 1992;327(2):70–5.

[68] Herve P, Humbert M, Sitbon O, et al. Pathobiology of pulmonary hypertension. The role of platelets and thrombosis. Clin Chest Med 2001;22(3):451–8.

[69] Giaid A. Nitric oxide and endothelin-1 in pulmonary hypertension. Chest 1998;114(3 Suppl):208S–12S.

[70] Giaid A, Saleh D. Reduced expression of endothelial nitric oxide synthase in the lungs of patients with pulmonary hypertension. N Engl J Med 1995; 333(4):214–21.

[71] Steiner MK, Preston IR, Klinger JR, et al. Pulmonary hypertension: inhaled nitric oxide, sildenafil and natriuretic peptides. Curr Opin Pharmacol 2005;5(3):245–50.

[72] Petkov V, Mosgoeller W, Ziesche R, et al. Vasoactive intestinal peptide as a new drug for treatment of primary pulmonary hypertension. J Clin Invest 2003;111(9):1339–46.

[73] Stewart DJ, Levy RD, Cernacek P, et al. Increased plasma endothelin-1 in pulmonary hypertension: marker or mediator of disease? Ann Intern Med 1991;114(6):464–9.

[74] Giaid A, Yanagisawa M, Langleben D, et al. Expression of endothelin-1 in the lungs of patients with pulmonary hypertension. N Engl J Med 1993;328(24): 1732–9.

[75] Barst RJ, Langleben D, Badesch D, et al. Treatment of pulmonary arterial hypertension with the selective endothelin-A receptor antagonist sitaxsentan. J Am Coll Cardiol 2006;47(10):2049–56.

[76] Martin KB, Klinger JR, Rounds SIS. Pulmonary arterial hypertension: new insights and new hope. Respirology 2006;11(1):6–17.

[77] Mauban JR, Remillard CV, Yuan JX. Hypoxic pulmonary vasoconstriction: role of ion channels. J Appl Physiol 2005;98(1):415–20.

[78] Burg ED, Remillard CV, Yuan JX. K+ channels in apoptosis. J Membr Biol 2006;209(1):3–20.

[79] Geraci MW, Moore M, Gesell T, et al. Gene expression patterns in the lungs of patients with primary pulmonary hypertension: a gene microarray analysis. Circ Res 2001;88(6):555–62.

[80] Yuan XJ, Wang J, Juhaszova M, et al. Attenuated K+ channel gene transcription in primary pulmonary hypertension. Lancet 1998;351(9104):726–7.

[81] Michelakis E. Anorectic drugs and vascular disease: the role of voltage-gated K+ channels. Vascul Pharmacol 2002;38(1):51–9.

[82] Michelakis ED, Weir EK. Anorectic drugs and pulmonary hypertension from the bedside to the bench. Am J Med Sci 2001;321(4):292–9.

[83] Yu Y, Sweeney M, Zhang S, et al. PDGF stimulates pulmonary vascular smooth muscle cell proliferation by upregulating TRPC6 expression. Am J Physiol Cell Physiol 2003;284(2):C316–30.

[84] Eddahibi S, Humbert M, Sediame S, et al. Imbalance between platelet vascular endothelial growth factor and platelet-derived growth factor in pulmonary hypertension. Effect of prostacyclin therapy. Am J Respir Crit Care Med 2000;162(4 Pt 1):1493–9.

[85] Humbert M, Monti G, Fartoukh M, et al. Platelet-derived growth factor expression in primary pulmonary hypertension: comparison of HIV seropositive and HIV seronegative patients. Eur Respir J 1998; 11(3):554–9.

[86] Barst RJ, McGoon M, Torbicki A, et al. Diagnosis and differential assessment of pulmonary arterial hypertension. J Am Coll Cardiol 2004;43(12 Suppl S): 40S–7S.

[87] Tuder RM, Groves B, Badesch DB, et al. Exuberant endothelial cell growth and elements of inflammation are present in plexiform lesions of pulmonary hypertension. Am J Pathol 1994;144(2):275–85.

[88] Achcar RO, Yung GL, Saffer H, et al. Morphologic changes in explanted lungs after prostacyclin therapy for pulmonary hypertension. Eur J Med Res 2006;11(5):203–7.

[89] Dorfmuller P, Perros F, Balabanian K, et al. Inflammation in pulmonary arterial hypertension. Eur Respir J 2003;22(2):358–63.

[90] Tamby MC, Chanseaud Y, Humbert M, et al. Anti-endothelial cell antibodies in idiopathic and systemic sclerosis associated pulmonary arterial hypertension. Thorax 2005;60(9):765–72.

[91] Nicolls MR, Taraseviciene-Stewart L, Rai PR, et al. Autoimmunity and pulmonary hypertension: a perspective. Eur Respir J 2005;26(6):1110–8.

[92] Montani D, Marcelin AG, Sitbon O, et al. Human herpes virus 8 in HIV and non-HIV infected patients with pulmonary arterial hypertension in France. AIDS 2005;19(11):1239–40.

[93] Archer SL, Michelakis ED. An evidence-based approach to the management of pulmonary arterial hypertension. Curr Opin Cardiol 2006;21(4): 385–92.

[94] Elliott CG, Glissmeyer EW, Havlena GT, et al. Relationship of BMPR2 mutations to vasoreactivity in pulmonary arterial hypertension. Circulation 2006; 113(21):2509–15.

[95] McGoon M, Gutterman D, Steen V, et al. Screening, early detection, and diagnosis of pulmonary arterial hypertension: ACCP evidence-based clinical practice guidelines. Chest 2004;126(1 Suppl): 14S–34S.

[96] Grunig E, Janssen B, Mereles D, et al. Abnormal pulmonary artery pressure response in asymptomatic carriers of primary pulmonary hypertension gene. Circulation 2000;102(10):1145–50.

[97] Grunig E, Dehnert C, Mereles D, et al. Enhanced hypoxic pulmonary vasoconstriction in families of adults or children with idiopathic pulmonary arterial hypertension. Chest 2005;128(6 Suppl): 630S–3S.

ELSEVIER
SAUNDERS

Clin Chest Med 28 (2007) 59–73

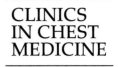

CLINICS
IN CHEST
MEDICINE

Diagnosis of Pulmonary Arterial Hypertension

Terence K. Trow, MD[a,b,*], John R. McArdle, MD[a,b]

[a]Section of Pulmonary and Critical Care Medicine, Division of Internal Medicine, Yale University School of Medicine,
333 Cedar Street, P.O. Box 208057, New Haven, CT 06520-8057, USA
[b]Pulmonary Hypertension Center, Yale University School of Medicine, 789 Howard Avenue, New Haven, CT 06519, USA

The accurate diagnosis of pulmonary arterial hypertension (PAH) is a challenging and complex process that requires a high index of clinical suspicion from even the most astute clinician, particularly early in the disease process. Because pulmonary vascular disease is not the exclusive domain of any given medical discipline, general internists and a broad range of medical specialists alike must be aware of the potential presentations of this disorder [1] and of the limitations and vagaries of noninvasive tests used to define patients in whom invasive testing is warranted. Ultimately right- and, often, concomitant left-heart catheterization is required to establish the diagnosis and to characterize the PAH phenotype before proper treatment can be initiated. This article reviews the fundamental evidence supporting the detection and diagnosis of PAH in patients at risk for or having symptoms suggestive of this disorder.

Patient history

The symptoms associated with PAH are nonspecific and often are confounded by the presence of comorbid conditions that might explain them. It is not surprising that the National Institutes of Health registry found that a median of 2 years transpired from the onset of symptoms before the correct diagnosis of PAH was finally established [2]. In that study of 187 patients, dyspnea (particularly with exertion) was the most common initial complaint (60%), followed by fatigue (19%), syncope (8%), chest pain (7%), near syncope (5%), palpitations (5%), and leg edema (3%) [2]. Idiopathic pulmonary arterial hypertension (IPAH) presentations occur more often in young women, often with normal examinations early in their course, making reassurance the most common initial intervention [2]. Because fatigue and exertional dyspnea commonly occur in active people, patients themselves often discount their symptoms often increasing the time before medical attention is sought [2]. For this reason, a high index of clinical suspicion should be maintained when a clear explanation for such symptoms is not readily evident. In addition, conditions with an increased incidence of associated PAH, such as connective tissue disease [3–7], cirrhosis of the liver [8–11], anorexigen use [12,13], and hemoglobinopathies [14–19], warrant increased concern on the part of the front-line practitioner.

Physical examination

Because the number of conditions associated with the development of PAH is extensive, a variety of examination clues may be present and should be sought out. These clues often are subtle, may occur later in the disease course, and may be overlooked [20]. Cardiac auscultation may reveal an accentuated pulmonic component to the second heart sound because of the delayed closure of the pulmonic valve (split "P2") in up to 90% of patients who have IPAH [2]. This accentuated component characteristically is fixed, without variation during inspiration and expiration, in cases of PAH associated with atrial septal defect [21]. Other signs may include a palpable left parasternal heave, a right ventricular S3 or S4 gallop,

* Corresponding author. Division of Internal Medicine, Section of Pulmonary and Critical Care, Yale University School of Medicine, 333 Cedar Street, LCI 105D, P.O. Box 208057, New Haven, CT 06520-8057.
    E-mail address: terence.trow@yale.edu (T.K. Trow).

prominence of the jugular "a" wave or "v" wave, hepatojugular reflux, and lower extremity edema [2]. A variety of murmurs also may be encountered on cardiac auscultation, including the high-pitched holosystolic murmur of tricuspid regurgitation heard best at the left sternal border [22], the crescendo-decrescendo systolic ejection murmur of pulmonic stenosis [23], or the early diastolic high-pitched Graham Steel murmur of pulmonic regurgitation [24]. Murmurs of ventricular septal defects are paradoxically louder for smaller defects and are characterized by a high-pitched sound at the 4th to 5th intercostal spaces that does not radiate and does not change with inspiration [25,26].

Aside from cardiac auscultation, cyanosis, seen in 20% of IPAH cases [2], suggests right-to-left shunting and severe reduction of cardiac output. The sequelae of liver disease such as testicular atrophy, palmar erythema, and spider telangiectasias should be sought. Also oral mucosal telangiectasias may suggest a diagnosis of hereditary hemorrhagic telangiectasia syndrome, now known to be associated with a mutation in the activin receptor-like kinase-1 gene in a minority of cases [27]. Calcinosis, sclerodactyly, mat telangiectasias, Raynaud's phenomenon, and digital ulcerations may be seen in scleroderma-associated PAH [20]. Because many women who have telangiectasias are self-conscious about the skin telangiectasias that appear on their faces, the examiner may need to ask for the removal of facial make-up to appreciate this finding. Digital clubbing is rare in IPAH [2] and when present should raise the possibility of congenital heart disease or pulmonary veno-occlusive disease [28].

Electrocardiography

Although electrocardiography (ECG) lacks sufficient sensitivity and specificity to serve as an effective screening tool [2,20,29,30], it can contribute important prognostic information, particularly when repeated over time, and should be performed. Right ventricular hypertrophy and right-axis deviation can be detected 87% and 79% of the time, respectively, in PAH [2]. Features of right ventricular hypertrophy suggestive of PAH include a tall R wave and small S wave (R/S ratio of >1) in lead V1, a large S wave and small R wave (R/S ratio <1) in lead V5 or V6, a qR complex in V1, and a rSR pattern in V1 (Fig. 1) [20,30]. The absence of these findings does not exclude PAH, however: one study of 61

patients who had PAH found 8 who had normal ECGs despite severe PAH by catheterization [30]. When both right and left chest leads are used to explore QTc and Tp-e (the interval from the peak of the T wave to the end of the T-wave), differences in QTc intervals between right and left leads are significantly shorter in patients who have PAH than in controls (3 ± 8 versus 40 ± 3 milliseconds, respectively) [31].

When ECG findings are present, however, they may be helpful prognostically because the presence of right atrial enlargement has been associated with a 2.8-fold greater risk of death over a 6-year period of observation, and right ventricular hypertrophy by World Heath Organization diagnostic criteria portended a 4.3-fold greater risk of death [32]. Greater degrees of right-axis deviation also have correlated with decreased survival, as did S1Q3 pattern in one retrospective study of patients who had IPAH [33].

Although ECG findings do not predictably follow the magnitude of pulmonary hypertension (PH), amplitude of the R forces in V1 of more than 1.2 mV or a R/SV1 greater than 7 indicated a pulmonary artery systolic pressure of more than 90 mm Hg with a sensitivity of 94% and specificity of 47% in one study of 47 patients who had IPAH [34]. Rarely, the dilated pulmonary artery trunk may cause angina and ischemic ECG changes as the result of mechanical compression [35].

Chest radiography

Like the ECG, a chest radiograph should be obtained in all patients suspected of having PAH even though it lacks sensitivity and specificity to establish the diagnosis [20,29]. Radiographic features of attenuated peripheral vascular markings, enlarged main and hilar pulmonary artery shadows, and obscuration of the retrosternal clear space on a lateral view because of the enlargement of the right ventricle may be noted, although these features may not be found in early PH (Fig. 2). An increase in the hilar thoracic index (defined as the ratio of the summed horizontal measurements of the pulmonary artery from the midline to their first division divided by the maximum transverse thorax diameter) of more than 38% was highly suggestive of PAH in one study of 50 patients [36], but this finding did not correlate well with the extent of pulmonary artery pressure (PAP) elevation seen. When patients who had chronic

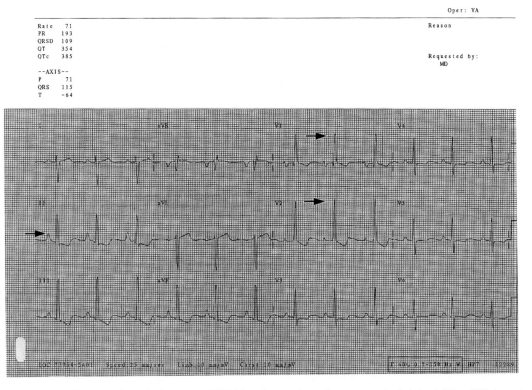

Oper: YA

Rate   71   Reason
PR   193
QRSD   109
QT   354
QTc   385   Requested by:
                                                        MD
--AXIS--
P   71
QRS   115
T   -64

Fig. 1. An ECG from a patient who has severe PAH. Note the prominent R wave magnitude in leads V1 and V2 (*arrow*) indicative of right ventricular hypertrophy. Vector forces for the QRS complex are 115° indicating right axis deviation. The presence of a P wave magnitude of greater than 2.5 mm in lead II (*arrow*) is indicative of significant right atrial enlargement.

obstructive pulmonary disease (COPD) were considered specifically, an increase of more than 16 mm in the diameter of the right descending pulmonary artery (RDPA) on a posterior-anterior projection and of more than 18 mm for the left descending pulmonary artery (also on a posterior-anterior film) permitted the correct diagnosis of PAH in the majority of these patients when right-heart catheterization was used to define PAP [37]. Chetty and colleagues [38] combined

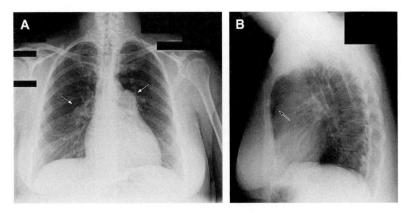

Fig. 2. A chest radiograph from a patient who has PAH. (*A*) Note the prominently enlarged right descending pulmonary artery (*arrow*) and left main pulmonary artery (*arrow*) seen on the posterior-anterior projection. Peripheral vasculature is attenuated. (*B*) The lateral view shows encroachment of the right ventricle on the retrosternal airspace (*arrow*).

the hilar thoracic index, RDPA branch diameter, hilar width, and cardiothoracic ratio in 34 patients who had COPD and found that 19 of 20 (95%) who had an elevated mean PAP had a hilar thoracic index of 36 or more, versus none of the 14 patients who had a normal mean PAP. Nineteen of 20 patients who had elevated mean PAP also had RDPA diameters of 20 mm, versus 3 of the 14 patients who had a normal mean PAP; they also found, however, that the chest radiograph could not be used to predict the actual PAP accurately [38].

The chest radiograph also may define concomitant parenchymal disease, pulmonary vascular congestion as may be seen in pulmonary veno-occlusive disease [39], hyperinflation changes of COPD, kyphosis, or findings suggestive of chronic thromboembolic disease such as mosaic oligemia, right ventricular hypertrophy, or an enlarged RDPA [40,41]. In general the extent of radiographic abnormalities and the degree of PAH in any given patient do not seem to be correlated [20,36,38]. In one study examining patients who had confirmed acute pulmonary emboli from the Prospective Investigation of Pulmonary Embolism Diagnosis trial, however, Stein and colleagues [42] did find correlation with mean PAP and a dilated heart or prominent central pulmonary arteries in patients who had no prior cardiac or pulmonary disease.

Pulmonary function testing and hypoxemia assessment

All patients who have PAH should have pulmonary function testing as a part of the initial evaluation. In IPAH, Rich and colleagues [2] found mild reductions in total lung capacity and forced vital capacity in both male and female subjects. Although roughly 20% of the 187 patients examined in their study demonstrated these findings, 50% of 79 patients in a more recent study had these restrictive changes in resting lung mechanics [43]. The diffusing capacity for carbon monoxide (DLCO) also measured significantly less than predicted in the National Institutes of Health registry trial [2], a finding confirmed by Sun and colleagues [43] in patients who had IPAH. Meyer and colleagues [44] also have recently observed respiratory muscle dysfunction in a cohort of 37 patients who had IPAH by noting significant impairment in maximum inspiratory and maximum expiratory pressures. Patients who

have chronic thromboembolic pulmonary hypertension (CTEPH) also show mild-to-moderate restrictive defects [45], a finding believed to result from parenchymal scarring from prior infarcts [46,47]. Often they also have mild DLCO reductions (60%–80% of the time), largely caused by abnormalities in pulmonary membrane diffusing capacity rather than by alterations in pulmonary capillary blood volume [48].

When other phenotypes of PH are examined, DLCO impairments are commonly seen in portopulmonary-associated PAH [49] and in sarcoidosis-related PH [50]. The latter study also showed more reductions in significant forced expiratory volume in the first second and in forced vital capacity in patients who had PH than in patients who had sarcoidosis but did not have PH [50]. Patients who have systemic sclerosis also frequently have DLCO abnormalities; such findings were seen in 20% of subjects in one study of 88 patients who had progressive systemic sclerosis [51]. When compared with patients who had limited scleroderma with calcinosis, Raynaud's phenomena, esophageal dysmotility, sclerodactyly, and telangiectasia (CREST), the patients who had CREST had lower mean DLCO values despite a higher mean vital capacity. Chang and colleagues [52] recently offered a retrospective cross-sectional review of 619 patients who had scleroderma and found that 18.1% had combined restrictive ventilatory defects and PH. When isolated DLCO impairments are seen in the limited cutaneous form of scleroderma, the likelihood of PH development is high [53,54]. Indeed, Scorza and colleagues [55] found that over 15 years of follow-up in a cohort of patients who had systemic sclerosis and a baseline DLCO less than 45% of predicted, 75% went on to develop PH defined by an echocardiographic systolic PAP above 40, and in these patients the DLCO correlated inversely with PAP measured by right-heart catheterization [56].

It is important to include measures of oxygen saturation with exercise in the work-up even when resting measures of oxygenation are normal, because supplemental oxygen may be warranted to prevent exertional desaturation with associated pulmonary arterial vasoconstriction [20]. Exercise saturations should be measured in all patients who have a DLCO less than 60% of predicted value. A surprisingly large percentage of patients who had IPAH (10/13) was found to have significant levels of nocturnal hypoxemia even in the absence of sleep-disordered breathing [57], and therefore all patients who have PAH should be assessed even when suspicion of sleep apnea is not high. Schulz and colleagues [58] discovered periodic (Cheyne-Stokes) breathing patterns in 30% in one study of 20 patients who had IPAH that seemed to be reversible with nocturnal oxygen supplementation.

Doppler echocardiography

The transthoracic echocardiogram (TTE) affords a widely available and noninvasive method to estimate PAP. It can only suggest (sometimes strongly) the presence of PH and cannot diagnose PAH (because it does not measure pulmonary capillary wedge or left-heart pressures) and should not a priori be used to do so. Although TTE remains the noninvasive tool of choice to assess which patients should go on to definitive invasive cardiac catheterization, certain vagaries inherent in acquisition of Doppler tricuspid jet velocity (TJV) envelopes define its limitations. Analyzable TJV can be obtained in anywhere from 39% [59] to 86% [60,61] of the time. This variability points out that the tenacity and experience of individual ultrasonographers can affect the usefulness of this tool. Additional error can be encountered when the estimates of right atrial pressure used in the modified Bernoulli equation are not based rigorously on inferior vena cava collapsibility [62], as is the case in many centers that arbitrarily assign a value of 10 mm Hg. Patients who have advanced lung disease pose a special challenge. In a cohort of 374 patients being assessed for lung transplantation [63], estimates of PAP were achievable in only 44% of 164; 48% of those were misclassified as having PAH, and 52% of the pressure estimates were inaccurate. Himelman and colleagues [64,65] have advocated the use of agitated saline contrast injection to improve Doppler envelope acquisition in patients who have COPD, but this procedure is not performed routinely in many centers unless specifically requested. Mildly elevated PAPs may result from the serendipitous observation of a nonrepresentative transient pressure elevation in an otherwise healthy individual (eg, TJV sampled after a premature ventricular contraction) [66] or from an overestimation in a patient who has normal pulmonary pressure (perhaps, in part, from an excessive estimate of right atrial pressure), a problem that is more likely in populations where the prevalence of disease is low [20,66,67]. This problem of false-positive TTE estimates of PAP is underscored by the experience of Penning and colleagues [68], who found that 32% of a cohort of pregnant patients suspected of having PAH by TTE did not have PAH on subsequent catheterization. In addition, normal variations in PAP have been observed in different populations and increase with age, gender (male sex), and body mass index [66,69] as well as degree of conditioning [70]. Taken together these findings support caution in overinterpreting incidental TTE elevated PAP estimates, especially when mild (< 50 mm Hg), to diagnose PAH [66–68].

Despite these caveats, Doppler echocardiography remains a generally sensitive if not always specific screening tool when properly done and when applied to appropriate populations. Sensitivity for estimates of PAP ranges from 0.79 to 1.0; estimates of specificity range from 0.68 to 0.98 [20,56,68,71–73]. When TTE correlation to right-heart catheterization is assessed, correlation coefficients of 0.57 [59], 0.76 [74], 0.78 [71], 0.83 [56], 0.89 [75], 0.90 [76], and 0.93 [77] have been reported. One study by Bossone and colleagues [78] reported poor correlation (r = 0.31) and noted that the largest discrepancies occurred when PAPs were 100 mm Hg or greater. Correlations in all these studies were most robust for PAPs greater than 50 mm Hg and less than 100 mm Hg.

The yield of TTE in screening depends on the sensitivity and specificity of the test and also on the prevalence of disease in the population. Current evidence-based guidelines support screening for patients who have known genetic mutations associated with PAH, first-degree relatives of patients who have familial PAH, patients who have scleroderma, patients who have portal hypertension before orthotopic liver transplantation, or patients who have congenital heart disease with systemic-to-pulmonary shunts [20,66]. When PAH is suspected by Doppler echocardiography, an agitated saline ("bubble") echocardiogram always should be obtained to assess for evidence of left-to-right shunting [20]. Transesophageal echocardiography can add additional information that may alter therapy, especially with the ability to diagnose atypically situated atrial septal defects of the sinus venosus type [79].

Aside from estimates of PAP, interpretation of possible PAH on TTE or transesophageal echocardiography must incorporate information about left ventricular size and function with special attention to diastolic relaxation characteristics, left atrial size, left-sided valvular disease, and right ventricular and atrial characteristics (Fig. 3).

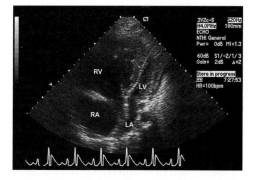

Fig. 3. A four-chamber echocardiographic view of a patient who has severe PAH. Note the massively dilated right ventricle (RV) and right atrium (RA) that have shifted the septa and narrowed the left ventricle (LV) and left atrium (LA).

Evidence of left atrial enlargement even in the absence of left ventricular dysfunction should raise the possibility of elevated left-sided pressures that may contribute to the pulmonary pressure elevation [20]. When present, right- and, often, left-heart catheterization to measure transpulmonary gradient and to assess for diastolic dysfunction is crucial, because treatments for PAH may make pulmonary venous hypertension worse, precipitating pulmonary edema [80,81]. The presence of pericardial effusion is a poor prognostic finding in PAH [82,83], but it rarely is associated with true tamponade physiology [84], and rarely should surgical drainage be considered, because the perioperative risks in this population are significant.

The role of stress echocardiography to uncover early PAH remains controversial. No clear consensus exists in the literature regarding the best exercise technique (eg, treadmill versus cycle ergometry) or protocols. Defining and marking a clear resting Doppler envelope of TJV in the left lateral decubitus position, often with the aid of agitated saline contrast, and acquisitioning the envelope quickly after exercise with the treadmill technique can represent logistical challenges causing some proponents to favor the more stable thoracic platform with real-time acquisition allowed by supine cycle ergometry [85,86]. Interpretation of elevations in PAP seen with exercise must be tempered by the physical conditioning of the patient [70]. Noninvasively measured PAP during exercise catheterization has been reported to correlate strongly (r = 0.86) with invasive measurement of PAP in one small study of 19 patients who had congestive heart failure

[87]. Stress echocardiography can be helpful in delineating effects of exercise on transmitral gradients in patients who have mitral stenosis when the resting severity of mitral stenosis does not seem to explain PAP or symptomatology [88–92]. Stress echocardiography also may be useful in assessing the exertional impact of relaxation abnormalities of the left ventricle (diastolic dysfunction) and of mitral regurgitation. In patients who have normal PAP estimates at rest in whom PAH with exercise is suspected, exercise echocardiography has been proposed as a useful tool [93]. In patients who have collagen-vascular disease, symptoms of exercise intolerance have been associated with exercise-induced PAH [94], and patients who do not report dyspnea also have been demonstrated to manifest PAP elevations with exercise [95–97]. In patients who had COPD, Himelman and colleagues [65] demonstrated that although 28% of 36 patients who had advanced lung disease had normal resting PAPs on TTE, nearly all showed abnormal increases in PAP with exercise. The significance of these observations and the implications for treatment remain unclear. Recent studies of IPAH family members suggest that supine bicycle exercise echocardiography may identify a subgroup of presently asymptomatic carriers of the PAH gene [98,99]; additional follow-up will be necessary to see if these individuals ultimately manifest clinical PAH.

Excluding thromboembolic disease

The presentation of CTEPH can mimic that of IPAH and often is not associated with an awareness of the original pulmonary embolus on the part of the patient or caregiver [100]. Although previous reports of CTEPH complicating acute pulmonary embolism suggested rates of 0.1% to 0.5% [100], more recent prospective evaluation suggests up to 4% of patients surviving the acute pulmonary embolism develop PH, usually within the first 2 years [101]. Because this form of PH is potentially curable by surgical intervention, all patients should undergo evaluation for this causation before being assigned an IPAH diagnosis [20]. A normal- or low-probability ventilation-perfusion (V/Q) scan effectively excludes the diagnosis of CTEPH [102–105], with sensitivities of 90% to 100% and a specificity of 94% to 100% [103–105]; therefore the V/Q scan is the screening method of choice for CTEPH [20]. Perfusion scans alone, however, tend to underestimate the severity of large- vessel obstruction [106]. Pulmonary angiography remains the diagnostic procedure of choice to evaluate suspected CTEPH and to define potential surgical candidates [20]. Although both contrast-enhanced CT angiography (CTPA) [107–109] and MRI [110–113] are useful in CTEPH and in defining alternative diagnoses (eg, sarcoma, vasculitis, mediastinal fibrosis) and may be complementary to V/Q scanning, these techniques are not applied with consistent algorithms and equipment at the current time in all centers and generally are not recommended as stand-alone techniques to exclude CTEPH [20]. Cases of false-negative CTPA in the authors' institution (Fig. 4) and others (Richard Channick, MD, 2004, and Harold Palevsky, MD, 2006, personal communication) have underscored the

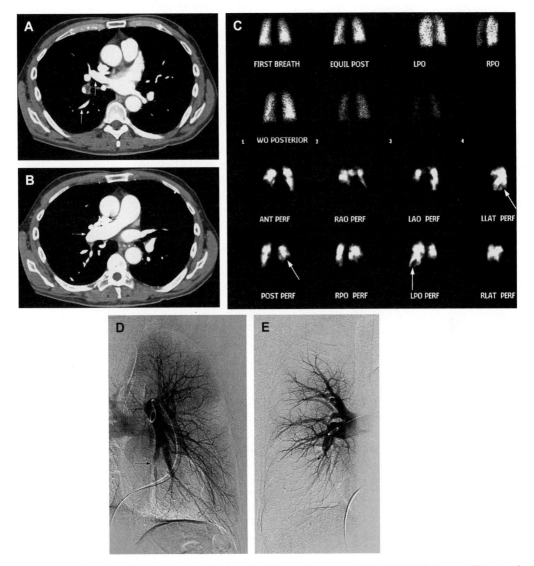

Fig. 4. Chronic thromboembolic pulmonary hypertension. The patient presented to the Yale Pulmonary Hypertension Center with 8 months of slowly increasing dyspnea with exertion without chest pain, pleurisy, or any recollection of an acute event. (A) CT angiography done at an outside institution was interpreted as normal without evidence of thromboemboli. The proximal right pulmonary artery appears normal (arrows). (A, B) Representative images. (C) Subsequent ventilation-perfusion scanning revealed multiple segmental and subsegmental unmatched defects (arrows). (D, E) Pulmonary angiography confirmed interlobar embolic occlusions (arrows).

dangers of substituting these modalities for V/Q scans in the screening assessment for CTEPH [114]. CTPA has been shown to be less sensitive than angiography for defining vascular distortions, stenoses, and webs in chronic pulmonary embolism [107].

Serologic testing

Selective testing of blood samples is appropriate in many instances of PAH [20]. The specific tests ordered depend on clinical suspicion as assessed by the history and physical examination, as well as by the absence of other clear causes of PAH in any individual patient. Although serologic tests may help focus diagnostic efforts aimed at PAH associated with connective tissue disease, it is important to note that up to 40% of patients who have IPAH have elevated antinuclear antibodies (usually of low titer) [115] and other autoantibodies such as anti-Ku [116]. Because the most common connective tissue disease associated with PAH, limited scleroderma, typically does not manifest interstitial lung disease on examination or chest radiograph, patients who have perceived IPAH should be assessed carefully for features of systemic sclerosis. Anti-centromere antibodies typically are positive in limited scleroderma [117], as are positive anti-nuclear antibodies including U3-RNP, B23, Th/To, and U1-RNP [118–120]. When PAH is associated with diffuse forms of scleroderma, U3-RNP usually is positive [121]. Anti-cardiolipin antibodies have been associated with PAH in systemic lupus erythematosus [122,123]. If any possibility of the HIV infection exists, testing is advised, because PAH is associated with HIV infection in up to 0.5% of cases [124]. It is equally important to assess for cirrhotic liver disease, because 2% of these patients will manifest PAH [8]. As such, measures of aminotransferases, alkaline phosphatase, bilirubin levels, and measures of synthetic function such as the activated partial thromboplastin time and prothrombin time, are advisable. Even when blood testing is unremarkable, liver-spleen scanning may be suggestive of portal hypertension and should be considered when suspicion is high. Thyroid disease has been implicated as a risk factor for PAH [125–130], although its exact relationship to PAH awaits definition [20]. Disorders of the thyroid gland should be sought and treated in PAH, because reversal of PAH with treatment has been reported [131,132].

MRI

Exquisite experimental work using MRI evaluation of right ventricular function and dysfunction has begun to appear in the literature [133]; some authors have proposed it may be superior to echocardiography in estimating PAP [134]. In CTEPH, reports suggest that good correlations with V/Q results can be expected with MRI in experienced hands [110,113] and that with proper breath holding MRI may be useful in identifying typical findings of CTEPH [112]. MRI can offer noninvasive measures of right ventricular chamber size, shape, thickness, and mass [135], and mean PAP has been shown to correlate with MRI measurement of right ventricular thickness, main pulmonary artery diameter [136], and right ventricular mass [137]. Not all reports support the accuracy of MRI in PH, however. One recent study concluded that accurate estimation of PAP in patients who had PH was not feasible with the set of MRI estimators they chose [138]. The incremental value of MRI to traditional echocardiographic assessments in PAH has not been reported.

Exercise testing

Measure of exercise intolerance may be helpful in the diagnosis of early PAH (before elevated pressures are present at rest) and in predicting survival and response to therapy [139,140]. Because patients who have PAH are limited in the extent to which they are able to raise cardiac output in response to tissue oxygen demands, small increases in workload can result in significant hypoxemia. Reductions in maximum peak oxygen consumption (VO_{2max}), anaerobic threshold, and ventilatory efficiency as assessed by cycle ergometry cardiopulmonary exercise testing (CPET) correlate well with New York Heart Association (NYHA) functional class [141]. In addition, end-tidal carbon dioxide in patients who have IPAH is significantly reduced at rest and with exercise in proportion to the severity of physiologic disease, and this finding on CPET when accompanied by arterial hypoxemia should trigger consideration of pulmonary vasculopathy [142]. CPET has been found reproducible and safe without complication or fatalities even in the most severely exercise-intolerant PAH patient [143]. When CPET measures of VO_{2max} were used as the primary endpoint in the Sitaxentan to Relieve Impaired Exercise trial, discrepancies between this and other measures previously validated in PAH trials (6-minute-walk test [6 MWT], functional class, pulmonary vascular resistance [PVR], and cardiac index) were observed, raising concern about the advisability of using CPET as a primary endpoint in future studies [144]. Great intercenter variability observed in that trial underscored the greater technical expertise required to conduct reliable CPET testing. VO_{2max} measures and ventilatory efficiency by CPET also show progressive improvement in response to surgical thromboendarterectomy [145].

A simple and practical substitute for full CPET is the 6 MWT. This validated test shows strong correlation between distance ambulated and VO_{2max} seen on CPET [146], as well as to total PVR, mean right atrial pressure, baseline cardiac output, and NYHA functional class [147]. The 6 MWT also can predict disease progression and patient response to therapy [148].

Measures of 6 MWT and CPET also have been shown to predict survival, with a 6 MWT distance of less than 380 m after 3 months of therapy [149] and peak oxygen uptake of less than 10.4 mL/min/kg [150] showing significantly worse survival outcomes. Combining these two measures to indicate when to add new therapies in an algorithm for combination therapy has been recently proposed [151].

Cardiac catheterization

Ultimately the diagnosis of PAH (as opposed to PH) requires right- and, often, left-heart catheterization [20,66,152]. Although purists point out that the fluid-filled thermodilution catheters are limited, in that only mean pressures and flows are determined, and that current methodology does not take into account the pulsatility of the pulmonary circulation in a dynamic fashion [67], right-heart catheterization is the standard for PAH diagnosis. Aside from excluding false-positive echocardiogram estimates of PAP [68], catheterization is crucial in assessing the transpulmonary gradient (pulmonary capillary wedge pressure), thereby excluding pulmonary venous hypertension [152]. Often exercise provocation or volume loading may be necessary in cases of diastolic dysfunction [153,154]. It also allows determination of oxygen saturation that maybe the only clue in diagnosing atrial septal defects with left-to-right shunting, especially of the sinus venosus type [152] or partial anomalous pulmonary venous return. In addition, measures of right atrial

pressure, cardiac index, and mean PAP have been shown to be useful in assessing prognosis and may influence therapeutic choices [155]. Vasodilator testing should be done in all cases of IPAH [156,157], although its role in other forms of PAH is controversial [152]. A positive vasodilator response has prognostic implications [158,159], and although recent work suggests that only 6.8% of patients who have IPAH may be long-term responders to calcium-channel blockers typically used for treatment in this group [157], this group should be sought out aggressively and treated with these agents [20]. Although previous investigators have defined a positive vasodilator response as decreases in PAP_{mean} and PVR of more than 20% without concomitant decreases in systemic pressure [160], the more recent work of Sitbon and colleagues [157] defines a positive vasodilator response as a decrease of a minimum of 10 mmHg in PAP_{mean} to an absolute PAP_{mean} of less than 40 mm Hg and a decrease in PVR of >30% to less than 6 Wood units (480 dynes/sec/cm^5) without decrease in the cardiac output, and these criteria are rapidly becoming the accepted ones for defining a clinically meaningful vasodilator response.

Right-heart catheterization represents a snapshot in time in a resting, supine (possibly sedated) patient, and variability by as much as 20 mm Hg in some subgroups of PAH has been seen over time [161]. Nonetheless, this technique is an indispensable part of the PAH evaluation and may need to be repeated over time.

Summary

The accurate diagnosis of PAH is a complex process. Initial clues from the history are nonspecific, and physical examinations often are subtle, requiring heightened acumen on the part of the front-line practitioner. Noninvasive testing that should be ordered in all cases of suspected PAH include the ECG, chest radiograph, pulmonary function tests (with DLCO), exercise and nocturnal oximetry, Doppler echocardiography with "bubble" contrast, and V/Q scanning to exclude CTEPH. The incremental diagnostic value of CTPA and MRI in the PH work-up (and especially in the evaluation of CTEPH) is not yet established, and at the present time these modalities should be used as adjuncts to V/Q scanning, echocardiography, and pulmonary angiography. Collagen vascular disease serologies, liver function testing, thyroid function testing,

HIV testing, and nocturnal polysomnography should be considered in all cases where a clear cause of PH is not readily apparent and when history and examination suggest the need. CPET may be helpful in clarifying prognosis and determining response to treatment but generally is reserved for use in specialized centers with expertise. The 6 MWT is a simple and reproducible validated test that correlates well with CPET measures and should be used to assess exercise capacity at diagnosis as well as serially with treatment of the patient who has PAH. Ultimately, cardiac catheterization is required to diagnose PAH and to exclude left-sided contributions to echocardiographically determined PAP elevations. Cardiac catheterization also is needed to exclude congenital heart defects, define vasoreactivity, and define a pulmonary vascular resistance of more than 280 dyne/sec/cm^5 (3 Wood units) required to establish true arteriopathy as the basis of elevated mean pulmonary artery pressure. Right-heart catheterization also can be useful in acquisition of prognostic information that may influence treatment decisions.

References

[1] Rubin LJ. Diagnosis and management of pulmonary arterial hypertension: ACCP evidence-based clinical practice guidelines. Chest 2004;126(1): 7S–10S.

[2] Rich S, Dantzker DR, Ayres SM, et al. Primary pulmonary hypertension. A national prospective study. Ann Intern Med 1987;107(2):216–23.

[3] Wigley FM, Lima JAC, Mayes M, et al. The prevalence of undiagnosed pulmonary arterial hypertension in subjects with connective tissue disease at the secondary health care level of community-based rheumatologists (the UNCOVER study). Arthritis Rheum 2005;52(7):453–9.

[4] MacGregor AJ, Canavan R, Knight C, et al. Pulmonary hypertension in systemic sclerosis: risk factors for progression and consequences for survival. Rheumatology 2001;40:453–9.

[5] Chang B, Schachna L, White B, et al. Natural history of mild-moderate pulmonary hypertension and the risk factors for severe pulmonary hypertension in scleroderma. J Rheumtol 2006;33(2): 269–74.

[6] Pan TLT, Thumboo J, Boey ML. Primary and secondary pulmonary hypertension in systemic lupus erythematosus. Lupus 2000;9:338–42.

[7] Johnson SR, Gladman DD, Urowitz MB, et al. Pulmonary hypertension in systemic lupus. Lupus 2004;13:506–9.

[8] Hadengue A, Behhayoun MK, Lebree D, et al. Pulmonary hypertension complicating portal hypertension: prevalence and relation to splanchnic hemodynamics. Gastroenterology 1991;100(2): 520–8.

[9] Ramsay MA, Simpson BR, Nguyen AT, et al. Severe pulmonary hypertension in liver transplant candidates. Liver Transpl Surg 1997;3(5):494–500.

[10] Starkel P, Vera A, Gunson B, et al. Outcome of liver transplantation for patients with pulmonary hypertension. Liver Transpl 2002;8(4):382–8.

[11] Krowka MJ. Hepatopulmonary syndrome and portopulmonary hypertension: implications for liver transplantation. Clin Chest Med 2005;26(4): 587–97.

[12] Brenot F, Herve P, Petitpretz P, et al. Primary pulmonary hypertension and fenfluramine use. Br Heart J 1993;70(6):537–41.

[13] Abenhaim L, Moride Y, Brenot F, et al. Appetite-suppressant drugs and the risk of primary pulmonary hypertension. N Engl J Med 1996;335(9): 609–16.

[14] Collins FS, Orringer EP. Pulmonary hypertension and cor pulmonale in the sickle hemoglobinopathies. Am J Med 1982;73:814–20.

[15] Gladwin MT, Sachdev V, Jison ML, et al. Pulmonary hypertension as a risk factor for death in patients with sickle cell disease. N Engl J Med 2004; 350(9):886–95.

[16] Minter K, Gladwin MT. Pulmonary complications of sickle cell anemia. A need for increased recognition, treatment, and research. Am J Respir Crit Care Med 2001;164:2016–9.

[17] Derchi G, Forni GL. Therapeutic approaches to pulmonary hypertension in hemoglobinopathies. Efficacy and safety of sildenafil in the treatment of severe pulmonary hypertension in patients with hemoglobinopathy. Ann N Y Acad Sci 2005; 1054:471–5.

[18] Aessopos A, Farmakis D, Deftereos S, et al. Thalassemia heart disease. A comparative evaluation of thalassemia major and thalassemia intermedia. Chest 2005;127(5):1523–30.

[19] Haque AK, Gokhale S, Rampy BA, et al. Pulmonary hypertension in sickle cell hemoglobinopathy: a clinicopathologic study of 20 cases. Hum Pathol 2002;33:1037–43.

[20] McGoon M, Gutterman D, Steen V, et al. Screening, early detection, and diagnosis of pulmonary arterial hypertension. ACCP evidence-based clinical practice guidelines. Chest 2004;126(1):14S–34S.

[21] Bull TM. Physical examination in pulmonary arterial hypertension. Advances in Pulmonary Hypertension 2005;4(3):6–10.

[22] Rios JC, Massumi RA, Breesman WT, et al. Auscultatory features of acute tricuspid regurgitation. Am J Cardiol 1969;23(1):4–11.

[23] Kaplan S, Adolph RJ. Pulmonic valve stenosis in adults. Cardiovasc Clin 1979;10:327–9.

[24] Braunwald E, editor. Heart disease: a textbook of cardiovascular medicine. New York: WB Saunders Company; 1997.

[25] Leatham A, Segal B. Auscultatory and phono-cardiographic signs of ventricular septal defect with left-to-right shunt. Circulation 1962;25: 318–27.

[26] Newburger JW, Rosenthal A, Williams RG, et al. Noninvasive tests in the initial evaluation of heart murmurs in children. N Engl J Med 1983;308(2): 61–4.

[27] Trembath RC, Thomson JR, Machado RD, et al. Clinical and molecular genetic features of pulmo-nary hypertension in patients with hereditary hem-orrhagic telangiectasia. N Engl J Med 2001;345(5): 325–34.

[28] Holcomb BW, Loyd JE, Ely EW, et al. Pulmonary veno-occlusive disease. A case series and new obser-vations. Chest 2000;118(6):1671–9.

[29] Alegro S, Morrison D, Ovitt T, et al. Noninvasive detection of pulmonary hypertension. Clin Cardiol 1984;7:148–56.

[30] Ahern GS, Tapson VF, Rebetz A, et al. Electrocar-diography to define clinical status of primary pul-monary hypertension and pulmonary arterial hypertension secondary to collagen vascular dis-ease. Chest 2002;122(2):524–7.

[31] Hlaing T, Donglin G, Zhao X, et al. The QT and Tp-e intervals in left and right chest leads: compar-ison between patients with systemic and pulmonary hypertension. Journal of Electrocardiography 2005;38:154–8.

[32] Bossone E, Pacioco G, Iarussi D, et al. The role prognostic role of the ECG in primary pulmonary hypertension. Chest 2002;121(2):513–8.

[33] Kanemoto N. Electrocardiogram in primary pul-monary hypertension. Eur J Cardiol 1980;12: 181–93.

[34] Kanemoto N. Electrocardiographic and hemody-namic correlations in primary pulmonary hyper-tension. Angiology 1988;39(9):781–7.

[35] Patrat JF, Jondeau G, Dubourg O, et al. Left main coronary artery compression during primary pul-monary hypertension. Chest 1997;112(3):842–3.

[36] Lupi E, Dumont C, Tejada VM, et al. A radiologic index of pulmonary arterial hypertension. Chest 1975;68:28–31.

[37] Matthay RA, Schwarz MI, Ellis JH, et al. Pulmo-nary artery hypertension in chronic obstructive pulmonary disease: determination by chest radiog-raphy. Invest Radiol 1981;16(2):95–100.

[38] Chetty KG, Brown SE, Light RW. Indentification of pulmonary hypertension in chronic obstructive pulmonary disease from routine chest radiographs. Am Rev Respir Dis 1982;126(2):338–41.

[39] Rich S, Pietra GG, Kieras K, et al. Primary pulmo-nary hypertension: radiographic and scintigraphic patterns of histologic subtypes. Ann Intern Med 1986;105(4):449–502.

[40] Woodruff WW, Hoeck BE, Chitwood WR, et al. Radiographic findings in pulmonary hypertension from unresolved embolism. AJR Am J Roentgenol 1985;144:681–6.

[41] Schmidt HC, Kauczor HU, Schild HH, et al. Pulmonary hypertension in patients with chronic pulmonary thromboembolism: chest radiograph and CT evaluation before and after surgery. Eur Radiol 1996;6:817–25.

[42] Stein PD, Anthanasoulis C, Greenspan RH, et al. Relation of plain chest radiographic findings to pulmonary arterial pressure and arterial blood oxygen levels in patients with acute pulmonary embolism. Am J Cardiol 1992;69:394–6.

[43] Sun XG, Hansen JE, Oudiz RJ, et al. Pulmonary function in primary pulmonary hypertension. J Am Coll Cardiol 2003;41:1028–35.

[44] Meyer FJ, Lozznitzer D, Kristen AV, et al. Respi-ratory muscle dysfunction in idiopathic pulmonary arterial hypertension. Eur Respir J 2005;25(1): 125–30.

[45] Viner SM, Bagg BR, Auger WR, et al. The manage-ment of pulmonary hypertension secondary to chronic thromboembolic disease. Prog Cardiovasc Dis 1994;37(2):79–92.

[46] Morris TA, Auger WR, Ysrael MZ, et al. Paren-chymal scarring is associated with restrictive spirometric defects in patients with chronic throm-boembolic pulmonary hypertension. Chest 1996; 110(2):399–403.

[47] Romano AM, Tomaselli S, Gualtieri G, et al. Respiratory function in precapillary pulmonary hypertension. Monaldi Arch Chest Dis 1993;48(3): 201–4.

[48] Steenhius LH, Groen HJM, Koeter GH, et al. Dif-fusion capacity and haemodynamics in primary and chronic thromboembolic pulmonary hyperten-sion. Eur Respir J 2000;16:276–81.

[49] Mohamed R, Freeman JW, Guest PJ, et al. Pulmo-nary gas exchange in liver transplant candidates. Liver Transpl 2002;8(9):802–8.

[50] Sulica R, Teirstein AS, Kakarla S, et al. Distinc-tive clinical, radiographic, and functional charac-teristics of patients with sarcoidosis-related pulmonary hypertension. Chest 2005;128(3): 1483–9.

[51] Owens GR, Fino GJ, Herbert DL, et al. Pulmonary function in progressive systemic sclerosis. Compar-ison of CREST syndrome variant with diffuse scleroderma. Chest 1984;84(5):546–50.

[52] Chang B, Wigley FM, White B, et al. Scleroderma patients with combined pulmonary hypertension and interstitial lung disease. J Rheumatol 2003; 30(11):2398–405.

[53] Steen VD, Graham G, Conte C, et al. Isolated diffusing capacity reduction in systemic sclerosis. Arthritis Rheum 1992;35(7):765–70.

[54] Stupi AM, Steen VD, Owens GR, et al. Pulmonary hypertension in the CREST syndrome variant of

systemic sclerosis. Arthritis Rheum 1986;29(4):
515–24.

[55] Scorza R, Caronni M, Bassi S, et al. Post-meno-
pause is the main risk factor for developing isolated
pulmonary hypertension in systemic sclerosis. Ann
N Y Acad Sci 2002;966:238–46.

[56] Denton CP, Cailes JB, Phillips GD, et al. Comparison of Doppler echocardiography and right heart
catheterization to assess pulmonary hypertension
in systemic sclerosis. Br J Rheumatol 1997;36(2):
239–43.

[57] Rafanan AL, Golish JA, Dinner DS, et al. Nocturnal hypoxemia is common in primary pulmonary
hypertension. Chest 2001;120(3):894–9.

[58] Schulz R, Baseler G, Ghofrani HA, et al. Nocturnal
periodic breathing in primary pulmonary hypertension. Eur Respir J 2002;19:658–63.

[59] Murata I, Kihara H, Shinohara S, et al. Echocardiographic evaluation of pulmonary arterial hypertension in patients with progressive systemic
sclerosis and related syndromes. Jpn Circ J 1992;
56:983–91.

[60] Borgenson DD, Seward JB, Miller FA Jr, et al. Frequency of Doppler measurable pulmonary artery
pressures. J Am Soc Echocardiogr 1996;9(6):832–7.

[61] Hinderliter AL, Willis PW, Barst RJ, et al. Effects
of long-term infusion of prostacyclin (epoprostenol) on echocardiographic measures of right ventricular structure and function in primary
pulmonary hypertension. Circulation 1997;95:
1479–86.

[62] Ommen SR, Nishimura RA, Hurrell DG, et al. Assessment of right atrial pressure with 2-dimensional
and Doppler echocardiography: a simultaneous
catheterization and echocardiographic study.
Mayo Clin Proc 2000;75(1):24–9.

[63] Arcasoy SM, Christie JD, Ferrari VA, et al. Echocardiographic assessment of pulmonary hypertension in patients with advanced lung disease. Am J
Respir Crit Care Med 2003;167:735–40.

[64] Himelman RB, Struve SN, Brown JK, et al. Improved recognition of cor pulmonale in patients
with severe chronic obstructive pulmonary disease.
Am J Med 1988;84:891–8.

[65] Himelman RB, Stulbarg M, Kircher B, et al. Noninvasive evaluation of pulmonary artery pressure
during exercise by saline-enhanced Doppler echocardiography in chronic pulmonary disease. Circulation 1989;79(4):863–71.

[66] Barst RJ, McGoon M, Torbicki A, et al. Diagnosis
and differential assessment of pulmonary arterial hypertension. J Am Coll Cardiol 2004;43(12 Suppl S):
40S–7S.

[67] Naeije R, Torbicki A. More on the noninvasive
diagnosis of pulmonary hypertension: Doppler
echocardiography revisited. Eur Respir J 1995;8:
1445–9.

[68] Penning S, Robinson KD, Major CA, et al. A comparison of echocardiography and pulmonary artery

catheterization for evaluation of pulmonary artery
pressures in pregnant patients with suspected pulmonary hypertension. Am J Obstet Gynecol 2001;
184(7):1568–70.

[69] McQuillan BM, Picard MH, Leavitt M, et al.
Clinical correlates and reference intervals for
pulmonary artery systolic pressure among echocardiographically normal subjects. Circulation
2001;104:2797–802.

[70] Bossone E, Rubenfire M, Bach DS, et al. Range of
tricuspid regurgitation velocity at rest and during
exercise in normal adult men: implications for the
diagnosis of pulmonary hypertension. J Am Coll
Cardiol 1999;33:1662–6.

[71] Kim WR, Krowka MJ, Plevak DJ, et al. Accuracy
of Doppler echocardiography in the assessment of
pulmonary hypertension in liver transplant candidates. Liver Transpl 2000;6:453–8.

[72] Pilatis ND, Jacobs LE, Rerkpattanapipat P, et al.
Clinical predictors of pulmonary hypertension in
patients undergoing liver transplant evaluation.
Liver Transpl 2000;6(1):85–91.

[73] Torregrosa M, Genesca J, Gonzalez A, et al. Role
of Doppler echocardiography in the assessment of
portopulmonary hypertension in liver transplantation candidates. Transplantation 2001;71(4):572–4.

[74] Shapiro SM, Oudiz RJ, Cao T, et al. Primary pulmonary hypertension: improved long-term effects
and survival with continuous intravenous epoprostenol infusion. J Am Coll Cardiol 1997;30(2):
343–9.

[75] Chan KL, Currie PJ, Seward JB, et al. Comparison
of three Doppler ultrasound methods in the prediction of pulmonary artery pressure. J Am Coll
Cardiol 1987;9(3):549–54.

[76] Currie PJ, Seward JB, Chan KL, et al. Continuous
wave Doppler determination of right ventricular
pressure: a simultaneous Doppler-catheterization
study in 127 patients. J Am Coll Cardiol 1985;
6(4):750–6.

[77] Yock PG, Popp RL. Noninvasive estimation of
right ventricular ultrasound in patients with tricuspid regurgitation. Circulation 1984;70(4):657–62.

[78] Bossone E, Duong-Wagner TH, Paciocco G, et al.
Echocardiographic features of primary pulmonary
hypertension. J Am Soc Echocardiogr 1999;12:
655–62.

[79] Gorscan J, Edwards TD, Ziady GM, et al. Transesophageal echocardiography to evaluate patients
with severe pulmonary hypertension for lung transplantation. Ann Thorac Surg 1995;59:717–22.

[80] Humbert M, Maitre S, Capron F, et al. Pulmonary
edema complicating continuous intravenous prostacyclin in pulmonary capillary hemangiomatosis.
Am J Respir Crit Care Med 1998;157:1681–5.

[81] Resten A, Maitre S, Humbert M, et al. Pulmonary
arterial hypertension: thin-section CT predictors of
epoprostenol therapy failure. Radiology 2002;
222(3):782–8.

[82] Mellins RB, Levine OR, Fishman AP. Effect of systemic and pulmonary venous hypertension on pleural and pericardial fluid accumulation. J Appl Physiol 1970;29(5):564–9.

[83] Raymond RJ, Hinderliter AL, Willis PW, et al. Echocardiographic predictors of adverse outcomes in primary pulmonary hypertension. J Am Coll Cardiol 2002;39(7):1214–9.

[84] Blanchard DG, Dittrich HC. Pericardial adaptation in severe chronic pulmonary hypertension. An intraoperative transesophageal echocardiographic study. Circulation 1992;85(4):1414–22.

[85] Himelman RB, Stulbarg MS, Lee E, et al. Noninvasive evaluation of pulmonary artery systolic pressures during dynamic exercise by saline-enhanced Doppler echocardiography. Am Heart J 1990; 119(3):685–8.

[86] Marwick TH. Progress in stress echocardiography. Application of stress echocardiography to the evaluation of non-coronary heart disease. Eur J Echocardiogr 2000;1(3):171–9.

[87] Kuecherer HF, Will M, da Silva KG, et al. Contrast-enhanced Doppler ultrasound for noninvasive assessment of pulmonary artery pressure during exercise in patients with chronic congestive heart failure. Am J Cardiol 1996;78(2):229–32.

[88] Voelker W, Jacksch R, Dittman H, et al. Validation of continuous-wave Doppler measurements of mitral valve gradients during exercise—a simultaneous Doppler-catheter study. Eur Heart J 1989; 10:737–46.

[89] Leavitt JI, Coats MH, Falk RH. Effects of exercise on transmitral gradient and pulmonary artery pressure in patients with mitral stenosis or a prosthetic mitral valve: a Doppler echocardiographic study. J Am Coll Cardiol 1991;17(7):1520–6.

[90] Cheriex EC, Pieters FAA, Janssen JHA, et al. Value of exercise Doppler-echocardiography in patients with mitral stenosis. Int J Cardiol 1994;45:219–26.

[91] Schwamenthal E, Vered Z, Agranat O, et al. Impact of atrioventricular compliance on pulmonary artery pressure in mitral stenosis. An exercise echocardiographic study. Circulation 2000;102:2378–84.

[92] Tunick PA, Freedberg RS, Gargiulo A, et al. Exercise echocardiography as an aid to clinical decision making in mitral valve disease. J Am Soc Echocardiogr 1992;5:225–30.

[93] Bossone E, Avelar E, Bach DS, et al. Diagnostic value of resting tricuspid regurgitation velocity and right ventricular ejection flow parameters for the detection of exercise induced pulmonary arterial hypertension. Int J Card Imaging 2000;16:429–36.

[94] Morelli S, Ferrante L, Sgreccia A, et al. Pulmonary hypertension is associated with impaired exercise performance in patients with systemic sclerosis. Scand J Rheumatol 2000;29:236–42.

[95] Mininni S, Diricatti G, Vono MC, et al. Noninvasive evaluation of right ventricle systolic pressure during dynamic exercise by saline-enhanced Doppler echocardiography in progressive systemic sclerosis. Angiology 1996;47(5):467–74.

[96] Winslow TM, Ossipov M, Redberg RF, et al. Exercise capacity and hemodynamics in systemic lupus erythematosus: a Doppler echocardiographic exercise study. Am Heart J 1993;126(2):410–4.

[97] Raeside DA, Chalmers G, Clelland J, et al. Pulmonary artery pressure variation in patients with connective tissue disease: 24 hour ambulatory pulmonary artery pressure monitoring. Thorax 1998; 53:857–62.

[98] Grunig E, Janssen B, Mereles D, et al. Abnormal pulmonary artery pressure response in asymptomatic carriers of primary pulmonary hypertension gene. Circulation 2000;102:1145–50.

[99] Rindermann M, Grunig E, von Hippel A, et al. Primary pulmonary hypertension may be a heterogeneous disease with a second locus on chromosome 2q31. J Am Coll Cardiol 2003;41(12):2237–44.

[100] Fedullo PF, Auger WR, Kerr KM, et al. Chronic thromboembolic pulmonary hypertension. N Engl J Med 2001;345(20):1465–72.

[101] Pengo V, Lensing AWA, Prins MH, et al. Incidence of chronic thromboembolic pulmonary hypertension after pulmonary embolism. N Engl J Med 2004;350(22):2257–64.

[102] Fishman AJ, Moser KM, Fedullo PF. Perfusion lung scans vs. pulmonary angiography in evaluation of suspected primary pulmonary hypertension. Chest 1983;84(6):679–83.

[103] D'Alonzo GE, Bower JS, Dantzker DR. Differentiation of patients with primary and thromboembolic pulmonary hypertension. Chest 1984;85(4):457–61.

[104] Chapman PJ, Bateman ED, Benatar SR. Primary pulmonary hypertension and thromboembolic pulmonary hypertension—similarities and differences. Respir Med 1990;84(6):485–8.

[105] Worsley DF, Palevsky HI, Alavi A. Ventilation-perfusion lung scanning in the evaluation of pulmonary hypertension. J Nucl Med 1994;35(5):793–6.

[106] Ryan KL, Fedullo PF, Davis GB, et al. Perfusion scan findings understate the severity of angiographic and hemodynamic compromise in chronic thromboembolic pulmonary hypertension. Chest 1988;93(6):1180–5.

[107] Tardivon AA, Musset D, Maitre S, et al. Role of CT in chronic pulmonary embolism: comparison with pulmonary angiography. J Comput Assist Tomogr 1993;17(3):345–51.

[108] Remy-Jardin M, Duhamel A, Deken V, et al. Systemic collateral supply in patients with chronic thromboembolic and primary pulmonary hypertension: assessment with multi-detector row helical CT angiography. Radiology 2005;235:274–81.

[109] Heinrich M, Uder M, Tscholl D, et al. CT findings in chronic thromboembolic pulmonary hypertension. Predictors of hemodynamic improvement after pulmonary thromboendarterectomy. Chest 2005;127(5):1606–13.

[110] Bergin CJ, Hauschildt J, Rios G, et al. Accuracy of MR angiography compared with radionuclide scanning in identifying the cause of pulmonary arterial hypertension. AJR Am J Roentgenol 1997; 168:1549–55.

[111] Ley S, Kauczor HU, Heussel CP, et al. Value of contrast-enhanced MR angiography and helical CT angiography in chronic thromboembolic pulmonary hypertension. Eur Radiol 2003;13: 2365–71.

[112] Kreitner KFJ, Ley S, Kauczor HU, et al. Chronic thromboembolic pulmonary hypertension: pre- and postoperative assessment with breath-hold MR imaging techniques. Radiology 2004;232: 535–43.

[113] Nikolaou K, Schoenberg SO, Attenberger U, et al. Pulmonary arterial hypertension: diagnosis with fast perfusion MR imaging and high-spatial-resolution MR angiography—preliminary experience. Radiology 2005;236:694–703.

[114] McLauglin VV, Channick R, Robbins IM, et al. Integrating current strategies for continuing assessment of pulmonary arterial hypertension. Advances in Pulmonary Hypertension 2005;4(3):26–30.

[115] Rich S, Kieras K, Hart K, et al. Antinuclear antibodies in primary pulmonary hypertension. J Am Coll Cardiol 1986;8(6):1307–11.

[116] Iserin RA, Yaneva M, Weiner E, et al. Autoantibodies in patients with primary pulmonary hypertension: association with anti-Ku. Am J Med 1992; 93:307–12.

[117] Steen VD, Ziegler GL, Rodnan GP, et al. Clinical and laboratory associations of anticentromere antibody in patients with progressive systemic sclerosis. Arthritis Rheum 1984;27(2):125–31.

[118] Okano Y, Steen VD, Medsger TA. Autoantibody to U3 nucleolar ribonucleoprotein (fibrillarin) in patients with systemic sclerosis. Arthritis Rheum 1992;35(1):95–100.

[119] Mitri GM, Lucas M, Fertig N, et al. A comparison between anti-Th/To and anticentromere antibody-positive systemic sclerosis patients with limited cutaneous involvement. Arthritis Rheum 2003;48(1): 203–9.

[120] Ulanet DB, Wigley FM, Gelber AC, et al. Autoantibodies against B23, a nucleolar phosphoprotein, occur in scleroderma and are associated with pulmonary hypertension. Arthritis Rheum 2003; 49(1):85–92.

[121] Sacks DG, Okano Y, Steen VD, et al. Isolated pulmonary hypertension in systemic sclerosis with diffuse cutaneous involvement: association with serum anti-U3RNP antibody. J Rheumatol 1996; 23(4):639–42.

[122] Falcao CA, Alves IC, Chahade WH, et al. Echocardiographic abnormalities and antiphospholipid antibodies in patients with systemic lupus erythematosus. Arq Bras Cardiol 2002;79(3):285–91.

[123] Asherson RA, Higgenbottam TM, Dinh Xuan AT, et al. Pulmonary hypertension in a lupus clinic: experience with twenty-four patients. J Rheumatol 1990;17(10):1292–8.

[124] Petitpretz P, Brenot F, Azarian R, et al. Pulmonary hypertension in patients with human immunodeficiency virus infection. Comparison with primary pulmonary hypertension. Circulation 1994;89(6): 2722–7.

[125] Ma RC, Chow CC. Thyrotoxicosis as a risk factor for pulmonary arterial hypertension. Ann Intern Med 2005;143(4):282–92.

[126] Ma RC, Cheng AY, So WY, et al. Thyrotoxicosis and pulmonary hypertension. Am J Med 2005; 1128(8):927–8.

[127] Roberts KE, Barst RJ, McElroy JJ, et al. Bone morphogenetic protein receptor 2 mutations in adults and children with idiopathic pulmonary arterial hypertension: association with thyroid disease. Chest 2005;128(6 Suppl):618S.

[128] Merce J, Ferras S, Oltra C, et al. Cardiovascular abnormalities in hyperthyroidism: a prospective Doppler echocardiographic study. Am J Med 2005;118(2):126–31.

[129] Chu JW, Kao PN, Faul JL, et al. High prevalence of autoimmune thyroid disease in pulmonary hypertension. Chest 2002;122(5):1668–73.

[130] Curnock AL, Dweik RA, Higgins BH, et al. High prevalence of hypothyroidism in patients with primary pulmonary hypertension. Am J Med Sci 1999;318(5):289–92.

[131] Nakchbandi IA, Wirth JA, Inzucchi SE. Pulmonary hypertension caused by Graves' thyrotoxicosis: normal pulmonary hemodynamics restored by (131) I treatment. Chest 1999;116(5):1483–5.

[132] Lozano HF, Sharma CN. Reversible pulmonary hypertension, tricuspid regurgitation and right-sided heart failure associated with hyperthyroidism: case report and review of the literature. Cardiol Rev 2004;12(6):299–305.

[133] Laffon E, Vallet C, Bernard V, et al. A computed method for noninvasive MRI assessment of pulmonary arterial hypertension. J Appl Physiol 2004;96: 463–8.

[134] Saba TS, Foster J, Cockburn M, et al. Ventricular mass index using magnetic resonance imaging accurately estimates pulmonary artery pressure. Eur Respir J 2002;20:1519–24.

[135] Boxt LM, Katz J, Kolb T, et al. Direct quantification of right and left ventricular volumes with nuclear magnetic resonance imaging in patients with primary pulmonary hypertension. J Am Coll Cardiol 1992;19(7):1508–15.

[136] Frank H, Globits S, Glogar D, et al. Detection and quantification of pulmonary hypertension with

MR imaging: results in 23 patients. AJR Am J Roentgenol 1993;161:27–31.

[137] Katz J, Whang J, Boxt LM, et al. Estimation of right ventricular mass in normal subjects and in patients with primary pulmonary hypertension by nuclear magnetic resonance imaging. J Am Coll Cardiol 1993;21(6):1475–81.

[138] Roeleveld RJ, Marcus JT, Boonstra A, et al. A comparison of noninvasive MRI-based methods of estimating pulmonary artery pressure in pulmonary hypertension. J Magn Reson Imaging 2005; 22:67–72.

[139] Waxman AB. Pulmonary function test abnormalities in pulmonary vascular disease and chronic heart failure. Clin Chest Med 2001;22(4):751–8.

[140] Janicki JS, Weber KT, Likoff MJ, et al. Exercise testing to evaluate patients with primary vascular disease. Am Rev Respir Dis 1984;129(2): S93–5.

[141] Sun XG, Hansen JE, Oudiz RJ, et al. Exercise pathophysiology in patients with primary pulmonary hypertension. Circulation 2001;104:429–35.

[142] Yasunobu Y, Oudiz RJ, Sun XG, et al. End-tidal PCO_2 abnormality in patients with primary pulmonary hypertension. Chest 2005;127(5):1637–46.

[143] Hansen JE, Sun XG, Yasunobu Y, et al. Reproducibility of cardiopulmonary exercise measurements in patients with pulmonary arterial hypertension. Chest 2004;126(3):816–24.

[144] Barst RJ, Langleben D, Frost A, et al. Sitaxentan therapy for pulmonary arterial hypertension. Am J Respir Crit Care Med 2004;169:441–7.

[145] Iwase T, Nagaya N, Ando M, et al. Acute and chronic effects of surgical thromboendarterectomy on exercise capacity and ventilatory efficiency in patients with chronic thromboembolic pulmonary hypertension. Heart 2001;86:188–92.

[146] Cahalin LP, Mathier MA, Semigran MJ, et al. The six-minute walk test predicts peak oxygen uptake and survival in patients with advanced heart failure. Chest 1996;110(2):325–32.

[147] Miyamoto S, Nagaya N, Satoh T, et al. Clinical correlates and prognostic significance of six-minute walk test in patients with primary pulmonary hypertension. Comparison with cardiopulmonary exercise testing. Am J Respir Crit Care Med 2000; 161:487–92.

[148] Wax D, Garofano R, Barst RJ. Effects of long-term infusion of prostacyclin on exercise performance in patients with primary pulmonary hypertension. Chest 1999;116(4):914–20.

[149] Sitbon O, Humbert M, Nunes H, et al. Long-term intravenous epoprostenol infusion in primary pulmonary hypertension. Prognostic factors and survival. J Am Coll Cardiol 2002;40(4):780–8.

[150] Wensel R, Opitz CF, Anker SD, et al. Assessment in patients with primary pulmonary hypertension. Importance of cardiopulmonary exercise testing. Circulation 2002;106:319–24.

[151] Hoeper MM, Markevych I, Spiekerkoetter E, et al. Goal-oriented treatment and combination therapy for pulmonary arterial hypertension. Eur Respir J 2005;26(5):858–63.

[152] Oudiz RJ, Langleben D. Cardiac catheterization in pulmonary arterial hypertension: an updated guide to proper use. Advances in Pulmonary Hypertension 2005;4(3):15–25.

[153] Nootens M, Wolfkiel CJ, Chomka EV, et al. Understanding right and left ventricular systolic function and interactions at rest and exercise in primary pulmonary hypertension. Am J Cardiol 1995;75: 374–7.

[154] Shapiro BP, Nishimura RA, McGoon M, et al. Diagnostic dilemmas: diastolic heart failure causing pulmonary hypertension and pulmonary hypertension causing diastolic dysfunction. Advances in Pulmonary Hypertension 2006;5(1):13–20.

[155] D'Alonzo GE, Barst RJ, Ayres SM, et al. Survival in patients with primary pulmonary hypertension. Results from a national prospective registry. Ann Intern Med 1991;115(5):343–9.

[156] Rich S, Brundage BH. High-dose calcium channel-blocking therapy for primary pulmonary hypertension: evidence for long-term reduction in pulmonary arterial pressure and regression of right ventricular hypertrophy. Circulation 1987; 76(1):135–41.

[157] Sitbon O, Humber M, Jais X, et al. Long-term response to calcium channel blockers in idiopathic pulmonary hypertension. Circulation 2005;111: 3105–11.

[158] McLaughlin VV, Shillington A, Rich S. Survival in primary pulmonary hypertension. The impact of epoprostenol therapy. Circulation 2002;106: 1477–82.

[159] Kawut SM, Horn EM, Berekashvili KK, et al. New predictors of outcome in idiopathic pulmonary arterial hypertension. Am J Cardiol 2005;95:199–203.

[160] Rich S, Kaufmann E, Levy PS. The effect of high dose calcium-channel blockers on survival in pulmonary hypertension. N Engl J Med 1992;327(2): 76–81.

[161] Rich S, D'Alonzo GE, Dantzker D, et al. Magnitude and implications of spontaneous hemodynamic variability in primary pulmonary hypertension. Am J Cardiol 1985;55(1):159–63.

ELSEVIER
SAUNDERS

Clin Chest Med 28 (2007) 75–89

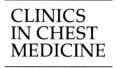

CLINICS
IN CHEST
MEDICINE

Surrogate End Points in Pulmonary Arterial Hypertension: Assessing the Response to Therapy

Jennifer L. Snow, MD[a], Steven M. Kawut, MD, MS[b,c],*

[a]Division of Pulmonary, Allergy, and Critical Care Medicine, Department of Medicine, University of Pennsylvania
School of Medicine, 844 West Gates Building, 3400 Spruce Street, Philadelphia, PA 19104, USA
[b]Division of Pulmonary, Allergy, and Critical Care Medicine, Department of Medicine, College of Physicians
and Surgeons, Columbia University, PH 8E, Room 101, 622 W. 168th Street, New York, NY 10032, USA
[c]Department of Epidemiology, Joseph L. Mailman School of Public Health, Columbia University,
722 W. 168th Street, New York, NY 10032, USA

The past several years have yielded an explosion of randomized clinical trials (RCTs) of several new medical therapies for pulmonary arterial hypertension (PAH). The hopes for these and all treatments for potentially fatal diseases are (1) to improve how a patient feels or functions and/or (2) to prolong survival. While simply stated, the assessment of progress toward these goals may be quite complex [1–6].

New PAH therapies have gained regulatory board approval based on studies with intermediate and surrogate end points as primary outcomes, believed to reflect the impact of these drugs on quality of life (QOL) and survival, respectively. While hemodynamic, plasma, cardiac imaging, exercise, functional, and QOL parameters are promising candidates, the reliability and validity of these measures are not clearly established. In addition, there are no RCTs addressing the use of such end points in guiding management decisions in PAH, such as changing, intensifying, escalating, or combining therapies. Despite this lack of evidence, clinicians who care for these patients frequently rely on end points measured in clinical practice and RCTs based on surrogate and intermediate end points to make important treatment decisions, warranting a review of their use.

Definitions

The National Institutes of Health define a surrogate as a characteristic that is objectively measured and evaluated as an indicator of a normal biologic process, pathogenic process, or pharmacologic response to a therapeutic intervention intended to substitute for a clinical end point [7]. The Food and Drug Administration defines a surrogate end point as "a laboratory measurement or physical sign that is used in therapeutic trials as a substitute for a clinically meaningful end point... and is expected to predict the effect of the therapy" [8]. Restrictive definitions require that a therapy's effect on the surrogate encompass, in its entirety, the impact on the clinical end point [9].

Alternatively, an intermediate end point is a parameter that directly reflects how a patient feels [10]. Intermediate end points are important to patients and physicians in and of themselves (unlike a surrogate) even without a validated relationship to survival. For example, a reduction in pulmonary vascular resistance (PVR) does not reflect how much farther a patient can walk without dyspnea but may have long-term implications regarding survival, making PVR a potential

Supported in part by NIH grants K23 HL67771, RO3 DK064103, RO1 HL086719, and RO1 HL082895.

* Corresponding author. Division of Pulmonary, Allergy, and Critical Care Medicine, Department of Medicine, Columbia University College of Physicians and Surgeons, PH 8E, Room 101, 622 W. 168th Street, New York, NY 10032.

E-mail address: sk2097@columbia.edu (S.M. Kawut).

surrogate end point for PAH. On the other hand, a reported increase in exercise capacity without dyspnea (ie, a decrease in New York Heart Association [NYHA] class) reflects improved patient function without any assumptions regarding long-term outcome, making this a potential intermediate end point. In addition, an intermediate end point (such as NYHA class) could concomitantly serve as a surrogate end point if treatment-induced changes in the measure predict differences in event-free survival (see below).

What are the "hard" clinical end points in PAH? Prolonging the time until death is the primary goal of treating PAH; however, there are other health states that patients and physicians wish to avoid. Lung transplantation is curative for PAH but entails a complicated surgical procedure, perioperative risk, multiple medications with side effects, and intensive follow-up. Patients therefore prefer to postpone this and other operative interventions (eg, atrial septostomy). Hospitalization is another end point that is uncomfortable and inconvenient for the patient and could itself serve as a surrogate end point for worse long-term outcome. Intravenous prostacyclin analog therapy is an important treatment for PAH, but drug delivery is suboptimal. As a result, both physicians and patients may view the initiation of parenteral prostacyclin analog therapy as an "undesirable" event (or at least a "trade-off") despite proven clinical efficacy [11–13]. A measurement made in the short term that reflected the long-term risk of reaching one or more of these end points would facilitate the assessment of treatment success.

Event-free survival is not the only end point of interest in PAH. Patients complain of dyspnea on exertion, fatigue, lower extremity edema, and limitation in performing daily tasks. A reliable metric incorporating these facets of disease activity (intermediate end point) would therefore be integral to developing drugs to ameliorate such symptoms. A therapy that successfully targeted intermediate end points but did not prolong time to clinical events would still be considered useful, as long as it did not significantly shorten event-free survival. In fact, most current therapies for PAH have been approved on this basis.

Regulatory issues

The Food and Drug Modernization Act permits approval for drugs for serious diseases without alternatives with a demonstrated "effect on a surrogate end point that is reasonably likely, based on epidemiologic, therapeutic, pathophysiologic, or other evidence, to predict clinical benefit or on the basis of an effect on a clinical end point other than survival or irreversible morbidity" [8]. The existence of multiple effective therapies for PAH may increase the pressure on sponsors to design RCTs that go beyond the "traditional" end points used for approval and focus on "harder" clinical end points to support more definitive claims, increasing confidence that new therapies result in incremental benefit over current drugs. Such Phase III trials based on definitive clinical end points could also serve to validate surrogates, reassuring investigators and clinicians that these end points are indeed appropriate for early-phase clinical testing and managing patients.

Strengths of surrogate end points

There are several advantages to using surrogate end points. Surrogates are often based on continuous variables that usually require smaller sample sizes for adequately powered studies than those required when using dichotomous end points (eg, dead/alive). Focusing on the mean changes in such measures over time usually reduces sample size requirements even further. For example, most clinical trials in PAH have compared changes in hemodynamics and 6-minute walk distance (6MWD) over time between drug and placebo groups, not the absolute values at study end. Usually surrogate end points can be measured sooner than the clinical outcomes they represent, shortening study duration and reducing costs. Measurements such as the 6-minute walk test (6MWT) may be serially repeated with minimal discomfort and expense, making them particularly useful for clinical management. Quantitative results from intermediate or surrogate end points may help to rank different therapies in terms of effectiveness, but differences between studies may significantly weaken comparability. Some researchers have proposed using surrogates as "auxiliary end points" to strengthen the analysis of ultimate clinical end points [14].

Weaknesses of surrogate end points

Dependence on surrogate end points may also be a liability. The smaller sample size, temporal immediacy, and narrow focus may increase the chances of missing uncommon, late, or extraneous adverse effects in RCTs, which could overshadow the drug benefits in clinical practice. For example, the short-term, apparently beneficial, effects of antiarrythmics on ventricular ectopy and of inotropes and vasodilators on hemodynamics and exercise function in patients with congestive heart failure (CHF) were trumped by an increased risk of death in the long term [15–17]. Similarly, it is possible (and perhaps even inevitable) to develop a PAH therapy that will decrease PVR, increase cardiac index (CI), and increase the 6MWD over the short term, yet also increase the long-term risk of adverse events.

The study population from a RCT is virtually always less heterogeneous than the actual clinical patient population; the effect of therapy on the surrogate in a study may therefore not translate to the definitive end point in clinical practice. The validation of a surrogate end point in a clinical trial does not apply to the patients who would have been excluded from that trial. Also, validation of a surrogate for one class of drugs does not guarantee that it will be applicable for other classes. For example, CI may be a valid surrogate for a PAH therapy that targets the pulmonary vasculature, reducing right ventricular afterload. However, an inotrope without pulmonary vascular effects may have the same (or greater) effect on the surrogate marker (CI) without necessarily affecting the disease course. In this case, CI may be a valid surrogate for drugs with a particular mechanism (ie, pulmonary vascular remodeling), but may not be appropriate for drugs with a different mechanism (ie, inotropic support).

Patients with PAH may refuse study procedures, drop out, become sicker, or die in RCTs, all resulting in missing end point data that are nonrandom. Even with complete assessments, technical difficulties in measurement may be related to clinical outcomes, leading to bias (eg, increased variability in plasma brain natriuretic peptide [BNP] levels in a decompensated patient).

Some clinical trials in PAH have used a range of values of an end point for an inclusion criterion, such as 6MWD. The subsequent truncation of the distribution of the measure in the study sample may lead to regression to the mean [18]. The observed mean change in the variable in the study is then not an unbiased estimate of the true change in the actual population of patients. This prevents the extrapolation of the findings of the study in terms of the surrogate to outcomes in clinical practice.

Last, there may not be a linear relationship between the value of a surrogate end point and the clinical implications. For example, a placebo-corrected difference in the change in 6MWD of +40 m in a RCT with Drug A does not necessarily mean that it is more effective than Drug B, which produces a placebo-corrected difference of +30 m. It is possible that any 6MWD increment more than +25 m or an absolute 6MWD after treatment more than 380 m results in improved QOL and survival, metrics by which both Drugs A and B may perform identically. Therefore, the differences in changes in 6MWD in the hypothetical trials may not have clinical significance. One recent study in fact supports such a "threshold effect" [19]. The temptation to compare clinical efficacy using surrogate and intermediate end points should therefore be resisted until the implications of such differences are better understood.

Criteria for a valid surrogate end point

The primary requirement for a surrogate or intermediate end point is reliability. Potential surrogates in PAH, such as cardiopulmonary exercise test (CPET) results, may be highly operator-, protocol-, equipment-, and reader-dependent, lessening their usefulness. A recent study implicated differential variability in hampering the use of CPET in a RCT [20]. Second, the surrogate should be in the causal pathway to the ultimate outcome or be closely related to a causal factor (Fig. 1). An intervention should target the disease pathway in which the surrogate lies, and alternative pathways to clinical end points should not exist. Additionally, extensive epidemiologic evidence should link the surrogate variable with outcome. While the strength and reproducibility of the relationship between the surrogate marker and the definitive clinical end point are necessary, "a correlate does not a surrogate make" [21]. Markers with powerful correlations with clinical outcomes or other end points may themselves be very poor surrogates of clinical efficacy. Therefore, RCTs of similar and different therapies must show that a quantitative modification of the surrogate is associated with a concomitant modification in the target outcome [22]. Such confirmatory trials must incorporate potential surrogate measures yet be sufficiently powered to show clinically significant effects of the therapy on ultimate end points. Adequate data satisfying this final most important criterion are severely lacking in PAH, ranking most potential PAH surrogates in the lowest category

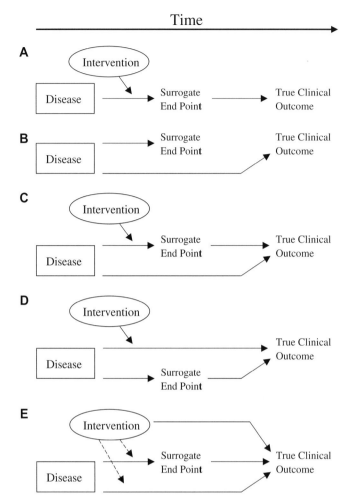

Fig. 1. (*A*) The intervention and surrogate act in the single causal pathway of PAH to morbidity or mortality. This setting has the greatest potential for the surrogate end point to be valid. Situations in which surrogates may fail include the following: (*B*) The surrogate is not in the causal pathway of PAH. (*C*) Of several causal PAH disease pathways to morbidity and mortality, the intervention affects only the pathway mediated through the surrogate. (*D*) The surrogate is not in the pathway of the intervention's effect or is insensitive to its effect. (*E*) The intervention has mechanisms of action (either beneficial or adverse) independent of the disease process of PAH. *Dotted lines*, mechanisms of action that might exist. (*Adapted from* Fleming TR, DeMets DL. Surrogate end points in clinical trials: are we being misled? Ann Intern Med 1996;125:605–613; with permission.)

of validation (ie, Level 4) in a recent hierarchical scheme (Table 1) [23].

Validating a surrogate-guided therapeutic approach

One recent observational study used a goal-oriented therapeutic strategy in PAH, using add-on combination therapy until patients met predefined 6MWD and peak exercise criteria [24]. With this approach, patients had a better overall event-free survival compared with a historical control group. The authors qualified their findings by highlighting the nonrandomized study design, the unvalidated nature of the end points used, the unproven efficacy of the combination therapy used, and the increased side effects and cost that could result from such a strategy. However, if it were true that a marker (or markers) captured all of the current and future effects of therapy, the optimal drug regimen would indeed be the one that maintained the surrogate at a low (or high) level.

Table 1
Hierarchy for outcome measures in pulmonary arterial hypertension

Level	Definition	Details	Examples
I	True clinical efficacy end point	Outcome directly reflects tangible benefit	Hospitalization
II	Validated surrogate end point	Outcome not reflecting tangible benefit but which reliably predicts the level of benefit	—
III	Nonvalidated surrogate end point	(1) Considerable evidence that intervention effect on the measure will accurately represent the intervention's effect on the predominant mechanism through which the disease process induces clinical events; (2) Considerable clinical evidence that the experimental intervention does not have important adverse effects on the clinical end point not captured by the surrogate end point; (3) Statistical analyses suggest that the net effect of the intervention on the true clinical-efficacy end point is consistent with what would be predicted by the level of effect on the measure; and (4) Targeted effect on the outcome measure is sufficiently strong and durable that, based on #1–3, this is reasonably likely to predict meaningful clinical benefit	Cardiac index, Pulmonary vascular resistance, Distance walked in 6 minutes
IV	Measure of biologic activity	Treatment effects on measure show that intervention is biologically active, but without sufficient evidence of translation to clinical benefit	Brain natriuretic peptide

Adapted from Fleming TR. Surrogate endpoints and FDA's accelerated approval process. Health Affairs 2005;24: 67–78.

To confirm the efficacy of such an approach requires a RCT of the surrogate measure(s) to guide therapy and escalation with a clearly effective established treatment algorithm for incomplete response or disease worsening. Patients would be randomized either to serial surrogate measurements with explicit therapeutic algorithms based on the results or to traditional care; such RCTs of surrogate end point–guided therapy are only recently being performed in CHF [25–27]. Without supportive evidence showing the incremental benefit of using goal-directed therapy, a surrogate end point–guided approach could result in significant overuse or underuse of therapies to the detriment of patients with PAH.

Potential surrogate and intermediate end points in PAH

Hemodynamics

Cardiopulmonary hemodynamic abnormalities not only are defining characteristics of PAH but are also the best-established indicators of the severity of illness. The earliest studies of PAH showed that increased right atrial (RA) pressure, decreased CI, and increased mean pulmonary artery (PA) pressure were predictors of death or lung transplantation [28–32]. While these findings were published in an era before effective therapy was available, they have generally (but not universally) been validated in more recent studies of patients at diagnosis or initiation of therapy [19,33–50]. Importantly, PAH patients with more severe cardiac dysfunction or history of heart failure at baseline continue to have a higher risk of death than those with less severe heart failure despite treatment with new therapies [33,34,36,38, 41,45,46,48,49].

Improvement in these characteristic hemodynamic abnormalities after therapy has been associated with better survival [19,49]. McLaughlin and colleagues [34] have shown that reductions in RA pressure and mean PA pressure and increases in CI after initiation of intravenous epoprostenol predicted a better survival. Similarly, Provencher and colleagues [49] and Sitbon and colleagues [19] demonstrated that the persistence of elevated total pulmonary resistance despite a few months of bosentan or epoprostenol therapy, respectively, was associated with an increased risk of death. Opitz and colleagues [48] showed that lower CI and higher RA pressure and PVR after 3 months of inhaled iloprost predicted an increased risk of death.

One study confirmed that hemodynamic measurements are valid surrogate end points in PAH. A RCT of continuous intravenous epoprostenol showed significant reductions in mean PA pressure and PVR and increases in CI [11]. This trial also showed significantly improved survival in the epoprostenol group. A subsequent RCT of intravenous epoprostenol in patients with PAH and systemic sclerosis demonstrated hemodynamic changes similar to those of the former study but no survival benefit over 12 weeks [51], suggesting that surrogate adequacy may depend on differences in disease states [46,52]. Other RCTs of prostacyclin analogs have shown smaller or no effects on hemodynamics in PAH and no differences in death, need for transplantation, or initiation of intravenous epoprostenol between drug and placebo groups [12,13,53–56]. Clinical trials of endothelin receptor antagonists and sildenafil have shown differences between drug and placebo in mean changes in hemodynamic measures similar to those found in the early epoprostenol study, but no effects on time to reaching ultimate clinical end points, such as initiation of parenteral therapy, septostomy, transplantation, or death [57–59]. This implies that surrogates that appeared promising in past studies need to be reevaluated in the current era before widespread use.

Integral to the causal pathway of PAH, hemodynamic measurements meet the epidemiologic criteria for surrogates, but the optimal parameter is not established. Only the first-mentioned RCT of epoprostenol found a concurrent effect on hemodynamics and differences in death or transplantation; that similar hemodynamic effects have not translated to survival differences in more recent RCTs is likely attributable to temporal changes in these studies and the participants. Hemodynamic criteria for "clinical improvement" may be applied to patients after the initiation of medical therapy for PAH; however, there are no data to support the institution of treatment changes based on the failure to meet certain goals. Strengths of hemodynamic measurements include standardization, availability, and strong biologic plausibility. The invasiveness, discomfort, risk, and expense of right heart catheterization pose significant drawbacks to its use in RCTs and in the clinical management of patients with PAH.

Plasma biomarkers

Biomarkers play an integral role in the diagnosis and management of more common cardiovascular diseases, but their clinical and investigative use has lagged in PAH. Optimal plasma biomarkers would be causal (or at least closely linked) to the extent of pulmonary vascular disease or degree of right heart dysfunction [10]. Circulating von Willebrand factor (vWF) and other substances are released by the vascular endothelium and are increased in PAH [60–62]. Higher vWF levels at baseline and despite therapy are independently associated with an increased risk of death in PAH [60]. Similarly, a variety of biomarkers tied to cardiac function have been investigated in PAH [38,50,63,64]. The best-studied, natriuretic peptides are produced by the cardiac atria and ventricles in response to myocyte stretch and may serve as endocrinologic indicators of heart function. Circulating levels of BNP and N-terminal proBNP (NT-proBNP) are increased in PAH and are closely tied to the causal pathway of disease progression [47,65–71]. Baseline and follow-up levels of BNP and NT-proBNP have been shown to be directly associated with the risk of death and other events in PAH [38,47,71,72].

One small RCT included BNP measurements [73]. This study randomized patients with PAH to either sildenafil or bosentan. Decreases in BNP levels were seen in both groups; however, BNP levels did not differ between drug groups, similar to other end points in this trial. Unfortunately, none of the recently published, placebo-controlled RCTs of new, effective therapies have included early assessment of BNP as a secondary end point, marking significant lost opportunities to advance the science of clinical trials and patient management in PAH.

As BNP and other plasma biomarker levels are assessed by phlebotomy, they may be obtained relatively noninvasively and safely, lending to serial evaluations over time. In addition, samples may be stored locally and transported for central analysis, potentially reducing measurement error in RCTs. The weaknesses of some biomarkers lie in their within-subject variability, which may be substantial, and the potential for therapies to directly affect them (endothelin receptor antagonists and endothelin-1, for example). RCTs demonstrating improvement in outcomes with the use of a biomarker-guided strategy are necessary before incorporating routine BNP or other measures into clinical practice in PAH [25–27].

Cardiac imaging

Considering the integral role of right ventricular function in the morbidity and mortality of PAH, cardiac imaging parameters might not only respond to effective therapies but also associate with outcome. It is well known that cardiac morphologic changes can long precede hemodynamic changes in left-sided heart disease. Similarly, imaging with echocardiography, radionuclide angiography, or magnetic resonance imaging (MRI) may capture subtle changes in right-sided cardiac function in PAH before hemodynamic decompensation occurs.

Echocardiography

Studies have shown that a variety of atrial, ventricular, and Doppler parameters have been associated with an increased risk of death or transplantation in patients with PAH [37,38, 44,63,74–76]. While pericardial effusion presence and size are also associated with death or transplantation, this parameter is unlikely to be sufficiently discriminating for research purposes [32,38,44,45,47,77]. It is notable that the estimate of right ventricular systolic pressure from echocardiography has not been found to be predictive of outcome [32,44,45,74].

In the RCT of intravenous epoprostenol for idiopathic PAH, differences in changes in ventricular and septal morphology were found between the epoprostenol and control groups, corresponding with a difference in survival [78]. A substudy of a RCT of bosentan versus placebo showed significant differences between groups in changes in ventricular morphology, the minimum diameter of the inferior vena cava, and Doppler measurements, including right ventricular ejection time and mitral valve peak velocity [37].

While the meaningfulness of echocardiography as a secondary end point in these RCTs shows the promise of this technique, the incremental prognostic value of echocardiography in monitoring patients after treatment has not been studied. Improvement in hemodynamics, exercise performance, and symptoms are often not reflected in routine echocardiographic measurements. In addition, many of the more specialized measurements are not regularly performed by most clinical echocardiography laboratories.

Strengths of echocardiography include noninvasiveness, plausibility, and incorporation in previous RCTs. Unfortunately, echocardiography is expensive and has varying availability. The operator-dependent nature of these highly technical measurements may impact reliability. In addition, the adequacy of echocardiographic measurements of the right ventricle depends on many patient factors (eg, body habitus), potentially introducing differential measurement error and bias.

Other cardiac imaging modalities

Radionuclide angiography measures the right ventricular ejection fraction (RVEF) [79], as does MRI, considered to be the "gold-standard" for assessing right atrial and ventricular dimensions, ventricular mass, and ventricular wall motion [80–85]. One study has shown an association between lower baseline RVEF and an increased risk of death, independent of other factors [45]. A single short-term RCT of bosentan and sildenafil used right ventricular mass by MRI as the primary end point [73]. Significant differences between the groups were not seen, although there were changes within groups over the study period. The requirement for radioactive agents for nuclear studies and the more complex technical issues and expense that accompany the use of these modalities to manage patients may limit their utility in clinical practice. However, as the most accurate technique to visualize the right ventricle, MRI may play a more prominent role in future RCTs of PAH.

Exercise testing

Six-minute walk test

The 6MWT is thought to reliably reflect the ability to perform activities of daily living in a quantitative manner in a variety of heart and lung diseases, making this an intermediate end point [86]. A recent report substantiated the impact of changes in 6MWD on health status and QOL [87]. However, 6MWD may also be linked to survival in PAH, making it a surrogate end point as well. Initially considered as a substitute for CPET to gauge maximal oxygen consumption, this deceivingly simple evaluation is one of the best-established and most often used tests in RCTs and clinical management of PAH. Doebeck and colleagues [88] have shown that the 6MWT was more metabolically demanding than CPET in PAH, whereas Provencher and colleagues [89] demonstrated that changes in 6MWD after therapy were closely linked to changes in cardiac function.

It is biologically plausible that interventions that improve exercise tolerance will improve survival in PAH (as it was in CHF before studies showed otherwise) [16]. Miyamoto and colleagues [90] found a direct association between 6MWD and survival, independent of other noninvasive measures. Almost all other studies of 6MWD in PAH have confirmed this association [19,35,38, 40–42,44,49,50,91]. Sitbon and colleagues [19] found inverse associations between 6MWD at baseline and after 3 months of epoprostenol therapy with the risk of death. An absolute 6MWD threshold of less than 380 m at 3 months after initiating therapy increased the risk of death, as opposed to the change in 6MWD after treatment (an often used end point in RCTs), which was not predictive. In another study, the change in and the absolute 6MWD 4 months after initiation of bosentan therapy predicted survival [49]. This suggests that absolute, incremental, or threshold values in 6MWD after treatment may reflect long-term outcomes depending on the patient severity of illness or type of therapy instituted.

The RCT of epoprostenol showed a significant difference in the mean changes of 6MWD from baseline and follow-up between the drug and control groups (+47 m) with a corresponding difference in survival [11]. RCTs of prostacyclin analogs, bosentan, sitaxsentan, and sildenafil have also shown statistically significant differences in changes in 6MWD, but no differences in survival, need for lung transplantation, or transition to intravenous epoprostenol [12,13,53,55,57–59,92], showing that the clinically significant increment in 6MWD may need to be redefined in the current era.

Advantages of the 6MWT include the ability to assess a global and integrated response of systems required for daily functioning, simplicity of performance, low cost, and evidence of reasonable reliability and validity in other chronic heart and lung diseases under standardized conditions [93,94]. Weaknesses of this test include variation in test conduct, a learning effect after repeated testing, variability based on other activities on the day of the testing, and the effect of musculoskeletal conditions on performance. The 6MWT is not within the causal pathway of PAH, but is likely closely related to causal factors (Fig. 1). The effort-dependent nature of this test may also be problematic, as it may be difficult to adequately

mask investigators and patients in studies of drugs with characteristic side effects, such as prostacyclin analogs. If the subject is able to discern the treatment assignment, test performance may be affected, similar to other volitional exercise assessments.

In addition, the inclusion of a permissible range of 6MWDs in the entry criteria of a RCT may truncate the distribution of this variable in the cohort, weakening the assumptions regarding even a validated surrogate measure in terms of clinical outcome [18]. Some have posited a "ceiling effect" specific to 6-minute walk testing [95]. As in other diseases, it is likely that healthier PAH patients tend to have smaller improvements after interventions than sicker patients. A final issue with the 6MWT is the prejudice that, because of its simplicity, the results must be less reliable or valid than other more invasive, sophisticated, or technical testing. However, this bias is not supported by the existing evidence.

Cardiopulmonary exercise testing

CPET quantifies the function of the many systems used in exercise, and therefore CPET could reflect cardiopulmonary benefits of effective therapies in PAH. Studies in other heart and lung diseases have shown relationships between oxygen consumption at peak exercise (VO_2max) and outcome and have used CPET measures as surrogate end points [96].

The sophisticated nature and sheer volume of the measurements produced by CPET offer an enticing insight into PAH. Test performance in RCT participants with PAH appears reliable [97]. VO_2max and the ventilatory equivalent for carbon dioxide with exercise are abnormal in patients with PAH, and these and other parameters are associated with hemodynamics [20,45,97–103].

Despite these findings, it is not clear which (if any) of the many parameters are predictive of long-term outcome in PAH. Wensel and colleagues [33] demonstrated that VO_2max corrected for weight as well as systolic and diastolic blood pressure at peak exercise were discriminating predictors of death in 70 patients undergoing initial evaluation for PAH. This study used treadmill testing for most of the subjects and showed a particularly high risk of death or transplantation at 1 year (32%), exceeding that of other centers during a similar time period and potentially limiting generalizability. These investigators subsequently published a cohort study of patients treated with inhaled iloprost in which VO_2max again predicted time until events [48]. However, in another study of 72 consecutive PAH patients, there was no association between VO_2max and survival, although lower systolic blood pressure and higher ventilatory equivalent for carbon dioxide at peak exercise did predict worse outcome [45].

A RCT of sitaxsentan used the change in VO_2max percent predicted as the primary end point [57]. While there were significant beneficial effects of the drug on hemodynamics and 6MWD (confirmed in a second trial) [92], similar benefits were not seen in CPET parameters. Further analysis of this cohort revealed that correlations of VO_2max with other measures differed between sites and changed over each patient's progress through the trial [20]. Similarly, VO_2max did not track with other more established surrogates in another RCT [54]. The lack of response of CPET to therapy that was otherwise effective in terms of more established end points should elicit caution in using CPET to guide treatment decisions or to study new therapies.

The strength of CPET is its biologic plausibility and its usefulness in other diseases. Weaknesses lie in the paucity and inconsistency of epidemiologic and RCT evidence of validity. CPET requires specialized, calibrated equipment and standardized test performance. The presence of a patent foramen ovale or uncorrected cardiac shunt affects test validity. Patients may be unable or unwilling to give a maximal effort on a cycle ergometer or treadmill. Last, CPET may not be safe or practical for severely ill patients.

Functional classification

The NYHA classification of functional status has been slightly altered for PAH in the form of the World Health Organization (WHO) classification (Table 2). Reliability has not been assessed in patients with PAH, however the validity of the NYHA/WHO classification is supported by the association with survival in a variety of cohort studies [19,29,33,34,40,42,46]. In addition, functional class correlates with QOL, underscoring its role as an intermediate end point [104]. Intravenous epoprostenol, endothelin receptor antagonists, and sildenafil improved functional class, forming an important basis for approval of these drugs for PAH [11,51,56–58,92,105]. The persistence of more limited functional class despite treatment predicted worse survival in some studies [19,46] but not in others [34,49].

Table 2
World Health Organization functional classification in pulmonary arterial hypertension

Class	
I	No limitation of physical activity. Ordinary physical activity does not cause undue dyspnea or fatigue, chest pain, or near syncope.
II	Slight limitation of physical activity. Patient is comfortable at rest. Ordinary physical activity causes undue dyspnea or fatigue, chest pain, or near syncope.
III	Marked limitation of physical activity. Patient is comfortable at rest. Less than ordinary activity causes undue dyspnea or fatigue, chest pain, or near syncope.
IV	Inability to carry out any physical activity without symptoms. Patient manifests signs of right-heart failure. Dyspnea and/or fatigue may be present at rest. Discomfort is increased by any physical activity.

Adapted from Rubin LJ. Diagnosis and management of pulmonary arterial hypertension: ACCP evidence-based clinical practice guidelines. Chest 2004;126(Suppl 1):9S; with permission.

Strengths of this end point include the convenience and ease of classification. A treatment-induced change in functional class translates to patient benefit, even without a confirmation of surrogacy for survival. Weaknesses lie in the self-report and interpretive role patients and investigators have in assignment. RCTs in which one or the other party is unmasked by side effects may result in bias. In addition, the blunt nature of this end point may mean that this classification is poorly discriminating and that subtle changes in clinical status will not be detected.

Quality of life

The improvement of QOL and health-related QOL are significant goals in the treatment of PAH. The assessment of the success of meeting these goals, however, is not straightforward. Although we look toward functional tests, such as the 6MWT, to provide this information, it is unlikely that a single physiologic test can capture all of the components that enter into the complex construct of satisfaction of the needs and desires of daily living. Investigators have therefore "asked" PAH patients in epidemiologic studies and RCTs about the components that comprise QOL, using instruments such as the Medical Outcome Study Short Form-36 (SF-36). More specific questionnaires focus on certain characteristics of the disease process under study, such as the Minnesota Living with Heart Failure (MLHF) questionnaire. These instruments are judged not only by content and criterion validity (reasonableness of the questions and correlation of the scale with another "gold standard" measure accepted in the field) but also convergent and discriminant validity (responses track with other assessments of similar constructs and not with unrelated variables). Last, change of the measurement in response to effective treatment testifies to the validity of the instrument.

Recent studies have initiated this validation process in PAH [87,104,106]. Taichman and colleagues [104] examined the SF-36 in reference to other components of disease activity in PAH. Higher WHO functional class and lower 6MWD were associated with a more affected (worse) physical activity summary score (convergent validity). On the other hand, hemodynamics had no association with either the physical or mental component scores (discriminant validity). Investigators have shown similar correlations between the physical subscore of the modified MLHF questionnaire with functional class, 6MWD, RA pressure, and CI [87,107]. The MLHF score was also associated with event-free survival [107]. Chua and colleagues [87] have shown that improvements in 6MWD over time translate to improvements in QOL measured by the SF-36.

One group has taken on the daunting but necessary task of creating a PAH-specific health-related QOL instrument, the Cambridge Pulmonary Hypertension Outcome Review (CAMPHOR) [108]. It appears that this instrument has good test-retest reliability and content, convergent, and discriminant validity. The responsiveness of this instrument to interventions, however, has not yet been assessed.

Strengths of these QOL instruments include content and criterion validity in PAH. Weaknesses include the few studies of convergent and discriminant validity and the limited use in PAH. The symptom constellation and treatment strategies of PAH likely make QOL questionnaires designed for other health conditions less sensitive and specific for the issues that face these patients.

Summary

The use of surrogate and intermediate end points is deeply ingrained in the clinical study of

PAH; however, few definitive, evidence-based statements may be made. New therapies for patients with PAH need to show beneficial hemodynamic effects in early phase trials. There may be a single hemodynamic parameter that is the "best" surrogate or different classes of therapies may warrant different surrogate measures. The literature suggests that an optimal time point for reassessment is at least 3 to 4 months after initiation of therapy, but earlier assessment of an end point might also predict treatment success. This could certainly vary based on the type of therapy under study. While beneficial drug effects on hemodynamic surrogates have not sufficed for regulatory approval, the validity of hemodynamics as surrogate end points should be reconsidered based on their merit in PAH, apart from their inadequacy in CHF.

While echocardiography and BNP hold promise as noninvasive surrogates, they are not ready for use as primary end points. Multiple long-term RCTs should incorporate BNP to validate this biomarker against definitive clinical end points with various drug classes. A RCT of BNP-guided medical management would assist clinicians in deciding if monitoring this biomarker benefits patients in clinical practice.

Differences in 6MWD between therapy and placebo groups over the short term may or may not be clinically meaningful. Future studies should better define the parameter(s) and increment of the 6MWD that reflect patient-perceived improved function. It would also be vitally important to extrapolate such findings to differences in event-free survival. The efficacy of therapies with prominent side effects and potential unmasking should be substantiated by non–effort-dependent tests. CPET measures should not be used as primary outcomes in RCTs until further examination of these metrics has been completed.

Functional status and QOL are important end points to include in RCTs of PAH therapy, as they reflect patient well-being. Longer-term trials with these end points would prove that such beneficial effects were durable. Validation of commonly used instruments and the further development of instruments specific for PAH (such as CAMPHOR) are necessary to achieve the goal of designing therapeutic approaches that definitively improve the QOL of patients with PAH.

The scientific discoveries and therapeutic advances in PAH require similar developments in clinical trial design. Many innovative technologies are changing how patients can be profiled and respond to therapy, including genetics, genomics, proteomics, metabolomics, and imaging. While these new techniques offer the opportunity to describe patients in more detail than ever, validation of the clinical utility of these technologies is less "high-tech" but no less difficult or important than the process of invention. Seemingly established surrogate and intermediate end points, such as hemodynamics and exercise testing, remain incompletely validated and poorly described in PAH; these priority candidates should be vetted before others are considered.

Therefore, future RCTs in PAH should abide by the recommendations and goals of the National Institutes of Health workshop on surrogate end points [109]. Progress in this area can only be made through incorporation of these measures into clinical trials powered to detect differences in time to clinically important end points. This makes for more expensive trials of longer duration, but this is necessary to gain confidence in these tests. Prospective planning for meta-analyses across RCTs of new and combination therapies would provide additional opportunities for sponsors and investigators to advance the science of clinical trials in PAH, while not distracting from the main hypotheses under study [110,111]. Such investments in the conduct of RCTs in PAH will pay great dividends in the future study and care of patients with PAH.

Acknowledgments

The authors are grateful for the administrative assistance of Tracey Huger and for the thoughtful review of the manuscript by Norman L. Stockbridge, MD, PhD.

References

[1] Hoeper MM, Oudiz RJ, Peacock A, et al. End points and clinical trial designs in pulmonary arterial hypertension: clinical and regulatory perspectives. J Am Coll Cardiol 2004;43:48S–55S.

[2] Peacock A, Naeije R, Galie N, et al. End points in pulmonary arterial hypertension: the way forward. Eur Respir J 2004;23:947–53.

[3] Kawut SM, Palevsky HI. Surrogate end points for pulmonary arterial hypertension. Am Heart J 2004; 148:559–65.

[4] Kawut SM, Palevsky HI. New answers raise new questions in pulmonary arterial hypertension. Eur Respir J 2004;23:799–801.

[5] Rich S. The current treatment of pulmonary arterial hypertension: time to redefine success. Chest 2006;130:1198–202.

[6] Roberts K, Preston I, Hill NS. Pulmonary hypertension trials: current end points are flawed, but what are the alternatives? Chest 2006;130:934–6.

[7] Biomarkers Definitions Working Group. Biomarkers and surrogate endpoints: preferred definitions and conceptual framework. Clin Pharmacol Ther 2001;69:89–95.

[8] New drug, antibiotic, and biological drug product regulations; accelerated approval; final rule. 57 FR 58958 as amended at 64 FR. 402; 1992.

[9] Prentice RL. Surrogate endpoints in clinical trials: definition and operational criteria. Stat Med 1989; 8:431–40.

[10] Temple R. Are surrogate markers adequate to assess cardiovascular disease drugs? JAMA 1999; 282:790–5.

[11] Barst RJ, Rubin LJ, Long WA, et al. A comparison of continuous intravenous epoprostenol with conventional therapy for primary pulmonary hypertension. N Engl J Med 1996;334:296–302.

[12] Olschewski H, Simonneau G, Galie N, et al. Inhaled iloprost for severe pulmonary hypertension. N Engl J Med 2002;347:322–9.

[13] Simonneau G, Barst RJ, Galie N, et al. Continuous subcutaneous infusion of treprostinil, a prostacyclin analogue, in patients with pulmonary arterial hypertension: a double-blind, randomized, placebo-controlled trial. Am J Respir Crit Care Med 2002;165:800–4.

[14] Fleming TR, Prentice RL, Pepe MS, et al. Surrogate and auxiliary endpoints in clinical trials, with potential applications in cancer and AIDS research. Stat Med 1994;13:955–68.

[15] Echt DS, Liebson PR, Mitchell LB, et al. Mortality and morbidity in patients receiving encainide, flecainide, or placebo. The Cardiac Arrhythmia Suppression Trial. N Engl J Med 1991;324:781–8.

[16] Cohn JN, Goldstein SO, Greenberg BH, et al. A dose-dependent increase in mortality with vesnarinone among patients with severe heart failure. Vesnarinone Trial Investigators. N Engl J Med 1998; 339:1810–6.

[17] Califf RM, Adams KF, McKenna WJ, et al. A randomized controlled trial of epoprostenol therapy for severe congestive heart failure: The Flolan International Randomized Survival Trial (FIRST). Am Heart J 1997;134:44–54.

[18] Wittes J, Lakatos E, Probstfield J. Surrogate endpoints in clinical trials: cardiovascular diseases. Stat Med 1989;8:415–25.

[19] Sitbon O, Humbert M, Nunes H, et al. Long-term intravenous epoprostenol infusion in primary pulmonary hypertension: prognostic factors and survival. J Am Coll Cardiol 2002;40:780–8.

[20] Oudiz RJ, Barst RJ, Hansen JE, et al. Cardiopulmonary exercise testing and six-minute walk correlations in pulmonary arterial hypertension. Am J Cardiol 2006;97:123–6.

[21] Fleming TR, DeMets DL. Surrogate end points in clinical trials: are we being misled? Ann Intern Med 1996;125:605–13.

[22] Bucher HC, Guyatt GH, Cook DJ, et al. Users' guides to the medical literature: XIX. Applying clinical trial results. A. How to use an article measuring the effect of an intervention on surrogate end points. Evidence-Based Medicine Working Group. JAMA 1999;282:771–8.

[23] Fleming TR. Surrogate endpoints and FDA's accelerated approval process. Health Aff (Millwood) 2005;24:67–78.

[24] Hoeper MM, Markevych I, Spiekerkoetter E, et al. Goal-oriented treatment and combination therapy for pulmonary arterial hypertension. Eur Respir J 2005;26:858–63.

[25] Lainchbury JG, Troughton RW, Frampton CM, et al. NTproBNP-guided drug treatment for chronic heart failure: design and methods in the "BATTLESCARRED" trial. Eur J Heart Fail 2006;8:532–8.

[26] Shah MR, Claise KA, Bowers MT, et al. Testing new targets of therapy in advanced heart failure: the design and rationale of the Strategies for Tailoring Advanced Heart Failure Regimens in the Outpatient Setting: BRain NatrIuretic Peptide Versus the Clinical CongesTion ScorE (STARBRITE) trial. Am Heart J 2005;150:893–8.

[27] Troughton RW, Frampton CM, Yandle TG, et al. Treatment of heart failure guided by plasma aminoterminal brain natriuretic peptide (N-BNP) concentrations. Lancet 2000;355:1126–30.

[28] Sandoval J, Bauerle O, Palomar A, et al. Survival in primary pulmonary hypertension. Circulation 1994; 89:1733–44.

[29] D'Alonzo GE, Barst RJ, Ayres SM, et al. Survival in patients with primary pulmonary hypertension. Results from a national prospective registry. Ann Intern Med 1991;115:343–9.

[30] Kanemoto N. Natural history of pulmonary hemodynamics in primary pulmonary hypertension. Am Heart J 1987;114:407–13.

[31] Glanville AR, Burke CM, Theodore J, et al. Primary pulmonary hypertension: length of survival in patients referred for heart-lung transplantation. Chest 1987;91:675–81.

[32] Eysmann SB, Palevsky HI, Reichek N, et al. Two-dimensional and Doppler-echocardiographic and cardiac catheterization correlates of survival in primary pulmonary hypertension. Circulation 1989; 80:353–60.

[33] Wensel R, Opitz CF, Anker SD, et al. Assessment of survival in patients with primary pulmonary hypertension: importance of cardiopulmonary exercise testing. Circulation 2002;106:319–24.

[34] McLaughlin VV, Shillington A, Rich S. Survival in primary pulmonary hypertension: the impact of epoprostenol therapy. Circulation 2002;106: 1477–82.

[35] Ewert R, Wensel R, Opitz C, et al. Prognosis in patients with primary pulmonary hypertension awaiting lung transplantation. Transplant Proc 2001;33:3574–5.

[36] Bossone E, Paciocco G, Iarussi D, et al. The prognostic role of the ECG in primary pulmonary hypertension. Chest 2002;121:513–8.

[37] Galie N, Hinderliter AL, Torbicki A, et al. Effects of the oral endothelin-receptor antagonist bosentan on echocardiographic and Doppler measures in patients with pulmonary arterial hypertension. J Am Coll Cardiol 2003;41:1380–6.

[38] Fijalkowska A, Kurzyna M, Torbicki A, et al. Serum N-terminal brain natriuretic peptide as a prognostic parameter in patients with pulmonary hypertension. Chest 2006;129:1313–21.

[39] Nunes H, Humbert M, Sitbon O, et al. Prognostic factors for survival in human immunodeficiency virus-associated pulmonary arterial hypertension. Am J Respir Crit Care Med 2003;167:1433–9.

[40] Williams MH, Das C, Handler CE, et al. Systemic sclerosis associated pulmonary hypertension: improved survival in the current era. Heart 2006;92: 926–32.

[41] Mahapatra S, Nishimura RA, Sorajja P, et al. Relationship of pulmonary arterial capacitance and mortality in idiopathic pulmonary arterial hypertension. J Am Coll Cardiol 2006;47:799–803.

[42] McLaughlin VV, Sitbon O, Badesch DB, et al. Survival with first-line bosentan in patients with primary pulmonary hypertension. Eur Respir J 2005; 25:244–9.

[43] Frank H, Mlczoch J, Huber K, et al. The effect of anticoagulant therapy in primary and anorectic drug-induced pulmonary hypertension. Chest 1997; 112:714–21.

[44] Raymond RJ, Hinderliter AL, Willis PW, et al. Echocardiographic predictors of adverse outcomes in primary pulmonary hypertension. J Am Coll Cardiol 2002;39:1214–9.

[45] Kawut SM, Horn EM, Berekashvili KK, et al. New predictors of outcome in idiopathic pulmonary arterial hypertension. Am J Cardiol 2005;95:199–203.

[46] Kuhn KP, Byrne DW, Arbogast PG, et al. Outcome in 91 consecutive patients with pulmonary arterial hypertension receiving epoprostenol. Am J Respir Crit Care Med 2003;167:580–6.

[47] Nagaya N, Nishikimi T, Uematsu M, et al. Plasma brain natriuretic peptide as a prognostic indicator in patients with primary pulmonary hypertension. Circulation 2000;102:865–70.

[48] Opitz CF, Wensel R, Winkler J, et al. Clinical efficacy and survival with first-line inhaled iloprost therapy in patients with idiopathic pulmonary arterial hypertension. Eur Heart J 2005;26:1895–902.

[49] Provencher S, Sitbon O, Humbert M, et al. Long-term outcome with first-line bosentan therapy in idiopathic pulmonary arterial hypertension. Eur Heart J 2006;27:589–95.

[50] Torbicki A, Kurzyna M, Kuca P, et al. Detectable serum cardiac troponin T as a marker of poor prognosis among patients with chronic precapillary pulmonary hypertension. Circulation 2003; 108:844–8.

[51] Badesch DB, Tapson VF, McGoon MD, et al. Continuous intravenous epoprostenol for pulmonary hypertension due to the scleroderma spectrum of disease. A randomized, controlled trial. Ann Intern Med 2000;132:425–34.

[52] Kawut SM, Taichman DB, Archer-Chicko CL, et al. Hemodynamics and survival in patients with pulmonary arterial hypertension related to systemic sclerosis. Chest 2003;123:344–50.

[53] Galie N, Humbert M, Vachiery JL, et al. Effects of beraprost sodium, an oral prostacyclin analogue, in patients with pulmonary arterial hypertension: a randomized, double-blind, placebo-controlled trial. J Am Coll Cardiol 2002;39:1496–502.

[54] Barst RJ, McGoon M, McLaughlin V, et al. Beraprost therapy for pulmonary arterial hypertension. J Am Coll Cardiol 2003;41:2119–25.

[55] McLaughlin VV, Gaine SP, Barst RJ, et al. Efficacy and safety of treprostinil: an epoprostenol analog for primary pulmonary hypertension. J Cardiovasc Pharmacol 2003;41:293–9.

[56] Rubin LJ, Mendoza J, Hood M, et al. Treatment of primary pulmonary hypertension with continuous intravenous prostacyclin (epoprostenol). Results of a randomized trial. Ann Intern Med 1990;112: 485–91.

[57] Barst RJ, Langleben D, Frost A, et al. Sitaxsentan therapy for pulmonary arterial hypertension. Am J Respir Crit Care Med 2004;169:441–7.

[58] Galie N, Ghofrani HA, Torbicki A, et al. Sildenafil citrate therapy for pulmonary arterial hypertension. N Engl J Med 2005;353:2148–57.

[59] Channick RN, Simonneau G, Sitbon O, et al. Effects of the dual endothelin-receptor antagonist bosentan in patients with pulmonary hypertension: a randomised placebo-controlled study. Lancet 2001;358:1119–23.

[60] Kawut SM, Horn EM, Berekashvili KK, et al. von Willebrand factor independently predicts long-term survival in patients with pulmonary arterial hypertension. Chest 2005;128:2355–62.

[61] Lopes AA, Maeda NY. Circulating von Willebrand factor antigen as a predictor of short-term prognosis in pulmonary hypertension. Chest 1998;114: 1276–82.

[62] Veyradier A, Nishikubo T, Humbert M, et al. Improvement of von Willebrand factor proteolysis after prostacyclin infusion in severe pulmonary arterial hypertension. Circulation 2000;102:2460–2.

[63] Nagaya N, Uematsu M, Satoh T, et al. Serum uric acid levels correlate with the severity and the mortality of primary pulmonary hypertension. Am J Respir Crit Care Med 1999;160: 487–92.

[64] Bendayan D, Shitrit D, Ygla M, et al. Hyperuricemia as a prognostic factor in pulmonary arterial hypertension. Respir Med 2003;97:130–3.

[65] Nagaya N, Nishikimi T, Okano Y, et al. Plasma brain natriuretic peptide levels increase in proportion to the extent of right ventricular dysfunction in pulmonary hypertension. J Am Coll Cardiol 1998;31:202–8.

[66] Williams MH, Handler CE, Akram R, et al. Role of N-terminal brain natriuretic peptide (N-TproBNP) in scleroderma-associated pulmonary arterial hypertension. Eur Heart J 2006;27: 1485–94.

[67] Leuchte HH, Holzapfel M, Baumgartner RA, et al. Clinical significance of brain natriuretic peptide in primary pulmonary hypertension. J Am Coll Cardiol 2004;43:764–70.

[68] Souza R, Bogossian HB, Humbert M, et al. N-terminal-pro-brain natriuretic peptide as a haemodynamic marker in idiopathic pulmonary arterial hypertension. Eur Respir J 2005;25: 509–13.

[69] Souza R, Jardim C, Julio Cesar Fernandes C, et al. NT-proBNP as a tool to stratify disease severity in pulmonary arterial hypertension. Respir Med 2007; 101:69–75.

[70] Mukerjee D, Yap LB, Holmes AM, et al. Significance of plasma N-terminal pro-brain natriuretic peptide in patients with systemic sclerosis-related pulmonary arterial hypertension. Respir Med 2003;97:1230–6.

[71] Andreassen AK, Wergeland R, Simonsen S, et al. N-terminal pro-B-type natriuretic peptide as an indicator of disease severity in a heterogeneous group of patients with chronic precapillary pulmonary hypertension. Am J Cardiol 2006;98: 525–9.

[72] Park MH, Scott RL, Uber PA, et al. Usefulness of B-type natriuretic peptide as a predictor of treatment outcome in pulmonary arterial hypertension. Congest Heart Fail 2004;10:221–5.

[73] Wilkins MR, Paul GA, Strange JW, et al. Sildenafil versus endothelin receptor antagonist for pulmonary hypertension (SERAPH) study. Am J Respir Crit Care Med 2005;171:1292–7.

[74] Yeo TC, Dujardin KS, Tei C, et al. Value of a Doppler-derived index combining systolic and diastolic time intervals in predicting outcome in primary pulmonary hypertension. Am J Cardiol 1998;81:1157–61.

[75] Bustamante-Labarta M, Perrone S, De La Fuente RL, et al. Right atrial size and tricuspid regurgitation severity predict mortality or transplantation in primary pulmonary hypertension. J Am Soc Echocardiogr 2002;15:1160–4.

[76] Forfia PR, Fisher MR, Mathai SC, et al. Tricuspid annular displacement predicts survival in pulmonary hypertension. Am J Respir Crit Care Med 2006;174:1034–41.

[77] Hinderliter AL, Willis PW, Long W, et al. Frequency and prognostic significance of pericardial effusion in primary pulmonary hypertension. Am J Cardiol 1999;84:481–4.

[78] Hinderliter AL, Willis PW, Barst RJ, et al. Effects of long-term infusion of prostacyclin (epoprostenol) on echocardiographic measures of right ventricular structure and function in primary pulmonary hypertension. Primary Pulmonary Hypertension Study Group. Circulation 1997;95:1479–86.

[79] Nichols K, Saouaf R, Ababneh AA, et al. Validation of SPECT equilibrium radionuclide angiographic right ventricular parameters by cardiac magnetic resonance imaging. J Nucl Cardiol 2002; 9:153–60.

[80] Saba TS, Foster J, Cockburn M, et al. Ventricular mass index using magnetic resonance imaging accurately estimates pulmonary artery pressure. Eur Respir J 2002;20:1519–24.

[81] Katz J, Whang J, Boxt LM, et al. Estimation of right ventricular mass in normal subjects and in patients with primary pulmonary hypertension by nuclear magnetic resonance imaging. J Am Coll Cardiol 1993;21:1475–81.

[82] Roeleveld RJ, Vonk-Noordegraaf A, Marcus JT, et al. Effects of epoprostenol on right ventricular hypertrophy and dilatation in pulmonary hypertension. Chest 2004;125:572–9.

[83] Blyth KG, Groenning BA, Martin TN, et al. Contrast enhanced-cardiovascular magnetic resonance imaging in patients with pulmonary hypertension. Eur Heart J 2005;26:1993–9.

[84] Boxt LM, Katz J, Kolb T, et al. Direct quantitation of right and left ventricular volumes with nuclear magnetic resonance imaging in patients with primary pulmonary hypertension. J Am Coll Cardiol 1992;19:1508–15.

[85] Hoeper MM, Tongers J, Leppert A, et al. Evaluation of right ventricular performance with a right ventricular ejection fraction thermodilution catheter and MRI in patients with pulmonary hypertension. Chest 2001;120:502–7.

[86] Sciurba F, Criner GJ, Lee SM, et al. Six-minute walk distance in chronic obstructive pulmonary disease: reproducibility and effect of walking course layout and length. Am J Respir Crit Care Med 2003;167:1522–7.

[87] Chua R, Keogh AM, Byth K, et al. Comparison and validation of three measures of quality of life in patients with pulmonary hypertension. Intern Med J 2006;36:705–10.

[88] Deboeck G, Niset G, Vachiery JL, et al. Physiological response to the six-minute walk test in pulmonary arterial hypertension. Eur Respir J 2005;26: 667–72.

[89] Provencher S, Chemla D, Herve P, et al. Heart rate responses during the 6-minute walk test in pulmonary arterial hypertension. Eur Respir J 2006;27: 114–20.

[90] Miyamoto S, Nagaya N, Satoh T, et al. Clinical correlates and prognostic significance of six-minute walk test in patients with primary pulmonary hypertension. Comparison with cardiopulmonary exercise testing. Am J Respir Crit Care Med 2000;161: 487–92.

[91] Paciocco G, Martinez FJ, Bossone E, et al. Oxygen desaturation on the six-minute walk test and mortality in untreated primary pulmonary hypertension. Eur Respir J 2001;17:647–52.

[92] Barst RJ, Langleben D, Badesch D, et al. Treatment of pulmonary arterial hypertension with the selective endothelin-A receptor antagonist sitaxsentan. J Am Coll Cardiol 2006;47: 2049–56.

[93] ATS Committee on Proficiency Standards for Clinical Pulmonary Function Laboratories. ATS statement: guidelines for the six-minute walk test. Am J Respir Crit Care Med 2002;166:111–7.

[94] Solway S, Brooks D, Lacasse Y, et al. A qualitative systematic overview of the measurement properties of functional walk tests used in the cardiorespiratory domain. Chest 2001;119:256–70.

[95] Frost AE, Langleben D, Oudiz R, et al. The 6-min walk test (6MW) as an efficacy endpoint in pulmonary arterial hypertension clinical trials: demonstration of a ceiling effect. Vascul Pharmacol 2005;43:36–9.

[96] American Thoracic Society; American College of Chest Physicians. ATS/ACCP statement on cardiopulmonary exercise testing. Am J Respir Crit Care Med 2003;167:211–77.

[97] Hansen JE, Sun XG, Yasunobu Y, et al. Reproducibility of cardiopulmonary exercise measurements in patients with pulmonary arterial hypertension. Chest 2004;126:816–24.

[98] Sun XG, Hansen JE, Oudiz RJ, et al. Gas exchange detection of exercise-induced right-to-left shunt in patients with primary pulmonary hypertension. Circulation 2002;105:54–60.

[99] Sun XG, Hansen JE, Oudiz RJ, et al. Exercise pathophysiology in patients with primary pulmonary hypertension. Circulation 2001;104:429–35.

[100] Rhodes J, Barst RJ, Garofano RP, et al. Hemodynamic correlates of exercise function in patients with primary pulmonary hypertension. J Am Coll Cardiol 1991;18:1738–44.

[101] Oudiz RJ. The role of exercise testing in the management of pulmonary arterial hypertension. Semin Respir Crit Care Med 2005;26:379–84.

[102] Yasunobu Y, Oudiz RJ, Sun XG, et al. End-tidal PCO2 abnormality and exercise limitation in patients with primary pulmonary hypertension. Chest 2005;127:1637–46.

[103] Yetman AT, Taylor AL, Doran A, et al. Utility of cardiopulmonary stress testing in assessing disease severity in children with pulmonary arterial hypertension. Am J Cardiol 2005;95: 697–9.

[104] Taichman DB, Shin J, Hud L, et al. Health-related quality of life in patients with pulmonary arterial hypertension. Respir Res 2005;6:92.

[105] Rubin LJ, Badesch DB, Barst RJ, et al. Bosentan therapy for pulmonary arterial hypertension. N Engl J Med 2002;346:896–903.

[106] Shafazand S, Goldstein MK, Doyle RL, et al. Health-related quality of life in patients with pulmonary arterial hypertension. Chest 2004;126:1452–9.

[107] Cenedese E, Speich R, Dorschner L, et al. Measurement of quality of life in pulmonary hypertension and its significance. Eur Respir J 2006;28:808–15.

[108] McKenna SP, Doughty N, Meads DM, et al. The Cambridge Pulmonary Hypertension Outcome Review (CAMPHOR): a measure of health-related quality of life and quality of life for patients with pulmonary hypertension. Qual Life Res 2006;15: 103–15.

[109] De Gruttola VG, Clax P, DeMets DL, et al. Considerations in the evaluation of surrogate endpoints in clinical trials. Summary of a National Institutes of Health workshop. Control Clin Trials 2001;22: 485–502.

[110] Buyse M, Molenberghs G, Burzykowski T, et al. The validation of surrogate endpoints in meta-analyses of randomized experiments. Biostatistics 2000;1:49–67.

[111] Daniels MJ, Hughes MD. Meta-analysis for the evaluation of potential surrogate markers. Stat Med 1997;16:1965–82.

ELSEVIER
SAUNDERS

Clin Chest Med 28 (2007) 91–115

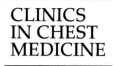

CLINICS
IN CHEST
MEDICINE

Standard Therapies for Pulmonary Arterial Hypertension

Shoaib Alam, MD[a],*, Harold I. Palevsky, MD[b,c,d]

[a]Division of Pulmonary, Allergy and Critical Care Medicine, Penn State University-Hershey Medical Center,
500 University Drive, Hershey, PA 17033, USA
[b]University of Pennsylvania School of Medicine, 3400 Spruce Street, Philadelphia, PA 19104-4283, USA
[c]Pulmonary, Allergy and Critical Care, Penn Presbyterian Medical Center, 51 N. 39th Street,
Philadelphia, PA 19104, USA
[d]Pulmonary Vascular Disease Program, Penn Presbyterian Medical Center, 51 N. 39th Street,
Philadelphia, PA 19104, USA

Pulmonary arterial hypertension (PAH) was first described in 1891 in a case report by Romberg [1]. The term "primary pulmonary hypertension" (PPH) was first used in 1951 when Dresdale and colleagues [2] reported clinical features and hemodynamics of 39 patients. Until approximately two decades ago, before the development of specific PAH therapies, such as prostacyclin analogs, endothelial receptor antagonists, and phosphodiestrase-5 inhibitors, PAH (especially idiopathic [IPAH] or PPH form of PAH) was considered a disease that was universally fatal with a median survival of 2.8 years [3]. An explosion of research and drug development has resulted in the development of several specific PAH therapies (see other articles elsewhere in this issue) [4–21]. Therapies such as oxygen supplementation, calcium channel blockers (CCBs), anticoagulation, digoxin, and diuretics have been in use since long before the development of the newer specific PAH agents. These therapies have been referred to as "standard PAH therapies" or "conventional PAH therapies" [22]. The concept of these standard therapies originated from the experience with other pulmonary and cardiac diseases with similar—but not identical—manifestations in terms of symptoms (eg, edema in congestive left heart failure and

use of diuretics) or physiologic observations (eg, hypoxemia in emphysema and use of oxygen supplementation therapy, low cardiac output in left ventricular [LV] systolic dysfunction and use of digoxin, high blood pressure in essential systemic hypertension and use of vasodilators, prothrombotic tendency in venous thromboembolism and use of anticoagulation). These practices were subsequently adopted in the treatment of PAH and right heart dysfunction and failure. None of these therapies is supported by well-designed placebo-controlled trials. Some of these practices are based on marked symptomatic relief or improvement with short-term use (eg, diuretics for edema) or by observations based on acute testing in the laboratory setting (eg, improvement in cardiac output by single administration of digoxin) [23] or from autopsy findings [24–26] (eg, in situ microthrombi in lungs of patients who have PAH and use anticoagulation). Therapies such as anticoagulation have been supported by a few retrospective studies [27,28] and an uncontrolled, single-center prospective study [29], especially in IPAH [30]. This raises the ethical question of the appropriateness of performing a placebo-controlled trial in these patients. On the other hand, the short-term benefits from diuretics are so obvious that it virtually obviates the need for a clinical trial to validate such benefit. For these reasons it seems unlikely that any large, prospective, clinical trials will examine the role of the standard therapies used in PAH in the near future. Such trials are needed, however.

* Corresponding author.
E-mail addresses: shoaibalam@yahoo.com;
salam1@psu.edu (S. Alam).

Especially lacking are data about use of standard therapies in PAH other than IPAH (associated [APAH]). It may be possible that in specific populations, these therapies may not be helpful, that they may be less helpful than they are currently considered, or that they may be even harmful.

In a prospective, controlled study of patients who had PAH and Eisenmenger syndrome, the use of oxygen supplementation in hypoxemic patients was not associated with any improvement in hematologic variables, quality of life, or survival [31]. A recent retrospective chart review of French patients who had IPAH showed that only 6.8% of all patients who had IPAH could be maintained on CCB therapy alone without any need for augmentation of therapy by a newer agent [32]. This is an example in which retrospective [33] and noncontrolled prospective [29,34] data led to enthusiasm, first about the use of acute vasoreactivity testing for assessing prognosis in PPH and second about the excessive use of CCBs in patients who have PAH. It should be noted that the initial studies [29,34], which reported that the "responders" had an excellent (94%) 5-year survival on CCBs, had mean fall in mean pulmonary artery pressure (mPAP) of 39% to 48% and mean fall in pulmonary vascular resistance (PVR) of 53% to 60%. The acceptance of relatively less stringent criteria for favorable acute vasoreactivity response [35–37] was at least partly caused by the fact that at that time the only alternative to CCB therapy was continuous intravenous prostacyclin therapy. Because currently several oral and inhaled therapies are available and it is known that as many as 46% of "acute responders" eventually will fail, CCB monotherapy [32], the need for and emphasis on performing acute vasoreactivity testing, and the use of CCBs as primary therapy for IPAH has changed [32]. Reliance on CCBs in such patients and not using specific PAH therapies may or may not be in patients' best interest.

This article reviews current recommendations and widely accepted practices regarding the use of standard therapies in PAH and presents the evidence available to support these practices. The primary purpose of this article is to provide clinicians with relevant information to be able to make informed therapeutic decisions in clinical situations in which data regarding standard therapies are lacking, relative contraindications to these therapies exist, or the therapies are poorly tolerated or adverse events occur.

Oxygen therapy

The value of long-term oxygen supplementation therapy in patients with PAH has not been evaluated by well-designed clinical trials. Recommendations and guidelines for oxygen therapy in patients who have PAH have been extrapolated from the clinical data available for chronic obstructive pulmonary disease (COPD). Pathophysiologically, hypoxemia is a potent stimulus for pulmonary vasoconstriction [38]. In COPD patients who have hypoxemia, two well-designed, prospective, randomized, non–placebo-controlled trials [39,40] have shown that there is marked improvement in long-term survival with the use of supplemental oxygen (Table 1) [31,39,40].

One trial [40] studied 87 patients who had COPD and a history of right heart failure (RHF) along with arterial oxygen partial pressure <60 mm Hg. Patients were randomly assigned to receive 15 h/d of oxygen supplementation therapy or no therapy. Five-year mortality rate in the oxygen treatment group was 46% versus 67% in control group (number needed to treat to save one life in approximately five). The study also showed an increase in PVR in the control group over the study period but no increase in PVR in the oxygen therapy group. The study was not powered to evaluate this parameter, however.

The other prospective, randomized, controlled study of 203 patients who had chronic hypoxemic COPD showed that in patients who were hypoxemic at rest during the daytime, the use of nocturnal oxygen supplementation (12 h/d) was associated with a higher 3-year mortality rate (42% versus 22%) when compared with the group that used continuous (at least 19 h/d) supplemental oxygen [39]. The number needed to treat to save one life was approximately five. The survival advantage was more pronounced in patients with less severe pulmonary hypertension at baseline (mean pulmonary arterial pressure <27 mm Hg). Continuous oxygen supplementation therapy improved long-term survival in patients who had COPD with significant hypoxemia ($PaO_2 <55$ mm Hg at rest) even if there was no significant improvement in pulmonary hemodynamics with acute oxygen supplementation. Patients with low baseline PVR had an improved mortality on continuous oxygen supplementation therapy, but the patient with high baseline PVR did not experience

Table 1
Clinical studies: oxygen therapy

Study [reference] (N)	Design, method	Follow-up duration, site	Study findings	Comments
Nocturnal Oxygen Therapy Trial Group, 1980 [39] (203)	Prospective, randomized, non–placebo-controlled trial, multicenter. Patients with chronic, hypoxic COPD. Patients received either continuous oxygen therapy or 12-h oxygen therapy	At least 12 months, at six centers in United States	Overall mortality in 12-h therapy group was 1.94 times greater than continuous group ($P = .01$). 1-y and 2-y mortality was 21% and 41%, respectively, in nocturnal therapy group versus 12% and 22%, respectively, in continuous therapy group	No placebo control and no blinding was used. NOTE: the trial involved COPD patients and not WHO I PAH patients; hence the results should be extrapolated with caution. The survival benefit was also present in patients with low mean pulmonary artery pressure and PVR and with relatively preserved exercise capacity. Survival advantage was pronounced in hypercapnic patients but was also present with relatively poor lung function, low mean nocturnal oxygen saturation
Medical Research Council Working Party, 1981 [40] (87)	Prospective, randomized, non–placebo-controlled trial, multicenter. Patients with chronic, hypoxic cor pulmonale secondary to COPD. 42 patients received oxygen at 2 L/min at least 15 h/d and 45 control patients received no oxygen	Five years, at three centers in U.K.	5-y mortality in treated group was significantly less than control (45% versus 67%). Survival advantage from oxygen did not emerge until 500 days of therapy	No placebo control and no blinding was used. NOTE: the trial involved COPD patients and not WHO I PAH patients; hence the results should be extrapolated with caution
Sandoval et al, 2001 [31] (23)	Prospective, randomized, non–placebo-controlled trial, single center. Patients with congenital heart disease and Eisenmenger's syndrome. 12 randomly assigned patients received nocturnal oxygen for at least 8 h at flow rate (mostly 2–3 L/min) that increased the oxyhemoglobin saturation from $79 \pm 6.5\%$ to $88 \pm 6.0\%$	Two years, at a center in Mexico	Nocturnal oxygen therapy did not improve hematologic variables, 6-minute walk distance, quality of life, or survival at 2-y follow-up	It is not known whether continuous oxygen therapy will be helpful in this patient population. Two patients died in oxygen therapy groups and three patients died in control group; probably the numbers were too small to reliably conclude "no difference" between the two groups. This study clearly highlights that similar interventions may have entirely different impact on different disease processes

N = Number of subjects.

a survival benefit. Patients who showed a large decrease in PVR on repeat right heart catheterization after 6 months of continuous oxygen therapy had greater mortality compared with patients with smaller decrease in PVR [39]. This finding suggests that mortality benefit in hypoxemic patients who have COPD and are on continuous long-term oxygen therapy is probably not derived from any reduction in PVR. This observation is important from the standpoint of oxygen therapy in patients who have PAH.

Because of the substantial survival (and hemodynamic) benefit observed in COPD patients who have hypoxemia, the oxygen supplementation therapy is widely used in PAH patients who have hypoxemia. The principles and criteria used for oxygen therapy in PAH are derived from the studies and practice guidelines for treatment of hypoxemic patients who have COPD [41].

Many patients who have PAH have hypoxemia at rest, with exertion, or during sleep. Hypoxemia in PAH is thought to be caused by low mixed-venous oxygen tension secondary to low cardiac output, altered diffusion capacity, and ventilation-perfusion mismatch. Some patients who have PAH present with relatively rapid worsening of hypoxemia secondary to opening of a patent foramen ovale, which results in right-to-left shunt. In such patients, hypoxemia is relatively refractory to oxygen supplementation. In most other patients, however, with the exception of patients with advanced disease, the hypoxemia at rest and at night can be corrected by oxygen supplementation at 2 to 6 L/min via nasal cannula, although increased oxygen supplementation is frequently required during activity or exertion.

Most current guidelines [29,32–34] from American or European professional societies recommend that all patients with PAH whose PaO_2 is consistently <55 mm Hg or in whom oxyhemoglobin saturation is ≤88% at rest, during sleep, or with ambulation should be prescribed sufficient supplemental oxygen therapy to keep the pulse oximetry oxyhemoglobin saturation >90% at all times. In patients with laboratory or clinical findings that suggest chronic hypoxemia (eg, hematocrit >55%), clinical signs of RHF, or suggestion of RHF on EKG or echocardiography, long-term oxygen supplementation therapy should be initiated at PaO_2 <60 mm Hg or oxyhemoglobin saturation of ≤89%. Such patients should be retested for oxygen requirement 3 months after the initiation of oxygen therapy. All patients with moderate to severely decreased diffusion capacity (DLCO

<60% of predicted) at rest should be tested for possibility of oxyhemoglobin desaturation with activity and while sleeping [42,43]. It should be noted that all such recommendations are based on expert opinion in the absence of any direct evidence in IPAH or any form of APAH except pulmonary hypertension (PH) associated with COPD.

Many patients with congenital heart disease have hypoxemia secondary to right-to-left shunt. Such hypoxemia is relatively refractory to oxygen supplementation therapy. The use of oxygen supplementation therapy in patients who have congenital heart disease and Eisenmenger syndrome remains controversial. A study of 15 pediatric patients with PAH associated with congenital heart disease and hypoxemia initially reported improved mortality with oxygen supplementation for a minimum of 12 h/d for 5 years [44]. A well-designed, prospective, randomized, controlled study of 23 adult patients who had hypoxemia and Eisenmenger syndrome showed that nocturnal oxygen supplementation had no effect on survival, quality of life, hematocrit, or 6-minute walking distance [31]. Some studies suggest that oxygen supplementation in these patients may reduce need for phlebotomy and may reduce neurologic complications [35]. Nocturnal oxygen supplementation in children who have PAH associated with congenital heart disease has been shown to decrease the rate of progression of polycythemia. Similarly in the PAH pediatric population, oxygen therapy has been shown to improve symptoms [44,45].

PaO_2 during sleep is almost always lower than PaO_2 while awake [46], which is probably secondary to sleep-induced hypoventilation and the resultant rise in PCO_2. In normal individuals with a normal wake PaO_2, nocturnal oxyhemoglobin desaturation is not seen because the oxyhemoglobin dissociation curve is relatively flat for PaO_2 above 90 mm Hg. Patients who are hypoxemic at rest while awake are always more hypoxemic during sleep, however [47]. This reduction in arterial oxygenation is even more pronounced during rapid eye movement sleep. The long-term value of treating nocturnal hypoxemia in patients who have PAH remains unclear, however. Screening with nocturnal oximetry may be performed to evaluate possibility of nocturnal hypoxemia when clinically suspected. Oxyhemoglobin saturation <90% for less than 5% of the recording time may be considered clinically insignificant regardless of the lowest recorded oxyhemoglobin saturation value. After initiation of oxygen supplementation, it is suggested that a repeat nocturnal oximetry study be obtained to assess the adequacy of nocturnal oxygen supplementation therapy.

In most patients without significant right-to-left shunt, a nocturnal oxygen supplementation at 2 to 3 L/min above the resting oxygen requirement is sufficient to maintain adequate oxygenation during sleep. The exception to this rule is presence of obstructive sleep apnea (OSA), in which nasal continuous positive airway pressure (CPAP) (or BiPAP) therapy is needed to correct the sleep-disordered breathing and hypoxemia. An overnight polysomnogram should be ordered for patients in whom OSA is suspected because of history of snoring, excessive daytime sleepiness, or witnessed apneas. Routine ordering of polysomnogram in all patients who have PAH is not indicated [48].

Prevalence of PH in OSA is much higher than the prevalence of IPAH in the general population; the reported prevalence of PH in OSA is 17% to 53% [48–60]. In contrast, the estimated incidence of IPAH in the general population is 1 to 2 new cases per million [61], which suggests a prevalence of <10 to 20 per million. Most of the studies [48–60] that estimated prevalence of PH in OSA used right heart catheterization for defining PAH. Data are difficult to interpret, however, because many of these studies defined PH as mPAP ≥20 mm Hg (less than the standard used to define PAH) or used estimated pressures by echocardiogram. Generally PH associated with OSA is mild in the absence of obesity-hypoventilation syndrome [47–59]. Any moderate or severe PH should not be attributed to OSA alone, no matter how severe the OSA. Modest improvement in PA pressures is expected from the treatment of OSA; the expected median decrease in pulmonary artery pressure is 3 to 6 mm Hg and expected median decrease in PVR is approximately 0.5 wood units [59,62,63]. Patients who have OSA and PH with hypoxemia who are treated with CPAP and oxygen supplementation have a more pronounced decrease in mPAP and PVR than patients who are treated with oxygen therapy alone. Resolution of PH is not an expected outcome of even the most successful therapy by CPAP, regardless of the severity of OSA and the duration of the CPAP therapy [59,62,63].

Obesity-hypoventilation syndrome (usually associated with body mass index >34 and always associated with the presence of daytime hypercapnia, ie, PCO_2 of ≥45 mm Hg) can be associated with severe PAH and RHF, regardless of presence or absence of concurrent OSA [64].

Oxygen supplementation or CPAP therapy or both combined are not adequate treatments for nocturnal hypoxemia in such patients; noninvasive positive pressure ventilation or bilevel positive pressure ventilation should be used. In patients who cannot tolerate this therapy (eg, because of claustrophobia), tracheostomy should be offered along with chronic outpatient mechanical ventilation. Near complete reversal of hypercapnia and signs of RHF within a few months with invasive or noninvasive mechanical ventilation therapy usually are seen in patients who do not have concurrent factors contributing to the development of PAH [65]. Weight loss after gastric surgery for morbid obesity also has been shown to substantially decrease the PCO_2 (mean, 52 mm Hg to 42 mm Hg) and mPAP (mean, 36 mm Hg to 23 mm Hg) at right heart catheterization [66]. In patients who have PH and a body mass index >34, an arterial blood gas analysis obtained on room air, should be performed to rule out possibility of obesity-hypoventilation syndrome (OHS) because the management principles of OHS associated PAH are different than those of OSA [65,66].

There is reluctance on the part of some physicians and many patients to consider oxygen supplementation as part of therapy. Oxygen supplementation is a major lifestyle change for patients (with the exception nocturnal oxygen supplementation therapy alone). Factors such as cost, the type of equipment required, and the inconvenience of many ambulatory oxygen systems impact on patients' acceptance and use of prescribed supplemental oxygen. In clinical practice most patients agree to the use of oxygen if prescribed by physician but do not like the oxygen tubing they need to wear in public. This has an impact on their perceptions of themselves and others' perceptions of them. Falls associated with long cords and tubing attached to oxygen concentrators and other oxygen delivery systems can occur.

Diuretics

The long-term role of diuretics in RHF and PAH has not been systematically studied. The use of diuretics in patients who have PAH with peripheral edema secondary to RHF is widespread and universally accepted. Almost all PAH patients with peripheral edema secondary to RHF are treated with diuretics, and the effect of the diuretics on edema is usually obvious. Most patients with edema report some improvement after "effective diuresis" as assessed by change in weight or pedal edema over relatively short periods of time. For many patients, maximal effects are only obtained when salt and fluid intake restrictions are used with diuresis. Whether diuretics alter mortality or morbidity in patients who have PAH with RHF is not known, however. Diuretics also can decrease the sensation of dyspnea in patients with enlarged right heart chambers compromising left heart function (see later discussion).

The effect of most diuretics (eg, furosemide) on mortality or morbidity either in left or right heart failure has not been evaluated by long-term trials. Spironolactone, an aldosterone antagonist used as a potassium-sparing diuretic, decreased mortality in a long-term prospective, randomized, placebo-controlled trial of patients with recent hospitalization for severe left heart failure with NYHA III or IV symptoms [67]. In this study, a relatively low dose of spironolactone (12.5 mg/d taken orally) was used as an add-on therapy to angiotensin-converting enzyme inhibitor therapy. Two-year mortality rate in the treatment group was 35% compared with 46% in controls, indicating 24% relative risk reduction (number needed to treat to save one life in approximately nine). The study also showed a 35% decrease in hospitalizations secondary to worsening of heart failure and improvement in functional class in treated patients. No studies have evaluated the long-term role of aldosterone antagonists in patients who have PAH and RHF. Secondary to convincing data regarding left heart failure, however, spironolactone is widely used in patients who have PAH and RHF as an adjunct to loop diuretics. Long-term value of spironolactone in such patients remains unknown. It should be noted that many interventions known to have a beneficial effect in LV failure (eg, angiotensin-converting enzyme inhibitors and beta adrenergic antagonists) have not been proven to be beneficial in patients who have PAH and RHF. Spironolactone should not be used in patients with serum creatinine >2.5 mg/dL or potassium >5.0 mEq/L or in patients with history of severe refractory hyperkalemia. Extreme caution should be observed in patients who have impaired renal function or diabetes, in elderly persons, and in patients with concurrent use of angiotensin-converting enzyme inhibitors or nonsteroidal anti-inflammatory agents [68].

Amiloride (a potassium-sparing diuretic) analogs have been shown to inhibit development of hypoxia-induced pulmonary hypertension in animal models [69]. The proposed mechanism is inhibition of sodium-proton ($Na+/H+$) exchange to prevent intracellular alkalinization, which seems to play a permissive role in pulmonary artery smooth muscle cell proliferation in the process of vascular remodeling [24]. There are no clinical studies in patients who have PAH to speculate the clinical significance of these observations.

In most recent trials of pharmacologic therapy for PAH [4–21], diuretics were used as adjunct therapy in a large proportion of patients, but the effect of diuretics was not tested as an end point in any of these trials. In severe RHF, large doses of diuretics may be required for effective diuresis. Some patients may require doses as high as furosemide, 600 mg/d, or bumetanide, 10 mg/d, or the addition of metolazone (up to 20 mg/d). Edema in many patients with severe RHF and impaired renal function may be disabling and can be refractory to even such high doses of diuretics (Box 1).

Right ventricular (RV) performance is preload dependant. Because of ventricular interdependence (ie, shared pericardium and septum), however, extreme RV dilatation may compromise LV filling in part by displacing the interventricular septum into the LV, which results in LV diastolic dysfunction and a decrease in cardiac output [70–72]. Patients who have PAH are likely to develop interstitial edema at relatively lower pulmonary capillary wedge pressures because the effective hydrostatic pressure to favor interstitial edema formation is equal to pulmonary capillary wedge pressure plus 40% of the gradient between mPAP and pulmonary capillary wedge pressure (Gaar's equation). Relatively minor fluctuations in fluid status may result in significant change in cardiac output or gas exchange, resulting in arterial hypoxemia. Caution should be observed when adjusting diuretic dose. There is no evidence or scientific rationale to urgently diurese patients or remove large volumes of fluid over a short period of time, except when there is cardiogenic pulmonary edema or acute worsening of arterial hypoxemia. "Optimal fluid status" in patients who have PAH and RHF is often a relatively narrow window in which patient's cardiac output is maintained, arterial hypoxemia is minimized, and signs of tissue perfusion (as assessed by renal function, presence or absence of peripheral cyanosis, or altered mentation) are optimal.

Severe passive hepatic congestion and bowel wall edema and ischemia may be present when patients who have severe RHF and reduced cardiac output present with significantly deranged

**Box 1. Management options
for refractory edema in pulmonary
arterial hypertension and severe chronic
right heart failure**

History and evaluation

- Carefully review compliance with salt and water intake restriction.
- Consider concurrent medications (eg, CCB, bosentan, sitaxsentan, or prostacyclin analogs) and temporal relation to the worsening of edema.
- Review possibility of worsening of underlying disease by other parameters (eg, 6-minute walking distance, oxygen requirement, RV hypertrophy on echocardiography).
- Reassess renal function.
- Consider discontinuing all nonsteroidal anti-inflammatory drugs.

Options

- Increase the dose of current loop diuretic (may use up to furosemide, 600 mg/d, or bumetanide, 10 mg/d).
- Add a diuretic from another class (metolazone, 2.5–5 mg twice daily, or spironolactone, 12.5–50 mg twice daily). Do not use spironolactone if serum creatinine is above 2.5 mg/dL or above 1.6 in patients older than 70 years. Do not use in patients who have diabetes or potassium above 4.5 or history of severe hyperkalemia.
- Change current loop diuretic to another loop diuretic.
- Consider hospitalization and intravenous diuretics.
- Consider hospitalization and ionotropic support by very low dose (2–3 ng/kg/min; avoid higher doses) IV dopamine or dobutamine.
- Consider atrial septostomy (if appropriate for patient).
- Consider lung transplantation (if appropriate for patient).
- Consider right ventricular assist device (if appropriate for patient).
- Tolerate current level of edema.
- Discuss end-of-life issues (if appropriate for patient).

liver function tests or a sepsis-like picture secondary to translocation of colonic micro-organisms as a consequence of bowel wall edema and bowel ischemia. Patients may present with abdominal pain, mild diffuse abdominal tenderness (without rebound or rigidity), and occult blood in the stools with or without gram-negative bacteremia. This may be a terminal event in patients who have PAH and severe RHF. The appropriate therapy may include use of diuretics or IV fluids. Depending on the individual patient, low-dose dopamine or dobutamine (2–3 µg/kg/min) and inhaled NO (10–40 ppm) or inhaled prostacyclin (started at 50 ng/kg/min and titrated down to lowest effective dose) IV antibiotics covering colonic flora (ie, covering gram-negative and anaerobic bacteria) should be considered. There are no published data to define the optimal way to manage acutely decompensated patients who have severe PAH and acute RHF.

Diuretic dosing should be revised if patients develop orthostatic dizziness, which temporally correlates with decreased edema, decreased weight, and recently increased diuretic dose. Charting of daily weights, use of written sliding scale for diuretics, and potassium use, based on edema or weight, may be useful strategies. Many patients who have severe PAH and RHF have relatively low systemic blood pressure. Diuretics should be used with caution in these patients. Concern over low blood pressure and subsequent underdosing of diuretics actually may result in worsening of edema or overall clinical worsening, however [68].

Potassium supplementation should be managed carefully, especially if there is worsening or fluctuation of renal function, addition or withdrawal of potassium-sparing diuretics, or concurrent use of digoxin. Arrhythmias, prolonged palpitations, or syncopal episodes may be secondary to PAH and RHF; however, in patients on diuretics, electrolyte and digoxin level testing should be considered.

Edema is a relatively common side effect of many PAH therapies (eg, CCBs [2%–15%], bosentan [4% 8%], sitaxsentan [7%], and less commonly, prostacyclin). Adjusting the dose of diuretics often can ameliorate such edema. In some instances, however, this medication-related edema is refractory to diuretics. Patients may benefit from scheduled elevation of legs, compression stockings, or, if possible, switching from the suspected causative agent to other alternatives. In other instances in which the PAH therapy is otherwise believed to be effective, patients are asked to tolerate increased pedal edema.

Digoxin

Cardiac glycosides such as digoxin increase myocardial contractility by blocking sodium-potassium adenosine triphosphatase pump (Na^+-K^+ ATPase) [73], which is present in the cell membrane of myocardial cells. In patients who have PAH and RHF, a single intravenous administration of digoxin has been shown to increase cardiac output and decrease circulating norepinephrine levels in a small, short-term, uncontrolled study (Table 2) [23]. This study included 17 patients who received a single dose of 1 mg IV digoxin over a 30-minute infusion; hemodynamic measurements were made 2 hours after the infusion and were compared with baseline hemodynamic values. A prospective, randomized, double-blind, placebo-controlled study [74] of 15 patients who had COPD and RHF and no clinical LV failure found that 8 weeks administration of digoxin did not improve RV ejection fraction in any

Table 2
Clinical studies: pulmonary arterial hypertension and digoxin

Study [reference] (N)	Design method	Follow-up duration, site	Study findings	Comments
Mathur et al, 1981 [74] (15)	Prospective, randomized, placebo-controlled trial, single center Patients who have RV failure secondary to COPD and no known LV failure	8 wk, McMaster University in Canada	At baseline, RV ejection fraction was reduced (on equilibrium radionuclide angiography) in all patients and reduced LVEF was seen in 4 patients 8 wk digoxin use, all the abnormal LVEF were normal; however, Digoxin increased RVEF only in patients who had reduced LVEF at baseline	It is not clear whether the reduced LVEF at baseline actually represents LV disease or simply reflects severely dilated RV causing LV dysfunction or coexisting LV disease; conversely, normalization of LV systolic function by 8-wk digoxin therapy in all 4 patients with low baseline LVEF is unusual for LV systolic dysfunction NOTE: the trial involved COPD patients with RV failure and not WHO I PAH patients; hence the results should be extrapolated with caution
Rich et al, 1998 [23] (17)	Prospective, single-center study; patients' baseline was used as control Patients with PPH diagnosis by NIH registry criteria and normal LV function on echocardiogram	Short-term study involving hemodynamic measurements before and after single administration of digoxin 1 mg IV over 30 min, University of Illinois	Single administration of 1 mg IV digoxin was associated with significant increase in cardiac out put (3.49 ± 1.2 to 3.81 ± 1.2 L/min) measured 2 hours after the completion on digoxin infusion	No placebo control was used NOTE: the study was short-term and no definitive conclusion can be drawn regarding effect on cardiac output after long-term use NOTE: the trials in LV systolic dysfunction did not show any prolongation of survival with long-term digoxin use (subgroup analysis, however, did show reduced mortality and hospitalizations in patients with LVEF below 25%, NYHA class III or IV functional class, or patients with cardiomegaly on chest radiograph)

N = Number of subjects.

patient who did not have reduced left ventricular ejection fraction (LVEF) on baseline equilibrium radionuclide angiography (see Table 2) [23,74]. The safety, efficacy, and impact on morbidity or mortality with long-term use of digoxin in patients who have PAH and RVF are not known. It should be noted that in patients with systolic LV dysfunction and NYHA class II and III symptoms, treatment with digoxin for 2 to 5 years did not have any impact on mortality [75]; there was some beneficial effect on rate of congestive heart failure-related hospitalizations, however.

Currently, digoxin is used in patients who have PAH and signs of RHF and in patients who have atrial rhythm abnormalities (eg, multifocal atrial tachycardia, atrial flutter, or atrial fibrillation). Some experts advocate using digoxin with calcium channel antagonists to counteract negative ionotropic effects of CCBs. Because most patients who have PAH and RHF are on digoxin and diuretics, it is important to take extreme caution to monitor digoxin levels and promptly recognize toxicity, especially in association with electrolyte disturbances that result from the use of diuretics. Paroxysmal atrial tachycardia with variable atrioventricular block and bidirectional tachycardia are well-known arrhythmias associated with digoxin toxicity. The half-life of digoxin is prolonged with worsening of renal function. Digoxin is renally cleared and is used in most US centers, whereas digitoxin is hepatically cleared and is mostly used in European centers.

There are no specific recommendations regarding how to monitor digoxin therapy in patients who have PAH, so guidelines developed for monitoring of digoxin therapy in patients with LV failure are relied upon [68]. Digoxin therapy may be started at 0.125 to 0.25 mg orally daily; however, many centers only use low-dose (ie, 0.125 mg/d) therapy. In patients with normal renal function the digoxin levels may be first checked after 1 week. In patients above age 70 with impaired renal function or low body weight, a reduced starting dose [76] (0.125 mg every other day) is more appropriate. When digoxin is used for positive ionotropic effect, it is generally recommended to keep the digoxin trough level between 0.5 and 1.0 ng/mL [68]. At a plasma concentration above 1.0 ng/mL, the risk-adjusted mortality increases, as shown by the Digitalis Investigation Group Trial [77]. In the absence of hypokalemia, hypomagnesemia, or hypothyroidism, digitalis

toxicity is generally not seen below a plasma digoxin concentration of 2.0 ng/mL (although digoxin toxicity may rarely be seen at lower concentrations) [78,79]. Digoxin should not be used in cases of suspected coronary ischemia or in patients with recent acute coronary syndrome because of increased risk of death from arrhythmia or myocardial infarction [68,75,80,81]. Concurrent use of clarithromycin, amiodarone, itraconazole, cyclosporine, and many other drugs can increase digoxin levels and increase the potential for toxicity [82–84].

Anticoagulation

Currently no prospective, randomized, placebo-controlled trials are available to provide evidence for or against the use of anticoagulation in patients who have PAH. Currently, it is a widely accepted practice to use anticoagulation in patients who have PAH (WHO group I [35]) unless there is a contraindication.

Patients who have significant PAH may have a sedentary lifestyle. Venous engorgement and stasis (as a result of elevated right atrial pressures) and poor flow through pulmonary and systemic circulations as a consequence of low cardiac output place them at increased risk for developing venous thromboembolism. The pulmonary vascular bed is already significantly compromised in patients who have PAH by the time they become symptomatic and the diagnosis is made. As a consequence, even a relatively minor pulmonary embolic event has more significant hemodynamic and gas exchange consequences and may be life threatening.

Substantial evidence from human studies of biochemical and serologic markers suggests presence of a prothrombotic state in patients who have PAH. Three key elements that influence existence of a prothrombotic state are endothelial function, platelet activation, and plasma proteins related to coagulation and fibrinolysis. Certain components of these three elements have been shown to have aberrant behavior favoring a prothrombotic state in several human studies involving patients with idiopathic and associated forms of PAH (Table 4) [85–93]. The evidence of these prothrombotic abnormalities is more robust in IPAH and chronic thromboembolic pulmonary hypertension (CTE-PHT) than most other forms of PAH. Some of these abnormalities have been shown to reverse with specific PAH therapies, such as intravenous prostacyclin [94–97] or bosentan [98].

Table 3
Clinical studies: pulmonary arterial hypertension and calcium channel antagonists

Study [reference] (N)	Design method	Follow-up duration, site	Study findings	Comments
Rich et al, 1987 [34] (13)	Prospective, single center, uncontrolled PPH patients who were "responders" as defined by patients who had a fall in PAP and PVR by 20% after acute CCB challenge (8 out of 13 patients) and were treated with high-dose CCB in long-term NOTE: acute vasoreactivity testing with CCB has been abandoned secondary to the high frequency of untoward events such as profound hypotension. Currently the testing is performed with inhaled nitric oxide, IV adenosine, IV or inhaled prostacyclin	1 y, University of Illinois	At 1 y, 5 patients returned for follow-up; 4 of these 5 patients had sustained reduction in PVR and PAP and regression of RV hypertrophy by echocardiogram and electrocardiogram NOTE: In the study once the effective dose was determined, the drug was administered in divided doses (every 4–8 h) to achieve total desired daily dose. More frequent and small doses (every 4 h) were used in patients who did not tolerate higher, less frequent dosing (every 8 h). Some patients were started at low dose of CCB (nifedipine, 20 mg, tid or diltiazem, 60 mg, tid) as outpatients and the dose was slowly titrated to desired dose (as determined at the time of acute CCB testing) over 6 wk. Digoxin was also started in these patients to counteract negative ionotropic effects of CCB.	Nifedipine was used if heart rate was > 100/min, diltiazem was used if heart rate < 100/min, starting dose 20 mg or 60 mg, respectively. This was followed by repeated doses every 1 h (all patients had PA catheter in place) until 50% fall in PVR, 33% fall in mPAP, or an untoward side effect [eg, hypotension, dizziness, or worsening of hypoxemia]) Long-term dose of CCB: Up to 720 mg/d diltiazem or 240 mg/d nifedipine No patient was treated with anticoagulants The responders in this study had fall in PAP by 48% and in PVR by 60%, which is much more pronounced than most current criteria for defining a positive acute vasoreactivity test
Rich et al, 1992 [29] (64)	Prospective, single center, uncontrolled (historical control from NIH PPH registry) High-dose CCBs were used in patients who were "responders" (Note: Mean dose of nifedipine was 172 ± 41 mg/d, and of diltiazem was 720 ± 208 mg/d)	Up to 5 y, University of Illinois	Patients who were "responders" as defined by patients who had a fall in PAP and PVR by 20% after acute CCB challenge (26% of all patients) were treated with high-dose CCB. Treated patients had much better 5-y survival rate (94% in treated responders versus 55% in nonresponders) Survival of responders was much better than historical control from NIH PPH registry patients (in which vasoreactivity status was not known) at the same institution	This study also involved use of warfarin in all PPH patients with nonuniform perfusion on V/Q scan (55% of all) 47% of responders and 57% of nonresponders had nonuniform perfusion of V/Q scans The responders in this study had fall in PAP by 39% and in PVR index by 53%, which is much more pronounced than most current criteria for defining a positive acute vasoreactivity test

Source	Study type	Patients	Results	Definition of responders
Barst et al, 1999 [33] (77)	Retrospective, single center Review of medical records of pediatric patients with PPH (mean age 7 years) (range: 7 mo–13 y)	All patients from 1982–1987, Columbia University, New York Median follow-up: 47 mo (range: 24–166 mo)	Patients who were "responders" (31 responders out of 74 tested; ie, 42%) were treated with high-dose CCB. Survival of responders was better than nonresponders (1-, 3-, and 5-y survival rates were 97%, 97%, and 97%, respectively, in responders versus 66%, 52%, and 35%, respectively, in nonresponders). 6 nonresponders were also treated with CCB in this study	"Responders" were defined as patients who had a fall in PAP and PVR by 20%, no change or increase in cardiac index, no change or decrease in PVR/SVR ratio, after acute testing with prostacyclin Warfarin was started in all the patients in mid-1980s when the adult studies showed survival benefit
Sitbon et al, 2005 [32] (557)	Retrospective, single center Review of medical records of patients with IPAH	All IPAH patients from 1984–2001, Universite Paris-Sud, Clamart France Median follow-up: 30 ± 28 mo in nonresponders and 7 ± 4.1 y in responders	Only 6.8% of all IPAH patients undergoing acute vasoreactivity testing are long-term CCB responders, defined as patients who were in NYHA class I or II after 1 y of CCB monotherapy Predictors of long-term CCB response: On multivariate analysis: (although the numbers are too small to reach sufficient power): Higher baseline mixed venous oxyhemoglobin saturation (69 ± 8 versus 61 ± 8), and lower PVR absolute value reached after acute vasoreactivity testing (5.2 ± 2.7 versus 8.6 ± 3.3 wood units) On univariate analysis: baseline SVO_2 <65% (OR: 19.18), absolute value of PVR reached post- acute vasoreactivity testing of <6.7 wood units (OR: 7.35), post- acute vasoreactivity testing fall in mPAP fall of >31% (OR: 7.35), absolute value of post-acute vasoreactivity testing on mPAP of <37 mm Hg (OR: 6.13), baseline PVR of <11.5 wood units (OR: 4.24), post-acute vasoreactivity testing fall in PVR of >45% (OR: 3.27), baseline cardiac index of <2.5 L/min/m sq. (OR: 3.21), absence of class III or IV dyspnea at baseline (OR: 3.02)	"Responders" were defined as patients who had a fall in both PAP and PVR by 20%, after acute testing with IV prostacyclin (until 1994) on inhaled NO (after 1994); 70 of 557 (12.6%) were vasoreactive; 38 of 70 (ie, 6.8% of all 557) were long-term CCB responders The long-term CCB responders had less severe baseline PAH (PVR 10.3 ± 4.6 versus 14.9 ± 5.3 wood units, CO 5.0 ± 1.5 versus 3.9 ± 1.1 L/min). At acute testing they had more pronounced fall in mPAP (−39 ± 11 versus −26 ± 7 mm Hg) and their mPAP reached a lower absolute value (33 ± 8 versus 46 ± 10 mm Hg) compared with nonresponders

N = Number of subjects.

Table 4
Prothrombotic abnormalities in pulmonary arterial hypertension

	Abnormalities	Subjects	Reference
I	**Platelets aggregation related**		
	↑ Urinary thromboxane metabolite (11 dehydroxy TxB2)	IPAH	[115]
	↓ Urinary PGI2 metabolite (PGI-M)	IPAH	[115]
	↑ Thromboxane A2	IPAH	[115]
	↓ Prostacyclin	IPAH	[115]
	↓ Nitric oxide (exhaled or urinary excretion)	IPAH, APAH	[85]
	↑ Circulating platelet aggregates	APAH	[86]
	↑ Plasma serotonin, ↓ platelet serotonin	IPAH	[87,88]
	↑ Plasma-P selectin	IPAH	[94]
	↓ Thrombomodulin	IPAH	[89,94,99]
II	**Endothelial function related**		
	↓ Endothelial NO synthase	IPAH	[90]
	↓ Prostacyclin synthase expression	IPAH	[116]
	↓ Urinary PGI2 metabolite (PGI-M)	IPAH	[115]
	↑ Urinary thromboxane metabolite (11 dehydroxy TxB2)	IPAH	[115]
	↓ Thrombomodulin	IPAH	[89,94,99]
	↑ VWF	IPAH, APAH	[91,99]
	↑ Fibrinogen inhibitor plasminogen activator 1	IPAH	[92,99]
III	**Coagulation and fibrinolytic proteins related**		
	↑ Prevalence of antiphospholipid antibody/lupus anticoagulant	IPAH, CTE-PHT	[93]
	↑ vWF antigen level	IPAH	[91,99]
	↑ Fibrinogen inhibitor plasminogen activator 1	IPAH	[92,99]
	↑ Euglobulin lysis time	IPAH	[99]
	↑ Fibrinogen level	APAH	[99]

Theoretical concerns about importance of thromboembolism are supported by various early observations (Table 5) [24–26,99,100].

Retrospective [27,28,101] clinical studies and a small prospective [29], noncontrolled, nonrandomized clinical study of PPH patients has shown that use of anticoagulation with warfarin seems to confer a survival advantage in patients who have PPH (Table 6) [27–29,101–103]. In PAH, other than IPAH, the evidence—either basic science or clinical—for or against the use of anticoagulation is even scarcer (with the exception of CTE-PHT, in which the need for chronic anticoagulation is well established). Because there are many similarities in the clinical course, hemodynamics, and histopathology of these and IPAH patients, the practice of anticoagulation has been extended to other forms of PAH. It should be noted, however, that the risk of bleeding complication (Table 7) and need for anticoagulation (Box 2) may differ in other causes of APAH [104].

There are no data from human studies as to whether there is any difference in terms of efficacy among various anticoagulation agents such as warfarin, unfractionated heparin, or low molecular weight heparins. Warfarin is the most commonly used agent for anticoagulation in patients who have PAH. Substantial data from animal studies suggest that heparin may have some additional therapeutic advantage in subjects with PAH. Human studies, however, have not been performed to support this theoretical superiority. Heparin has been shown to prevent development of PAH and RV hypertrophy in animal models (hypoxic mice or guinea pig model of PAH) [105,106]. The mechanism of action of heparin on pulmonary vasculature is not completely understood. Proposed mechanisms include inhibition of platelet-derived growth factor [105] and inhibition of pulmonary artery smooth muscle cell growth, probably by upregulation of expression of cell cycle regulation of gene p27, which influences the level of cyclin-dependent kinase inhibitor [107]. Cyclin-dependent kinase and cyclin-dependent kinase inhibitor play key roles in the balance between cell proliferation and cell quiescence. Research also has shown in animal models that anticoagulation with warfarin does not have the same effect as that of heparin to protect animals from developing PAH upon prolonged exposure to hypoxia [108]. O-hexanoyl low-molecular-weight heparin derivatives have been shown to be more effective in growth inhibition of bovine pulmonary artery smooth muscle cells in culture than heparin [109]. Because of such observations, the authors concluded that heparin derivatives may be envisioned as potential future PAH therapy. Currently, there are no human clinical data to support the use of heparin or heparin derivatives instead of warfarin in patients who have PAH.

In clinical practices, warfarin has been the agent most frequently used. Target international normalized ratio (INR) in most US centers is between 1.5 and 2.5 and in many European centers it is 2.0 to 3.0. Both approaches are based on expert opinions, weighing potential benefits of therapy versus risk of bleeding complications with higher target INR [110]. It may be appropriate to keep INR > 2.0 in the following situations:

1. In any patient in whom there exists a clinical indication for anticoagulation (eg, atrial fibrillation, CTE-PHT, acute recent venous thromboembolism, or prosthetic valve)
2. In patients with remote history of idiopathic venous thromboembolism
3. In patients in whom ventilation-perfusion (V/Q) scans or PA angiograms are not consistent with chronic pulmonary thromboembolic disease (CPTED) but who have at least one subsegmental mismatched defect or diffusely decreased tracer uptake in certain subsegments or in whom PA angiograms are unequivocal for the absence of CPTED
4. In patients with history of ischemic stroke or transient ischemic attack with known right-to-left shunt

The role of antiplatelet agents such as aspirin and clopidogrel has not been thoroughly evaluated. A recent preliminary randomized, double-blind, placebo-controlled, crossover study of 19 patients who have IPAH explored the biochemical effects of clopidogrel and aspirin on inhibition of platelet aggregation eicosanoid metabolism [111]. The study represents the first well-structured, placebo-controlled trial to evaluate biochemical effects of antiplatelet agents in patients who have IPAH. The study showed that both drugs inhibit platelet aggregation in patients who have IPAH. Arachidonic acid–induced platelet inhibition was more completely blocked by aspirin, whereas ADP-induced platelet aggregation was more effectively blocked by clopidogrel. Only aspirin inhibited thromboxane metabolite production without affecting prostaglandin I2 metabolite synthesis, thus restoring normal eicosanoid balance.

Empiric anticoagulation may be considered if clinical suspicion of PAH is moderate to high and an echocardiogram shows an estimated pulmonary artery pressure >60 while the patient is undergoing evaluation [112]. When an interruption in anticoagulation therapy is required, such as before a surgical procedure, in the absence of any other indication for anticoagulation warfarin may be stopped 5 to 7 days before the procedure and restarted after the procedure when the increased risk of bleeding has resolved, without any overlap with intravenous heparin or subcutaneous low molecular weight heparin. When the INR is <1.5, appropriate deep venous thrombosis prophylaxis should be instituted when patients are hospitalized or as appropriate for the patient's clinical status [113].

Calcium channel blockers

The hallmark of PAH is increased PVR, which compromises the ability of the right ventricle to maintain cardiac output [3]. Increased RV stroke work (volume of blood pumped × pressure against which the volume is pumped) against the abnormally increased PVR has been thought to be the cause of RV hypertrophy and dilatation and, eventually, failure to pump effectively

---

Box 2. Pulmonary arterial hypertension–associated conditions in which anticoagulation management is dictated by principals of the associated disease

CTE-PHT (also consider inferior vena-caval [IVC] filter)
Mitral or other valve prosthesis
High-risk atrial fibrillation
Osler-Weber Rendu syndrome and similar diseases with history of ischemic strokes or transient ischemic attacks
Lupus anticoagulant syndrome or other procoagulant states

Table 5
Observations suggesting role of thrombosis in patients who have idiopathic pulmonary arterial hypertension

Study [reference] (N)	Design method	Study findings	Comments
Wagenvoort, 1980 [24] (72)	Retrospective Review of lung biopsy specimens from patients with pulmonary vascular disease	12/40 (30%) patients with unexplained PAH had evidence of CPTED (ie, severe eccentric intimal fibrosis) in the absence of concentric lesions	The criteria for calling a biopsy consistent with CPTED may or may not correctly identify CPTED cases It is not clear whether all of these patients were evaluated by V/Q scan or pulmonary artery angiogram before the biopsy
Bjornsson et al, 1985 [25] (85)	Retrospective Review of lung biopsy specimens from patients with clinical diagnosis of PPH from 1930–1983 at Mayo Clinic	56% of the patients had biopsies consistent with thromboembolic disease	Mean age for primary pulmonary arteritis on biopsy was 16 years and 21–34 years for plexogenic pulmonary arteriopathy, primary medial arteriopathy, and pulmonary veno-occlusive disease versus 41 years for patients with thromboembolic disease Biopsy specimens were taken from tissue registry (73 autopsies, 6 open lung biopsies, 1 both)
Loyd et al, 1988 [100] (Familial PAH: 23)	Retrospective Review of histopathology of postmortem lung sections 23 members of 13 families with familial PAH; pathologists were blinded to patient and family identity; every artery and abnormal vein was categorized by adopted WHO classification that was used in pathology core NIH PPH registry 2516 vessels (28–264 with mean of 109 ± 62 SD per patient) were described Quantitative description was reported	18/23 (78%) patients from 12/13 (92%) families had vessels with organized thrombi 18/23 (78%) patients from 12/13 (92%) families had plexiform lesions 2.7% of all arteries had organized thrombi 3.4 of all arteries had plexiform lesions 15/23 (65%) patients had coexisting plexiform and thrombotic lesions There was no correlation between type of lesion or percent of arteries with plexiform lesions between age of patient or survival in this study	The study represents one of the most insightful reviews of pathologic changes in PAH Authors concluded that coexistence of thrombotic and plexiform lesions within the same family and individual represents that these lesions are not specific but they represent different manifestations of the same initial pathologic process These lesions are probably two different outcomes of a single starting pathologic process in a disease caused by autosomal dominant inheritance pattern The differentiation of these lesions may depend on the anatomic location of the lesion, other factors in the local lung environment, or a random phenomenon

| Pietra et al, 1989 [26] (58) | Retrospective (although patients were identified prospectively) Review of histopathology of lung biopsy, pneumonectomy, or autopsy specimens from PPH patients in NIH/NHLBI registry of PPH patients | 19/48 (40%) patients who had luminal or intimal lesions had thrombotic lesions as defined by both recanalized thrombi and eccentric intimal fibrosis without plexiform lesions 9/25 (36%) patients with plexiform lesions also had recanalized thrombi | Prognosis of patients with thrombotic lesions was much better than for patients with plexiform lesions or veno-occlusive disease NOTE: the NIH registry only included patients with low probability V/Q scans or normal pulmonary artery angiogram; all patients were required to have V/Q scan or pulmonary angiogram |
| Welsh et al, 1996 [99] (PPH: 12, SPH: 25, Control: 15) | Cross-sectional Plasma samples of PPH, SPH, and age-matched controls were collected and multiple coagulation related parameters were studied | Compared with the control group: *In PPH patients:* • Thrombomodulin levels were decreased • Fibrinolytic inhibitor plasminogen activator-I was increased • Euglobulin lysis time was increased *In SPH patients:* • Von Willebrand factor was increased • Fibrinogen level was increased | Lower fibrinolytic activity correlated with higher mean pulmonary artery pressures Whether decreased fibrinolytic activity is an effect of or cause of elevated mean pulmonary artery pressure is not clear |

N = Number of subjects.

(maintain cardiac output) against increasing resistance. The idea of attempting to decrease PVR in PAH by vasodilation has always been tempting [114]. Multiple basic science experiments and clinical studies suggest that in animal models of PAH and in patients who have PAH, the mediators of pulmonary vasodilation are decreased, whereas the mediators of vasoconstriction are overexpressed [115–117]. Clinical studies indicated that the ability to successfully produce vasodilation by certain agents with known vasodilator properties (eg, CCBs [118], IV prostacyclin [119,120], inhaled NO [121–124], IV adenosine [125], or inhaled iloprost [126]) in patients with PPH identifies the patients who have much better prognosis [29,32–34,127], particularly if they are treated with high-dose CCBs (Table 3) [29,32–34]. Such testing (known as acute vasoreactivity testing [Table 8]) became a routine for almost all patients who have PAH and are undergoing initial diagnostic right heart catheterization, except patients with low cardiac output or concurrent left heart failure, as indicated by elevated pulmonary capillary wedge pressure. Patients who have significant (see Table 6) pulmonary vasodilation without a significant systemic vasodilation (as assessed by change in PVR/SVR ratio or clinically unacceptable fall in systemic blood pressure) in acute vasoreactivity testing are called "responders" and are candidates for long-term CCB therapy. The current definition of a responder is a decrease in mean pulmonary arterial pressure of >10 mm Hg to a mean pulmonary artery pressure of ≤40 mm Hg with a maintained (or increased) cardiac output. "Responders" comprise 10% to 26% of IPAH patients undergoing such testing; unfortunately, the proportion of patients who are responders among APAH (eg, scleroderma or CTE-PHT) is even lower [128]. The role of acute vasoreactivity testing and the use of CCBs in patients who have APAH who demonstrate acute vasodilation are not known.

There are reports of patients who have IPAH and who were initially nonresponders to acute vasoreactivity testing, transforming to responders at repeat right heart catheterization after prolonged use of IV prostacyclin [129]. No data are available to define the safety or role of CCBs in such patients. A recent report suggests that only a small minority (6.8%) of all patients who have PAH can be managed by CCBs in the long-term without need for additional specific PAH therapy, because as many as half of the patients on CCBs deteriorate in the subsequent years [32]. Because

Table 6
Clinical studies: anticoagulation and pulmonary arterial hypertension

Study [reference] (N)	Design method	Follow-up duration, site	Study findings	Comments
Fuster et al, 1984 [27] (120)	Retrospective, single center Review of medical records of patients with PPH diagnosis by clinical and hemodynamic criteria	PPH patients from 1955–1977 who were followed up until 1983 at Mayo Clinic, with minimum follow-up of 5 y (median 14 y, longest 27 y) or up to death	Of 56 patients who underwent autopsy, 57% patients had changes consistent with only thromboembolic PH in the absence of plexogenic pulmonary arteriopathy Patients who were treated with anticoagulation as defined by initiation within 1 y of diagnosis had significantly better 3-y survival (49% versus 21%) compared with those who were not anticoagulated	Improved survival on anticoagulation was noted in thromboembolic and plexogenic arteriopathy, but numbers were too small to reach statistical significance (to ascertain statistical power) The criteria for deciding not to anticoagulate are not clear and might have introduced a selection bias
Rich et al, 1992 [29] (64)	Prospective, uncontrolled, single center (historical control from NIH PPH registry) Warfarin was given to all PPH patients with nonuniform perfusion on V/Q scan (55% of all)	Up to 5 y, University of Illinois	Warfarin use was associated with improved survival, particularly in patients who were nonresponders to high-dose CCB (1-y survival: 91% versus 62%, 3-y survival: 47% versus 31%) when compared with historical control from NIH PPH registry	This study also involved use of high-dose CCB in patients who were "responders" as defined by patients who had a fall in PAP and PVR by 20% after acute CCB challenge 47% of responders and 57% of nonresponders had nonuniform perfusion of V/Q scans Patients with high probability V/Q scans were excluded from the study
Frank et al, 1997 [101] (173)	Retrospective, two centers were involved Review of medical records of patients with PPH (total 64, 24 received warfarin) and anorectic drug-induced PAH (total 104, 56 received warfarin)	Approximately up to 10 y, University of Vienna and University of Bern	Anticoagulated aminorex-treated patient had better mean survival compared with nonanticoagulated aminorex-treated patients (8.3 versus 6.1 y) Aminorex PHT patients who started receiving anticoagulation therapy sooner had better mean survival compared with patients who stated treatment 2 y after diagnosis (10.9 versus 5.9 y) Overall, patients treated with aminorex had better mean survival compared with PPH patients (7.5 versus 3.9 y)	Contrary to most studies cited in this table, this study showed no difference in survival in first 5 y of follow-up of anticoagulated and nonanticoagulated PPH patients. In the following 5 y, some survival advantage was noted in anticoagulated PPH group that did not reach statistical significance. NOTE: the study included only 24 PPH patients who received anticoagulation

| Kawut et al, 2005 [28] (84) | Retrospective, single center Review of medical records of patients with IPAH (66), familial PAH (14), anorexogen-related PAH (4) | All consecutive adult patients with initial evaluation between 1994 and 2002, Columbia University, New York (median follow-up, 764 d) | Among the patients treated with anticoagulation (94% of all), transplant-free survival was improved (hazard ratio: 0.35, 95% CI: 0.12–0.90, $P = .05$). | 1-, 3-, and 5-y transplant-free survival rates were 87%, 75%, and 61%, respectively, for the whole cohort The criteria for deciding not to anticoagulate are not clear and might have introduced a selection bias[a] |

N = Number of subjects.

[a] Note: There are other less structured retrospective studies or case series, some of which favor anticoagulation [102,127] and others [103] that reported no difference in survival among anticoagulated and non-anticoagulated patients who have PAH.

of such reports and the availability of newer safe and effective oral and inhaled (rather than parenteral) PAH therapies, the enthusiasm to support the necessity of acute vasoreactivity testing as an essential part of PAH evaluation has somewhat decreased. Currently, however, acute vasoreactivity testing continues to be part of the algorithm for the evaluation of patients who have PAH (particularly IPAH). The predictors of long-term response to CCBs without the need for additional agent are listed in Table 3 [32].

It should be noted that 80% to 90% of all patients who have IPAH and a greater percentage of patients who have APAH are nonresponders at acute vasoreactivity testing, and these patients are treated with specific PAH therapies (eg, prostacyclin analogs, endothelial receptor antagonists, or 5-phosphodiestrase inhibitors). Importantly, the lack of response to acute vasoreactivity testing (ie, the administration of inhaled or IV prostacyclin, NO, or adenosine) does not rule out the likelihood of improvement with long-term use of prostacyclins or other specific PAH therapies [4–21].

The primary purpose of acute vasoreactivity testing is to determine whether CCBs could be used as PAH therapy. The CCBs are not used in patients who have significant acute RHF because of cardiodepressor effects. There is no role of acute vasoreactivity testing in patients who have PAH who are hospitalized with acute worsening of RHF. Similarly, if at the time of right heart catheterization (RHC) the cardiac output is determined to be low (CI <2.0) acute vasoreactivity should not be performed because it will have no impact on the treatment and it may be associated with an undesirable fall in systemic blood pressure or cardiac output. In any patient, acute vasoreactivity testing may precipitate acute pulmonary edema and marked worsening of hypoxemia [130]. It should be done with caution in patients who have a pulmonary capillary wedge pressure of ≥ 15 cm H_2O. In the event of any sudden worsening in oxyhemoglobin saturation during acute vasoreactivity testing, acute pulmonary edema should be considered. The vasodilator agent should be discontinued and treatment with intravenous morphine, intravenous nitroglycerine, and furosemide may be considered [130]. It should be noted that acute severe pulmonary edema during acute vasoreactivity testing is not a contraindication to the use of pulmonary vasodilator agents, such as intravenous prostacyclin. This should be done with extreme caution, and dose escalation should be done slowly [130]. Some authorities favor testing

Table 7
Associated pulmonary arterial hypertensive conditions and clinical circumstances with increased rate of complications from anticoagulation

Diseases/circumstances	Caution	Management comments
Congenital heart disease	Massive hemoptysis is cause of death in many patients	Extreme caution; discontinue anticoagulation if more than minimal hemoptysis
Scleroderma	Risk of gastrointestinal bleed secondary to telangiectesias	Extreme caution; monitor for hypochromic microcytic anemia, occult blood, or malena; discontinue anticoagulation if significant gastrointestinal bleed; consider restarting anticoagulation after a few months if bleed was minor and endoscopic findings are not alarming
Portopulmonary hypertension	Many patients have coagulopathy and/or thrombocytopenia; many have varices	Extreme caution; do not anticoagulate patients with significant varices, history of significant variceal bleed, or moderate to severe coagulopathy (INR > 1.4) or thrombocytopenia (platelet count <40, 000/mL); drug interactions may be more pronounced
HIV	Many patients have thrombocytopenia; many have concurrent advanced liver disease; HAART therapy may have drug interaction	Similar cautions apply as in portopulmonary hypertension
Bosentan therapy	Increases warfarin dose requirement	Increase warfarin dose by 30%–40%; recheck INR in 7–10 days and monitor INR more frequently until INR becomes stable, only at the initiation or termination of Bosentan therapy
Sitaxsentan therapy	Decreases warfarin dose requirement	Decrease warfarin dose by 80%, recheck INR in 7–10 days, and monitor INR more frequently until INR becomes stable, only at the initiation or termination of Sitaxsentan therapy
Intravenous prostacyclin or treprostinil	Risk of central venous catheter–related clot and risk of clogging of the catheter lumen secondary to low flow rate of infusion	It is generally recommended that all patients receiving PAH therapies via central venous catheter should be anticoagulated. NOTE: prostacyclins also have antiplatelet aggregation properties, and direct evidence to support such recommendation is lacking
Severe RHF	Passive hepatic congestion may cause coagulopathy or ischemic bowl	Check INR and hemoglobin more frequently, hold anticoagulation if necessary; patient may become bactremic secondary to ischemic colonic ulcerations (as many terminal patients with severe RHF do); consider broad-spectrum antibiotics covering enteric gram-negative rods and anaerobes
Syncope	Syncopal and presyncopal episodes are common in patients who have severe PAH	Anticoagulation should be continued at any cost in patients with CTE-PHT or in whom PE is suspected cause of an isolated syncope; in all other patients, risks and benefits should be carefully weighed; advising patients to pace themselves may be the initial advice

Pregnancy	Warfarin is teratogenic and is contraindicated (Class D) in pregnancy	Pregnancy carries a high risk of mortality (30%–50%) in patients with moderate to severe PAH; all female PAH patients of reproductive potential should be advised to observe strict contraception; termination of pregnancy should be strongly advised in patients who do become pregnant; if, however, a patient does insist on continuing pregnancy, LMWH should be used
Acute illness, antibiotic use, sepsis	Relative vitamin K deficiency related to antibiotic use or poor oral intake may prolong INR; sepsis may cause coagulopathy and/or thrombocytopenia	Consider transiently holding anticoagulation while using systemic compression devices (SCDs) for deep venous thrombosis prophylaxis; consider oral or subcutaneous vitamin K supplementation

with IV nitroprusside [131] in patients with high pulmonary capillary wedge pressure. A fall in systemic arterial blood pressure with IV nitroprusside causing increase in cardiac output and drop in pulmonary capillary wedge pressure highly suggests the possibility of concurrent LV diastolic dysfunction. Similarly, in patients with pulmonary veno-occlusive disease, the acute vasoreactivity testing may result in massive pulmonary edema, which may even be fatal. Death has been reported in a patient with pulmonary veno-occlusive disease as a result of administration of IV prostacyclin [132] at 2 ng/kg/min for only 5 minutes.

Inhaled NO, inhaled prostacyclin, IV prostacyclin, or IV adenosine may be used for acute testing [35–37]. These agents are short acting, easily administered and titrated, have minimal systemic effects at doses that can result in pulmonary arterial vasodilation, and demonstrate rapid reversal of effects if complications ensue. The CCBs should not be used for this testing because they are longer acting and their use may be associated with complications such as systemic hypotension and worsening of hypoxemia. These reactions to CCBs were primarily seen in patients who were actually nonresponders. Because of little likelihood of benefit and a risk of side effects and complications, empiric use of CCBs in all patients who have PAH without knowing acute vasoreactivity status is not indicated, is dangerous, and may be fatal.

In only a small subset (10%–26%) of patients who are responders and have no specific contraindication to CCBs, these agents may be started as an inpatient treatment with PA catheter in place (acute CCB dose escalation) or by slowly increasing the dose on an outpatient basis (see Table 8). The choice of agent depends on the resting heart rate of the patient [29,32–34]. If the patient's heart rate is > 100 beats/min, diltiazem is used; if the heart rate is < 100 beats/min, nifedipine is used. Verapamil is generally not used because of its strong cardiodepressor properties. Amlodipine is another choice, especially for patients who cannot tolerate the other CCBs secondary to side effects, such as worsening of peripheral edema, systemic hypotension, or abnormally low or high heart rate.

Summary

After half a century of clinical experience and research, PAH management remains a challenge. Currently, data to support the use of standard PAH therapies (eg, oxygen supplementation, diuretics, digoxin, anticoagulation, and CCBs) are

Table 8
Use of calcium channel blockers in pulmonary arterial hypertension

Indications
- PAH patients with WHO group I and
- PAH diagnosis confirmed on right heart catheterization (ie, PVR above 3.0 wood units by Fick's method) and
- "Responder" on "acute vasoreactivity testing"

Contraindications
- Low cardiac output, cardiac index <2.0
- Severe RHF
- Hypotension, systolic BP below 90 mm Hg
- History of adverse reaction or intolerance to CCB

Cautions
- Empiric trial of CCB without acute vasoreactivity testing should not be performed. It is unsafe and may cause hypotension [125] and even death [124]
- Acute vasoreactivity testing should not be performed with CCB because it is unsafe and may cause profound hypotension, acute pulmonary edema, and potentially death
- Patients who are acutely decompensated with RHF are not candidates for CCB therapy. There is no real reason to perform acute vasoreactivity testing in such patients

Acute vasoreactivity testing
A. Agents used [121–127]
- Inhaled NO: 20 ppm for 6–10 minute by face mask
- IV prostacyclin: Start 1 ng/kg/min; increase by 1–2 ng/kg/min every 5–15 min to maximum of 12 ng/kg/min or untolerable side effects or 2.5 ng/kg/min, increase by 2.5 ng/kg/min every 10 min to maximum of 12 ng/kg/min; mean tolerated dose: 8 ng/kg/min
- Inhaled prostacyclin:50 ng/kg/min via nebulizer for 15 min
- IV adenosine: fast IV bolus 50 mg/kg/min; increase by 50 mg/kg/min every 2 min to maximum of 500 mg/kg/min

B. Criteria for significant response ("acute responder")
- Drop in mPAP >10 mm Hg or Attaining an mPAP <40 mm Hg or Decrease in PVR by ≥20% or Attaining a PVR <8 wood units
- and Increase or no decrease in cardiac output
- and No or only clinically acceptable fall in systemic blood pressure
- NOTE: there are no universally accepted criteria [35–37]

Practical use of CCBs
Choice and dose of calcium channel blockers
- Chose nifedipine if baseline resting heart rate <100/min and diltiazem if >100/min
- Amlodipine may be used if significant side effects from other agents (eg, worsening edema, significant tachycardia, bradycardia, or hypotension)
- Verapamil should not be used secondary to strong cardiodepressor effects
- Generally high doses are required (eg, nifedipine up to 240 mg/d and diltiazem 720 mg/d, both in three divided doses, amlodipine up to 5 mg twice a day
- Only oral administration is used

Initiation of CCB
CCB may be started in either inpatient setting or outpatient setting (there are no rigid recommendations, and approaches may vary among different centers)
A. Inpatient setting: rapid CCB dose escalation
- All rapid CCB dose escalations are generally performed with PA catheter in place
- Patients receive initial dose of nifedipine 10–20 mg orally or diltiazem 60 mg orally; hemodynamic measurements are obtained in 1 h
- The dose and hemodynamic measurements are repeated every hour until a "threshold" response (fall in PVR by 50% and, not or, fall in mPAP by 33%) is achieved or significant side effects are experienced (eg, hypotension [mBP <90 mm Hg], gastrointestinal upset [nausea, vomiting])
- Total daily dose is calculated by adding up total amount of drug administered during this testing. The goal is to achieve this in three divided doses (four to six divided doses if significant side effects)
- Patient is then given nifedipine 20 mg orally three times daily or diltiazem 60 mg orally three times daily next day and is discharged
- The dose is then gradually increased to the desired level (as estimated previously) over a period of 6–12 wk while frequently monitoring BP and heart rate

B. Outpatient setting: slow CCB dose escalation
- Patients are started on initial dose of nifedipine 10–20 mg orally three times daily or diltiazem 60 mg orally three times daily
- The dose is then gradually increased with a goal to ultimately achieve the maximum dose (nifedipine 240 mg/d or diltiazem 720 mg/d, both in three divided doses; amlodipine up to 5 mg twice daily) over a period of 6–12 wk, while frequently monitoring the BP and heart rate. If patient experiences limiting side effects (as mentioned previously) before the maximum dose is reached, either the dose is kept at that level or further increase is achieved by increasing the dose frequency to every 4–6 h

Follow-up, when to use additional therapies
- Only 6.8% of all patients who have PAH are long-term responders to CCB (ie, who will be in NYHA I or II on monotherapy with CCB for 1 y) [32]
- Approximately half of the patients who are responders at initial acute vasoreactivity testing and are placed on CCB require an additional PAH therapy within 1 y
- Secondary to this risk of failure of CCB monotherapy, such patients should be closely followed (every 3–6 mo) and should be started on an additional therapy if there is clinical worsening or worsening of 6-minute walking distance.
- Secondary to this risk of failure of CCB monotherapy, some experts consider adding a specific PAH agent at the beginning, especially in patients who have poor predictors of long-term response at baseline hemodynamics and vasoreactivity testing [32]

mostly retrospective, uncontrolled prospective, or derived from other diseases with similar but not identical manifestations. In the absence of any further prospective, controlled studies, it is reasonable to use these therapies when they are tolerated. When these therapies are poorly tolerated, however, the threshold for discontinuation should be low.

References

[1] Romberg E. Über sklerose der lungen arterie. Dtsch Arch Klin Med 1891;48:197–206 [in German].

[2] Dresdale DT, Schultz M, Michtom RJ. Primary pulmonary hypertension. I: clinical and hemodynamic study. Am J Med 1951;11(6):686–705.

[3] Rich S, Dantzker DR, Ayres SM, et al. Primary pulmonary hypertension: a national prospective study. Ann Intern Med 1987;107(2):216–23.

[4] Rubin LJ, Mendoza J, Hood M, et al. Treatment of primary pulmonary hypertension with continuous intravenous prostacyclin (epoprostenol): results of a randomized trial. Ann Intern Med 1990;112(7): 485–91.

[5] Barst RJ, Rubin LJ, McGoon MD, et al. Survival in primary pulmonary hypertension with long-term continuous intravenous prostacyclin. Ann Intern Med 1994;121(6):409–15.

[6] Barst R, Rubin LJ, Long WA, et al. A comparison of continuous intravenous epoprostenol (prostacyclin) with conventional therapy for primary pulmonary hypertension: the Primary Pulmonary Hypertension Study Group. N Engl J Med 1996; 334(5):296–302.

[7] Rich S, McLaughlin VV. The effects of chronic prostacyclin therapy on cardiac output and symptoms in primary pulmonary hypertension. J Am Coll Cardiol 1999;34(4):1184–7.

[8] Badesch DB, Tapson VF, McGoon MD, et al. Continuous intravenous epoprostenol for pulmonary hypertension due to the scleroderma spectrum of disease: a randomized, controlled trial. Ann Intern Med 2000;132(6):425–34.

[9] Hoeper MM, Schwarze M, Ehlerding S, et al. Long-term treatment of primary pulmonary hypertension with aerosolized iloprost, a prostacyclin analogue. N Engl J Med 2000;342(25):1866–70.

[10] Channick RN, Simonneau G, Sitbon O, et al. Effects of the dual endothelin-receptor antagonist bosentan in patients with pulmonary hypertension: a randomised placebo-controlled study. Lancet 2001;358(9288):1119–23.

[11] Rubin LJ, Badesch DB, Barst RJ, et al. Bosentan therapy for pulmonary arterial hypertension. N Engl J Med 2002;346(12):896–903.

[12] Simonneau G, Barst RJ, Galie N, et al. Continuous subcutaneous infusion of treprostinil, a prostacyclin analogue, in patients with pulmonary arterial hypertension: a double-blind, randomized, placebo-controlled trial. Am J Respir Crit Care Med 2002;165(6):800–4.

[13] Sitbon O, Humbert M, Nunes H, et al. Long-term intravenous epoprostenol infusion in primary pulmonary hypertension: prognostic factors and survival. J Am Coll Cardiol 2002;40(4):780–8.

[14] McLaughlin VV, Shillington A, Rich S. Survival in primary pulmonary hypertension: the impact of epoprostenol therapy. Circulation 2002;106(12): 1477–82.

[15] Ghofrani HA, Wiedemann R, Rose F, et al. Combination therapy with oral sildenafil and inhaled iloprost for severe pulmonary hypertension. Ann Intern Med 2002;136(7):515–22.

[16] Sitbon O, Gressin V, Speich R, et al. Bosentan for the treatment of human immunodeficiency virus-associated pulmonary arterial hypertension. Am J Respir Crit Care Med 2004;170(11):1212–7.

[17] Mikhail GW, Prasad SK, Li W, et al. Clinical and haemodynamic effects of sildenafil in pulmonary hypertension: acute and mid-term effects. Eur Heart J 2004;25(5):431–6.

[18] Wilkins MR, Paul GA, Strange JW, et al. Sildenafil versus Endothelin Receptor Antagonist for Pulmonary Hypertension (SERAPH) study. Am J Respir Crit Care Med 2005;171(11):1292–7.

[19] McLaughlin VV, Sitbon O, Badesch DB, et al. Survival with first-line bosentan in patients with primary pulmonary hypertension. Eur Respir J 2005; 25(2):244–9.

[20] Galie N, Ghofrani HA, Torbicki A, et al. Sildenafil citrate therapy for pulmonary arterial hypertension. N Engl J Med 2005;353(20):2148–57.

[21] Barst RJ, Langleben D, Badesch D, et al. Treatment of pulmonary arterial hypertension with the selective endothelin-A receptor antagonist sitaxsentan. J Am Coll Cardiol 2006;47(10):2049–56.

[22] Naeije R, Vachiery JL. Medical therapy of pulmonary hypertension: conventional therapies. Clin Chest Med 2001;22(3):517–27.

[23] Rich S, Seidlitz M, Dodin E, et al. The short-term effects of digoxin in patients with right ventricular dysfunction from pulmonary hypertension. Chest 1998;114(3):787–92.

[24] Wagenvoort CA. Lung biopsy specimens in the evaluation of pulmonary vascular disease. Chest 1980;77(5):614–25.

[25] Bjornsson J, Edwards WD. Primary pulmonary hypertension: a histopathologic study of 80 cases. Mayo Clin Proc 1985;60(1):16–25.

[26] Pietra GG, Edwards WD, Kay JM, et al. Histopathology of primary pulmonary hypertension: a qualitative and quantitative study of pulmonary blood vessels from 58 patients in the National Heart, Lung, and Blood Institute, Primary Pulmonary Hypertension Registry. Circulation 1989; 80(5):1198–206.

[27] Fuster V, Steele PM, Edwards WD, et al. Primary pulmonary hypertension: natural history and the importance of thrombosis. Circulation 1984;70(4): 580–7.

[28] Kawut SM, Horn EM, Berekashvili KK, et al. New predictors of outcome in idiopathic pulmonary arterial hypertension. Am J Cardiol 2005;95(2): 199–203.

[29] Rich S, Kaufmann E, Levy PS. The effect of high doses of calcium-channel blockers on survival in primary pulmonary hypertension. N Engl J Med 1992;327(2):76–81.

[30] Johnson SR, Granton JT, Mehta S. Thrombotic arteriopathy and anticoagulation in pulmonary hypertension. Chest 2006;130(2):545–52.

[31] Sandoval J, Aguirre JS, Pulido T, et al. Nocturnal oxygen therapy in patients with the Eisenmenger syndrome. Am J Respir Crit Care Med 2001; 164(9):1682–7.

[32] Sitbon O, Humbert M, Jais X, et al. Long-term response to calcium channel blockers in idiopathic pulmonary arterial hypertension. Circulation 2005;111(23):3105–11.

[33] Barst RJ, Maislin G, Fishman AP. Vasodilator therapy for primary pulmonary hypertension in children. Circulation 1999;99(9):1197–208.

[34] Rich S, Brundage BH. High-dose calcium channel-blocking therapy for primary pulmonary hypertension: evidence for long-term reduction in pulmonary arterial pressure and regression of right ventricular hypertrophy. Circulation 1987;76(1): 135–41.

[35] Badesch DB, Abman SH, Ahearn GS, et al. Medical therapy for pulmonary arterial hypertension: ACCP evidence-based clinical practice guidelines. Chest 2004;126(1 Suppl):35S–62S.

[36] Galie N, Torbicki A, Barst R, et al. Guidelines on diagnosis and treatment of pulmonary arterial hypertension: the task force on diagnosis and treatment of pulmonary arterial hypertension of the European Society of Cardiology. Eur Heart J 2004;25(24):2243–78.

[37] British Cardiac Society Guidelines and Medical Practice Committee, Gibbs JS, Higenbottam TW. Recommendations on the management of pulmonary hypertension in clinical practice. Heart 2001; 86(Suppl 1):11–3.

[38] Weissmann N, Hassell KL, Badesch DB, et al. Hypoxic vasoconstriction in intact lungs: a role for NADPH oxidase-derived H(2)O(2)? Am J Physiol Lung Cell Mol Physiol 2000;279(4): L683–90.

[39] Nocturnal Oxygen Therapy Trial Group. Continuous or nocturnal oxygen therapy in hypoxemic chronic obstructive lung disease: a clinical trial. Nocturnal Oxygen Therapy Trial Group. Ann Intern Med 1980;93(3):391–8.

[40] Long term domiciliary oxygen therapy in chronic hypoxic cor pulmonale complicating chronic bronchitis and emphysema: report of the Medical Research Council Working Party. Lancet 1981; 1(8222):681–6.

[41] Global strategy for the diagnosis, management and prevention of chronic obstructive pulmonary disease: NHLBI/WHO workshop report. In: Global initiative for chronic obstructive pulmonary lung disease. Bethesda (MD): National Heart, Lung and Blood Institute; 2005 Available at: http://www.goldcopd.com/Guidelineitem.asp?l1=2&l2=1&intId=989. Accessed January 25, 2007.

[42] Owens GR, Rogers RM, Pennock BE, et al. The diffusing capacity as a predictor of arterial oxygen desaturation during exercise in patients with chronic obstructive pulmonary disease. N Engl J Med 1984;310(19):1218–21.

[43] Kelley MA, Panettieri RA Jr, Krupinski AV. Resting single-breath diffusing capacity as a screening test for exercise-induced hypoxemia. Am J Med 1986;80(5):807–12.

[44] Bowyer JJ, Busst CM, Denison DM, et al. Effect of long term oxygen treatment at home in children with pulmonary vascular disease. Br Heart J 1986;55(4):385–90.

[45] Widlitz A, Barst RJ. Pulmonary arterial hypertension in children. Eur Respir J 2003;21(1): 155–76.

[46] Douglas NJ, White DP, Pickett CK, et al. Respiration during sleep in normal man. Thorax 1982; 37(11):840–4.

[47] Koo KW, Sax DS, Snider GL. Arterial blood gases and pH during sleep in chronic obstructive pulmonary disease. Am J Med 1975;58(5):663–70.

[48] Atwood CW Jr, McCrory D, Garcia JG, et al. Pulmonary artery hypertension and sleep-disordered breathing: ACCP evidence-based clinical practice guidelines. Chest 2004;126(1 Suppl):72S–7S.

[49] Podszus T, Bauer W, Mayer J, et al. Sleep apnea and pulmonary hypertension. Klin Wochenschr 1986;64(3):131–4.

[50] Weitzenblum E, Krieger J, Apprill M, et al. Daytime pulmonary hypertension in patients with obstructive sleep apnea syndrome. Am Rev Respir Dis 1988;138(2):345–9.

[51] Krieger J, Sforza E, Apprill M, et al. Pulmonary hypertension, hypoxemia, and hypercapnia in obstructive sleep apnea patients. Chest 1989;96(4): 729–37.

[52] Apprill M, Weitzenblum E, Krieger J, et al. Frequency and mechanism of daytime pulmonary hypertension in patients with obstructive sleep apnoea syndrome. Cor Vasa 1991;33(1):42–9.

[53] Laks L, Lehrhaft B, Grunstein R, et al. Pulmonary hypertension in obstructive sleep apnoea. Eur Respir J 1995;8(4):537–41.

[54] Chaouat A, Weitzenblum E, Krieger J, et al. Pulmonary hemodynamics in the obstructive sleep apnea syndrome: results in 220 consecutive patients. Chest 1996;109(2):380–6.

[55] Sajkov D, Wang T, Saunders N, et al. Daytime pulmonary hemodynamics in patients with obstructive sleep apnea without lung disease. Am J Respir Crit Care Med 1999;159(5 Pt 1):1518–26.

[56] Sanner BM, Doberauer C, Konermann M, et al. Pulmonary hypertension in patients with obstructive sleep apnea syndrome. Arch Intern Med 1997;157(21):2483–7.

[57] Niijima M, Kimura H, Edo H, et al. Manifestation of pulmonary hypertension during REM sleep in obstructive sleep apnea syndrome. Am J Respir Crit Care Med 1999;159(6):1766–72.

[58] Bady E, Achkar A, Pascal S, et al. Pulmonary arterial hypertension in patients with sleep apnoea syndrome. Thorax 2000;55(11):934–9.

[59] Alchanatis M, Tourkohoriti G, Kakouros S, et al. Daytime pulmonary hypertension in patients with obstructive sleep apnea: the effect of continuous positive airway pressure on pulmonary hemodynamics. Respiration 2001;68(6):566–72.

[60] Yamakawa H, Shiomi T, Sasanabe R, et al. Pulmonary hypertension in patients with severe obstructive sleep apnea. Psychiatry Clin Neurosci 2002; 56(3):311–2.

[61] Abenhaim L, Moride Y, Brenot F, et al. Appetite-suppressant drugs and the risk of primary pulmonary hypertension: International Primary Pulmonary Hypertension Study Group. N Engl J Med 1996;335(9):609–16.

[62] Sajkov D, Wang T, Saunders NA, et al. Continuous positive airway pressure treatment improves pulmonary hemodynamics in patients with obstructive sleep apnea. Am J Respir Crit Care Med 2002;165(2):152–8.

[63] Arias MA, Garcia-Rio F, Alonso-Fernandez A, et al. Pulmonary hypertension in obstructive sleep apnoea: effects of continuous positive airway pressure. A randomized, controlled cross-over study. Eur Heart J 2006;27(9):1106–13.

[64] Kessler R, Chaouat A, Schinkewitch P, et al. The obesity-hypoventilation syndrome revisited: a prospective study of 34 consecutive cases. Chest 2001; 120(2):369–76.

[65] Masa JF, Celli BR, Riesco JA, et al. The obesity hypoventilation syndrome can be treated with non-invasive mechanical ventilation. Chest 2001;119(4): 1102–7.

[66] Sugerman HJ, Baron PL, Fairman RP, et al. Hemodynamic dysfunction in obesity hypoventilation syndrome and the effects of treatment with surgically induced weight loss. Ann Surg 1988;207(5): 604–13.

[67] Pitt B, Zannad F, Remme WJ, et al. The effect of spironolactone on morbidity and mortality in patients with severe heart failure: Randomized Aldactone Evaluation Study Investigators. N Engl J Med 1999;341(10):709–17.

[68] Hunt SA. ACC/AHA 2005 guideline update for the diagnosis and management of chronic heart failure in the adult: a report of the American College of Cardiology/American Heart Association Task Force on Practice guidelines (Writing Committee to Update the 2001 Guidelines for the Evaluation and Management of Heart Failure). J Am Coll Cardiol 2005;46(6):e1–e82.

[69] Quinn DA, Du HK, Thompson BT, et al. Amiloride analogs inhibit chronic hypoxic pulmonary hypertension. Am J Respir Crit Care Med 1998;157(4 Pt 1):1263–8.

[70] Krayenbuehl HP, Turina J, Hess O. Left ventricular function in chronic pulmonary hypertension. Am J Cardiol 1978;41(7):1150–8.

[71] Dittrich HC, Chow LC, Nicod PH. Early improvement in left ventricular diastolic function after relief of chronic right ventricular pressure overload. Circulation 1989;80(4):823–30.

[72] Gan CT, Lankhaar JW, Marcus JT, et al. Impaired left ventricular filling due to right-to-left ventricular interaction in patients with pulmonary arterial hypertension. Am J Physiol Heart Circ Physiol 2006; 290(4):H1528–33.

[73] Akera T, Baskin SI, Tobin T, et al. Ouabain: temporal relationship between the inotropic effect and the in vitro binding to, and dissociation from, (Na + + K +)- activated ATPase. Naunyn Schmiedebergs Arch Pharmacol 1973;277(2):151–62.

[74] Mathur PN, Powles P, Pugsley SO, et al. Effect of digoxin on right ventricular function in severe chronic airflow obstruction: a controlled clinical trial. Ann Intern Med 1981;95(3):283–8.

[75] The Digitalis Investigation Group. The effect of digoxin on mortality and morbidity in patients with heart failure. N Engl J Med 1997;336(8):525–33.

[76] Jelliffe RW, Brooker G. A nomogram for digoxin therapy. Am J Med 1974;57(1):63–8.

[77] Rathore SS, Curtis JP, Wang Y, et al. Association of serum digoxin concentration and outcomes in patients with heart failure. JAMA 2003;289(7): 871–8.

[78] Fogelman AM, La Mont JT, Finkelstein S, et al. Fallibility of plasma-digoxin in differentiating toxic from non-toxic patients. Lancet 1971;2(7727): 727–9.

[79] Ingelfinger JA, Goldman P. The serum digitalis concentration: does it diagnose digitalis toxicity? N Engl J Med 1976;294(16):867–70.

[80] Leor J, Goldbourt U, Rabinowitz B, et al. Digoxin and increased mortality among patients recovering from acute myocardial infarction: importance of digoxin dose. The SPRINT Study Group. Cardiovasc Drugs Ther 1995;9(5):723–9.

[81] Eichhorn EJ, Gheorghiade M. Digoxin. Prog Cardiovasc Dis 2002;44(4):251–66.

[82] Hager WD, Fenster P, Mayersohn M, et al. Digoxin-quinidine interaction pharmacokinetic evaluation. N Engl J Med 1979;300(22):1238–41.

[83] Bizjak ED, Mauro VF. Digoxin-macrolide drug interaction. Ann Pharmacother 1997;31(9):1077–9.

[84] Juurlink DN, Mamdani M, Kopp A, et al. Drug-drug interactions among elderly patients hospitalized for drug toxicity. JAMA 2003;289(13): 1652–8.

[85] Archer SL, Djaballah K, Humbert M, et al. Nitric oxide deficiency in fenfluramine- and dexfenfluramine-induced pulmonary hypertension. Am J Respir Crit Care Med 1998;158(4):1061–7.

[86] Lopes AA, Maeda NY, Almeida A, et al. Circulating platelet aggregates indicative of in vivo platelet activation in pulmonary hypertension. Angiology 1993;44(9):701–6.

[87] Herve P, Launay JM, Scrobohaci ML, et al. Increased plasma serotonin in primary pulmonary hypertension. Am J Med 1995;99(3):249–54.

[88] Kereveur A, Callebert J, Humbert M, et al. High plasma serotonin levels in primary pulmonary hypertension: effect of long-term epoprostenol (prostacyclin) therapy. Arterioscler Thromb Vasc Biol 2000;20(10):2233–9.

[89] Cacoub P, Karmochkine M, Dorent R, et al. Plasma levels of thrombomodulin in pulmonary hypertension. Am J Med 1996;101(2):160–4.

[90] Giaid A, Saleh D. Reduced expression of endothelial nitric oxide synthase in the lungs of patients with pulmonary hypertension. N Engl J Med 1995;333(4):214–21.

[91] Collados MT, Sandoval J, Lopez S, et al. Characterization of von Willebrand factor in primary pulmonary hypertension. Heart Vessels 1999;14(5): 246–52.

[92] Hoeper MM, Sosada M, Fabel H. Plasma coagulation profiles in patients with severe primary pulmonary hypertension. Eur Respir J 1998;12(6): 1446–9.

[93] Wolf M, Boyer-Neumann C, Parent F, et al. Thrombotic risk factors in pulmonary hypertension. Eur Respir J 2000;15(2):395–9.

[94] Sakamaki F, Kyotani S, Nagaya N, et al. Increased plasma P-selectin and decreased thrombomodulin in pulmonary arterial hypertension were improved by continuous prostacyclin therapy. Circulation 2000;102(22):2720–5.

[95] Boyer-Neumann C, Brenot F, Wolf M, et al. Continuous infusion of prostacyclin decreases plasma levels of t-PA and PAI-1 in primary pulmonary hypertension. Thromb Haemost 1995;73(4):735–6.

[96] Veyradier A, Nishikubo T, Humbert M, et al. Improvement of von Willebrand factor proteolysis after prostacyclin infusion in severe pulmonary arterial hypertension. Circulation 2000;102(20): 2460–2.

[97] Friedman R, Mears JG, Barst RJ. Continuous infusion of prostacyclin normalizes plasma markers of endothelial cell injury and platelet aggregation in primary pulmonary hypertension. Circulation 1997;96(9):2782–4.

[98] Girgis RE, Champion HC, Diette GB, et al. Decreased exhaled nitric oxide in pulmonary arterial hypertension: response to bosentan therapy. Am J Respir Crit Care Med 2005;172(3):352–7.

[99] Welsh CH, Hassell KL, Badesch DB, et al. Coagulation and fibrinolytic profiles in patients with severe pulmonary hypertension. Chest 1996;110(3): 710–7.

[100] Loyd JE, Atkinson JB, Pietra GG, et al. Heterogeneity of pathologic lesions in familial primary pulmonary hypertension. Am Rev Respir Dis 1988; 138(4):952–7.

[101] Frank H, Mlczoch J, Huber K, et al. The effect of anticoagulant therapy in primary and anorectic drug-induced pulmonary hypertension. Chest 1997;112(3):714–21.

[102] Roman A, Rodes-Cabau J, Lara B, et al. Clinico-hemodynamic study and treatment of 44 patients with primary pulmonary hypertension. Med Clin (Barc) 2002;118(20):761–6.

[103] Storstein O, Efskind L, Muller C, et al. Primary pulmonary hypertension with emphasis on its etiology and treatment. Acta Med Scand 1966;179(2): 197–212.

[104] Ansell J, Hirsh J, Poller L, et al. The pharmacology and management of the vitamin K antagonists: the seventh ACCP conference on antithrombotic and thrombolytic therapy. Chest 2004;126(3 Suppl):204S–33S.

[105] Hales CA, Kradin RL, Brandstetter RD, et al. Impairment of hypoxic pulmonary artery remodeling by heparin in mice. Am Rev Respir Dis 1983; 128(4):747–51.

[106] Hassoun PM, Thompson BT, Hales CA. Partial reversal of hypoxic pulmonary hypertension by heparin. Am Rev Respir Dis 1992;145(1):193–6.

[107] Yu L, Quinn DA, Garg HG, et al. Gene expression of cyclin-dependent kinase inhibitors and effect of heparin on their expression in mice with hypoxia-induced pulmonary hypertension. Biochem Biophys Res Commun 2006;345(4):1565–72 [Epub 2006].

[108] Hassoun PM, Thompson BT, Steigman D, et al. Effect of heparin and warfarin on chronic hypoxic pulmonary hypertension and vascular remodeling in the guinea pig. Am Rev Respir Dis 1989; 139(3):763–8.

[109] Garg HG, Hales CA, Yu L, et al. Increase in the growth inhibition of bovine pulmonary artery smooth muscle cells by an O-hexanoyl low-molecular-weight heparin derivative. Carbohydr Res 2006;341(15):2607–12.

[110] Levine MN, et al. Hemorrhagic complications of anticoagulant treatment: the seventh ACCP conference on antithrombotic and thrombolytic therapy. Chest 2004;126(3 Suppl):287S–310S.

[111] Robbins IM, et al. A study of aspirin and clopidogrel in idiopathic pulmonary arterial hypertension. Eur Respir J 2006;27(3):578–84.

[112] Rubin LJ. Pulmonary arterial hypertension. Proc Am Thorac Soc 2006;3(1):111–5.

[113] Geerts WH, et al. Prevention of venous thrombo-embolism: the seventh ACCP conference on antithrombotic and thrombolytic therapy. Chest 2004; 126(3 Suppl):338S–400S.

[114] Dresdale DT, Michtom RJ, Schultz M. Recent studies in primary pulmonary hypertension, including pharmacodynamic observations on pulmonary vascular resistance. Bull N Y Acad Med 1954;30(3): 195–207.

[115] Christman BW, McPherson CD, Newman JH, et al. An imbalance between the excretion of thromboxane and prostacyclin metabolites in pulmonary hypertension. N Engl J Med 1992;327(2):70–5.

[116] Tuder RM, Cool CD, Geraci MW, et al. Prostacyclin synthase expression is decreased in lungs from patients with severe pulmonary hypertension. Am J Respir Crit Care Med 1999;159(6):1925–32.

[117] Stewart DJ, Levy RD, Cernacek P, et al. Increased plasma endothelin-1 in pulmonary hypertension: marker or mediator of disease? Ann Intern Med 1991;114(6):464–9.

[118] Olivari MT, Levine TB, Weir EK, et al. Hemodynamic effects of nifedipine at rest and during exercise in primary pulmonary hypertension. Chest 1984;86(1):14–9.

[119] Higenbottam T, Wheeldon D, Wells F, et al. Long-term treatment of primary pulmonary hypertension with continuous intravenous epoprostenol (prostacyclin). Lancet 1984;1(8385):1046–7.

[120] Groves B, Badesch DB, Turkevich D, et al. Correlation of acute prostacyclin response in primary (unexplained) pulmonary hypertension and efficacy of treatment with calcium channel blockers and survival. In: Weir K, editor. Ion flux in pulmonary vascular control. New York: Plenum Press; 1993. p. 317–30.

[121] Sitbon O, Brenot F, Denjean A, et al. Inhaled nitric oxide as a screening vasodilator agent in primary pulmonary hypertension: a dose-response study and comparison with prostacyclin. Am J Respir Crit Care Med 1995;151(2 Pt 1):384–9.

[122] Sitbon O, Humbert M, Jagot JL, et al. Inhaled nitric oxide as a screening agent for safely identifying responders to oral calcium-channel blockers in primary pulmonary hypertension. Eur Respir J 1998; 12(2):265–70.

[123] Pepke-Zaba JH, Dinh-Xuan AT, Stone D, et al. Inhaled nitric oxide as a cause of selective pulmonary vasodilatation in pulmonary hypertension. Lancet 1991;338(8776):1173–4.

[124] Ricciardi MJ, Knight BP, Martinez FJ, et al. Inhaled nitric oxide in primary pulmonary hypertension: a safe and effective agent for predicting response to nifedipine. J Am Coll Cardiol 1998; 32(4):1068–73.

[125] Schrader BJ, Inbar S, Kaufmann L, et al. Comparison of the effects of adenosine and nifedipine in pulmonary hypertension. J Am Coll Cardiol 1992; 19(5):1060–4.

[126] Opitz CF, Wensel R, Bettmann M, et al. Assessment of the vasodilator response in primary pulmonary hypertension: comparing prostacyclin and iloprost administered by either infusion or inhalation. Eur Heart J 2003;24(4):356–65.

[127] Ogata M, Ohe M, Shirato K, et al. Effects of a combination therapy of anticoagulant and vasodilator on the long-term prognosis of primary pulmonary hypertension. Jpn Circ J 1993;57(1): 63–9.

[128] Humbert M, Sitbon O, Chaouat A, et al. Pulmonary arterial hypertension in France: results from a national registry. Am J Respir Crit Care Med 2006;173(9):1023–30.

[129] Ziesche R, Petkov V, Wittmann K, et al. Treatment with epoprostenol reverts nitric oxide non-responsiveness in patients with primary pulmonary hypertension. Heart 2000;83(4):406–9.

[130] Preston IR, Klinger JR, Houtchens J, et al. Pulmonary edema caused by inhaled nitric oxide therapy in two patients with pulmonary hypertension associated with the CREST syndrome. Chest 2002; 121(2):656–9.

[131] Zakliczynski M, Zebik T, Maruszewski M, et al. Usefulness of pulmonary hypertension reversibility test with sodium nitroprusside in stratification of early death risk after orthotopic heart transplantation. Transplant Proc 2005;37(2): 1346–8.

[132] Palmer SM, Robinson LJ, Wang A, et al. Massive pulmonary edema and death after prostacyclin infusion in a patient with pulmonary veno-occlusive disease. Chest 1998;113(1):237–40.

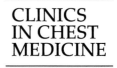
CLINICS
IN CHEST
MEDICINE

ELSEVIER
SAUNDERS

Clin Chest Med 28 (2007) 117–125

Endothelin Receptor Antagonists in the Treatment of Pulmonary Arterial Hypertension

David Langleben, MD, FRCPC[a,b,*]

[a]McGill University, Montreal, Quebec, Canada
[b]Center for Pulmonary Vascular Disease, Division of Cardiology, Sir Mortimer B. Davis Jewish General Hospital, 3755 Cote Ste Catherine, Montreal, Quebec, Canada H3T 1E2

Endothelin-1 in pulmonary arterial hypertension

Since its discovery in 1988, endothelin-1 (ET-1) has been increasingly recognized as an important mediator in the pathogenesis of pulmonary arterial hypertension (PAH) [1]. Although recent theories suggest that PAH may result from dysregulated proliferation and abnormal apoptosis of endothelial cells [2–4], the actions of ET-1 as a vasoconstrictor and its actions on the growth of endothelial cells, smooth muscle cells, fibroblasts, and pericytes probably contribute to the ongoing vascular remodeling seen in PAH. Endothelial cells are the principal source of ET-1, but the link between the abnormal endothelial growth pattern and excess synthesis of ET-1 in PAH is not understood at this time. ET-1, however, does have antiapoptotic effects on endothelial cells and smooth muscle cells [5,6], and these effects might in some way contribute to the abnormalities in apoptosis seen in PAH. Previous studies have established that plasma ET-1 levels are increased in PAH [7] and that pulmonary expression and synthesis of ET-1 is increased in PAH, particularly in the remodeled precapillary pulmonary microvasculature that is the site of the increased pulmonary vascular resistance in PAH [1]. With the recognition of these abnormalities, the development of clinically useful endothelin receptor antagonists was begun [8].

Receptors for endothelin-1

Two G protein–coupled receptors for ET-1, termed "ET_A" and "ET_B," have been described [9,10]. Activation of the ET_A receptor on smooth muscle cells, pericytes, and fibroblasts results in vasoconstriction and proliferation in vitro [11]. The in vitro effects of activation of the ET_B receptor on these cells are inconsistent, and vary with the cell type, the receptor-specific agonist used, and its concentration [12]. The relevant molecule for disease states, however, is ET-1, not an agonist, and the burden of evidence from experimental studies supports a much greater role for the ET_A receptor than for the ET_B receptor in the constrictive and proliferative responses of cells of mesenchymal origin to the levels of endogenous ET-1 seen in disease states [13]. In human pulmonary hypertension, two studies describe the increased expression of smooth muscle ET_B receptors, but the physiologic significance of this finding is unclear [14,15]. Those studies could not resolve the effects of the disease on the endothelial ET_B receptor.

In endothelial cells, ET_B receptors are abundantly present, particularly in the distal lung

This work was supported in part by the Canadian Institutes for Health Research and the Fonds de la Recherche en Sante du Quebec. Dr. Langleben has received financial support in the form of grants, consultancies, or speakers' fees from Actelion, Encysive, Myogen, Glaxo-Smith-Kline, and United Therapeutics. He has a minor equity holding in Encysive and United Therapeutics.

* Center for Pulmonary Vascular Disease, Division of Cardiology, Sir Mortimer B. Davis Jewish General Hospital, 3755 Cote Ste Catherine, Montreal, Quebec, Canada H3T 1E2.

E-mail address: david.langleben@mcgill.ca

microvasculature [14]. There is no evidence for ET$_A$ receptor expression on endothelial cells. The interaction of ET-1 with the endothelial ET$_B$ receptor may moderate some of the detrimental effects of ET-1 within the circulation, in that it leads to release of the vasodilators and antiproliferative molecules nitric oxide and prostacyclin from the endothelium [16]. Also, clearance of ET-1 from the circulation occurs principally through the pulmonary endothelial ET$_B$ receptor, which may offer another measure of protection in disease states by lowering ET-1 levels [17,18]. It has been proposed elsewhere that a diseased, dysfunctional endothelium in PAH might have reduced expression or dysfunction of the endothelial ET$_B$ receptor [19,20]. Contrary to this hypothesis, the author and colleagues have demonstrated recently that most patients who have idiopathic PAH or PAH related to connective tissue disease have intact or only modestly reduced endothelial ET$_B$–mediated clearance, despite a reduced microvascular surface area from vascular remodeling [21]. Thus, in PAH, selective ET$_A$ receptor antagonists, which preserve endothelial ET$_B$ receptor vasodilatory and clearance activity, may offer more benefit than nonselective ET$_A$ plus ET$_B$ antagonists. This question will be resolved only by clinical trials.

Selectivity of endothelin receptor antagonists

The receptor selectivity of the various antagonists has been determined using standardized in vitro assays that allow comparison between compounds. The degree of selectivity also relates to the concentration of the antagonist, so even a selective antagonist will become relatively less selective at very high doses. Agents with an ET$_A$:ET$_B$ selectivity ratio greater than approximately 2500:1 generally are considered to be selective, and, although it is not used clinically, BQ-123 (ET$_A$:ET$_B$, 2465:1) has served as a useful antagonist in studies of the effects of receptor selectivity. Three endothelin receptor antagonists are approved or are in the late stages of the approval process. All are orally active, and all carry some risk of hepatotoxicity (elevated transaminases and/or bilirubin levels), possibly through effects on the hepatic cytochrome P-450 enzyme system or other mechanisms [22]. Bosentan (ET$_A$:ET$_B$, 20:1) and ambrisentan (ET$_A$:ET$_B$, 77:1) are nonselective; sitaxsentan (ET$_A$:ET$_B$, 6500:1) is highly selective.

Clinical trials of endothelin receptor antagonists in pulmonary arterial hypertension

Table 1 summarizes all the studies listed below.

Bosentan

The initial study of bosentan in a cohort of seven patients who had PAH showed that an infusion could lower pulmonary vascular resistance. Several of the patients in this study died or suffered clinical deterioration during the second phase of the trial, possibly related to their poor clinical status at the time of entry into the trial. In this study, plasma ET-1 levels were measured serially after the administration of bosentan and rose, demonstrating that bosentan was blocking the endothelial ET$_B$ receptor.

A subsequent randomized, double-blind, placebo-controlled 12-week trial showed that oral bosentan (62.5 mg twice daily for 4 weeks, then 125 mg twice daily) improved 6-minute-walk distance, pulmonary vascular resistance, and World Health Organization functional class in patients who had idiopathic PAH or PAH related to scleroderma [23]. All patients were in World Health Organization functional class 3 at baseline. The incidence of hepatotoxicity in bosentan-treated patients was 10% and resolved on discontinuation of the drug. Plasma ET-1 levels were not measured in this study.

This initial trial was followed by a larger 16-week, double-blind, placebo-controlled study, the Bosentan Randomized Trial of Endothelin Antagonist Therapy (BREATHE-1) [24]. Two hundred thirteen patients were assigned randomly to placebo or to bosentan (62.5 mg twice daily for 4 weeks, then either 125 mg or 250 mg twice daily). Almost all patients were in functional class 3 at baseline. As compared with placebo, bosentan-treated patients had improved 6-minute-walk distance, functional class, and delayed time to clinical worsening. There was a 9% incidence of hepatotoxicity in the combined bosentan group, with a greater risk of hepatotoxicity at the dose of 250 mg twice daily. The improvement in 6-minute-walk distance was apparent in the idiopathic PAH group but not in the patients who had PAH related to scleroderma. An echocardiographic substudy showed that bosentan improved right ventricular size and systolic function as well as left ventricular filling [25]. The BREATHE-1 study provided the first broadly applicable oral therapy for PAH.

The current recommended dose for bosentan in adults is 62.5 mg orally twice daily for 1 month and then increased to 125 mg orally twice daily long-term if there is no evidence of hepatotoxicity.

A subsequent 1-year follow-up study of patients receiving open-label bosentan showed that the improvement in 6-minute-walk distance, pulmonary hemodynamics, and functional class was sustained for many patients [26]. By 12 months, only 55% of patients were in functional class 3, whereas 38% were in class 2. The incidence of hepatotoxicity was 9%.

In a different cohort of 169 bosentan-treated patients who had idiopathic PAH, 2-year survival was approximately 92% [27]. Nine percent of these patients were in functional class 2 at baseline, however, and would have an expected high survival rate, and another 10% of the patients failed bosentan therapy alone and required concurrent epoprostenol therapy. Another analysis of a large cohort of patients who had idiopathic PAH, were in functional class 3 at baseline, and then were treated with bosentan or epoprostenol showed 1- and 2-year gross survival rates of 97% and 91%, respectively, for the bosentan group, but addition of a second therapy was required by 13% of patients in year 1 and by 15% of patients in year 2 [28]. Nonetheless, all these results are impressive for an oral agent.

An open-label 12-week trial of weight-adjusted bosentan therapy (BREATHE-3) in 19 pediatric patients who had PAH, including PAH related to congenital heart disease, showed improvement in pulmonary hemodynamics [29]. Approximately half the patients were receiving concomitant epoprostenol. In a 16-week, open-label study of bosentan in 16 patients who had HIV-related PAH (BREATHE-4), there were significant improvements in 6-minute-walk distance, functional class, hemodynamics, Doppler echocardiographic variables, and quality of life [30]. There was a 9% incidence of hepatotoxicity, and there were no adverse interactions related to antiretroviral medications. The authors could not comment on survival benefit in this relatively small, short-term trial. In the BREATHE-5 trial, 54 patients who had functional class 3 PAH and Eisenmenger's syndrome from congenital heart disease were assigned randomly in a double-blind fashion to placebo or bosentan for 16 weeks [31]. Bosentan therapy significantly reduced pulmonary vascular resistance and pulmonary artery pressure and increased exercise capacity.

Sitaxsentan

An initial 12-week open-label study of sitaxsentan, 100 to 500 mg twice daily, demonstrated significant increases in 6-minute-walk distances and improved hemodynamics in patients who had functional class 2, 3, and 4 PAH [32]. Two cases of acute hepatitis, one fatal, occurred during the extension phase, however. These cases were related to the then-unrecognized nonlinear pharmacokinetics of sitaxsentan at high doses; subsequent studies have used lower doses.

The subsequent placebo-controlled, double-blind Sitaxsentan To Relieve Impaired Exercise (STRIDE-1) trial studied lower doses (100 mg and 300 mg once daily) of sitaxsentan for 12 weeks [33]. In addition to including patients who had functional class 3 and 4 idiopathic or connective tissue disease–related PAH, and with a baseline 6-minute-walk distance no greater than 450 m, as in BREATHE-1 [24], STRIDE-1 included patients in functional class 2 and patients who had PAH related to congenital heart disease, and there was no ceiling on the 6-minute-walk distance. Change in peak oxygen consumption on cardiopulmonary exercise testing was the primary endpoint. This parameter subsequently has been shown to have excessive interhospital variability, and its use as an endpoint in multicenter trials is problematic [34,35]. Despite this variability, in STRIDE-1 the 6-minute-walk distance, functional class, and pulmonary hemodynamics all improved significantly [33], and the trial has been considered as pivotal by the US Food and Drug Administration. Unlike BREATH-1, STRIDE-1 showed significant improvement with therapy in patients who have PAH related to connective tissue disease. Elevation of hepatic transaminases above three times the upper limit of normal (ULN) was 0% at a dosage of 100 mg daily and 10% at a dosage of 300 mg daily, and a pharmacokinetic study revealed nonlinearity of sitaxsentan elimination at a dosage of 300 mg daily. During the study extension trial (STRIDE-1X), at a median exposure of 26 weeks, there was a 5% incidence of elevated transaminases with the 100-mg daily dosage and a 21% incidence with 300-mg daily dosage. Sitaxsentan inhibits the hepatic cytochrome P450 enzyme CYP2C9, resulting in altered metabolism of warfarin and a need for a substantial warfarin dose reduction. A long-term continuation study of 11 patients who had completed STRIDE-1 has shown sustained improvement in functional class, pulmonary vascular resistance, and cardiac output over

incidence was less than 5% in the 100-mg sitaxsentan group and 11% in the bosentan group.

Another dose-ranging trial comparing sitaxsentan, 50 mg or 100 mg daily, with placebo, STRIDE-4, has been completed in Latin America, Poland, and Spain [38]. The study results were unusual in that the 6-minute-walk distance in the placebo group increased by 34 m. This improvement was ascribed to perception of improved medical care after enrollment among patients who otherwise might not have had access to that level of care. The 100-mg dose showed improvement in walk distance, functional class, and Borg dyspnea scale. The 50-mg dose showed no significant efficacy. The drug was well tolerated, with only one patient in each group (3%) experiencing elevated liver enzymes.

STRIDE-2X continued patients who received sitaxsentan (100 mg) or bosentan (125 mg) twice daily during STRIDE-2 on their respective therapies, in an open-label fashion [39]. Patients receiving sitaxsentan (50 mg daily) during STRIDE-2 then were given sitaxsentan (100 mg daily), and the STRIDE-2 placebo patients were assigned to sitaxsentan (100 mg daily) or bosentan (125 mg twice daily). Prespecified analysis of results for patients treated for as long as 1 year revealed significant differences between the treatment arms, with consistently better outcomes for the sitaxsentan-treated patients in such objective parameters as risk of discontinuation of monotherapy, discontinuation for adverse events, and abnormal liver enzymes. There were strong trends in favor of sitaxsentan for risk of clinical worsening and survival. The most impressive results were seen in the group that had PAH related to connective tissue disease. Because of the open-label nature of the study and potential pitfalls in including the STRIDE 2 50-mg group in the STRIDE-2X sitaxsentan group, a more conservative analysis, which excludes the 50-mg group, has been performed. In addition, this analysis only considers endpoints such as death, hospitalization, transplantation, change in functional class and exercise duration, and need for epoprostenol rescue therapy. Even in this analysis, the trends all favor sitaxsentan over bosentan, suggesting a consistent clinical advantage. Until the data are published, these interpretations must be considered preliminary. Most of the patients continuing on sitaxsentan therapy after one or more of the clinical trials or starting sitaxsentan de novo have entered STRIDE-3, a long-term safety trial. No results have been reported to date for the over 800 patients in the study.

To study whether patients who had discontinued bosentan therapy because of hepatotoxicity or loss of efficacy could tolerate or benefit from therapy with another endothelin receptor antagonist, a 12-week study, STRIDE-6, was performed [40]. After 3 months, only 1 patient of the 13 who had previously experienced hepatotoxicity when taking bosentan developed elevation of liver enzymes while taking sitaxsentan. Thirty-three percent of the patients who experienced loss of efficacy with bosentan had an improvement in 6-minute-walk distance of more than 15% while taking sitaxsentan. No longer-term data are available yet. Thus, at least in the short term, sitaxsentan may be a useful and safe alternative for patients who do not respond to bosentan therapy or develop hepatotoxicity while taking bosentan.

Ambrisentan

A 12-week blinded-to-dose but not placebo-armed study has been reported for ambrisentan [41]. Patients at all doses (1, 2.5, 5, or 10 mg daily) had improved 6-minute-walk distance as compared with baseline, with improved functional class, Borg score, and pulmonary hemodynamics. Elevated liver transaminases were seen in 3% of patients. In the subgroup that had idiopathic PAH, there seemed to be a dose–response relationship for 6-minute-walk distance.

In the subsequent 12-week trial, Ambrisentan in PAH—A Phase III, Randomized, Double-Blind, Placebo-Controlled, Multicenter, Efficacy Study of Ambrisentan in Subjects With Pulmonary Arterial Hypertension (ARIES-1), 202 patients were assigned randomly to placebo, ambrisentan (5 mg), or ambrisentan (10 mg), once daily. Preliminary results show statistically significant improvements in 6-minute-walk distance, functional class, Borg dyspnea score, and quality-of-life score. In the 12-week ARIES-2 trial, patients were assigned randomly to placebo, ambrisentan (2.5 mg), or ambrisentan (5 mg), once daily [42]. Preliminary results show improvement in 6-minute-walk distance and time to clinical worsening. None of the ambrisentan-treated patients had liver transaminases more than three times the ULN, but there was an extremely low incidence in the placebo group as well, suggesting that the populations of the studies had a low risk for liver abnormalities. There were no interactions with warfarin. These results are extremely promising.

Determining the success of endothelin antagonist therapy

The ease of use of these oral agents and the understandable desire to avoid parenteral therapy for as long as possible may lead to a patient-driven or physician-driven tolerance for a level of response that might otherwise have been judged inadequate. Until recently, there were no criteria that might indicate a successful response to endothelin antagonist therapy. In a review of a large database of patients who had PAH, Provencher and colleagues [43] have identified factors that predict a better long-term prognosis after bosentan therapy. They found that patients in functional class 4 are better off if they initially receive epoprostenol instead of bosentan. Other factors that predict a poorer prognosis or requirement for addition of epoprostenol include remaining in functional class 3 after 4 months of bosentan treatment, a 6-minute-walk distance shorter than 250 m, a decrease of more than 10% in 6-minute-walk distance on two consecutive tests performed at least 2 weeks apart, and a cardiac index of less than 2.2 L/min/m^2.

Transitioning from other pulmonary arterial hypertension therapy to endothelin antagonists

The attractiveness of an oral therapy for PAH has prompted efforts to transition patients from parenteral PAH therapy to an endothelin receptor antagonist. In an initial study, four patients who had normal pulmonary arterial pressure while taking epoprostenol transitioned successfully to oral bosentan and remained stable [44]. Another group of three children who had normal pulmonary arterial pressure while taking epoprostenol were switched to bosentan, with subsequent stability for a 1-year study period [45]. The common feature for success in these two studies is the normalization or near-normalization of pulmonary arterial pressure during the prostaglandin therapy. By contrast, in a larger study of adults in whom pulmonary artery pressure had not normalized during the prostaglandin therapy, only 65% transitioned successfully to bosentan over a 3-month period, and in 61% bosentan therapy failed within 3 to 16 months after the prostaglandin was stopped [46]. Therefore, the current recommendation is that transition from prostaglandins to bosentan be considered only in patients whose pulmonary artery pressure has normalized during prostaglandin therapy and take place under close observation.

Combination therapy with endothelin receptor antagonists

The recognition that monotherapy for PAH yields inadequate improvement for many patients has led to attempts to combine several classes of therapies, including endothelin receptor antagonists. In an initial trial involving patients already receiving either inhaled iloprost or oral beraprost, the addition of open-label bosentan significantly improved the 6-minute-walk distance after 3 months of combined therapy [47]. In the 16-week BREATH-2 study of patients already receiving intravenous epoprostenol, bosentan or placebo was added [48]. Hemodynamics improved, but not significantly; there was no improvement in exercise tolerance or functional class. There were serious adverse events, including death, in the group that received the active combination, and a negative interaction of the combined therapy could not be excluded. In the recent 12-week safety and pilot efficacy trial in combination with bosentan for evaluation in pulmonary arterial hypertension (STEP) trial, inhaled iloprost or placebo was given to patients who had taken bosentan for at least 4 months [49]. As compared with patients taking placebo, patients receiving iloprost had significant improvements in 6-minute-walk distance, mean pulmonary artery pressure, and time to clinical worsening. The authors correctly point out that the ideal design for combination trials would have three arms, one for each therapy alone, and one for the combination. In many instances, this design will not be feasible.

Summary

The nearly 20 years since the description of endothelin-1 have seen a rapid translation of basic knowledge into therapies that have improved and possibly lengthened the lives of thousands of patients who have PAH. Soon there will be three approved therapies. The choice for a particular patient will be individualized based on the type of PAH, comorbidities such as liver disease, convenience, drug interactions, and effectiveness. In the short-term studies, the therapies have similar efficacy. Despite the limitations in its design, the only trial that studied two endothelin receptor antagonists, STRIDE-2X, provides some evidence that over a 1-year period sitaxsentan therapy may be less hepatotoxic and more effective than bosentan therapy. Monthly monitoring of liver enzymes probably will be required for all three medications. Warfarin dose must be reduced significantly with sitaxsentan. Issues for the future include understanding the pharmacogenomics of responders versus nonresponders, demonstration of long-term (>5-year) durability of effect, further resolving the relative benefits of selectivity versus nonselectivity, identifying effective combination therapy, expanding the indications for use, and understanding the contribution of endothelin to the altered patterns of apoptosis that are thought to occur early and later in PAH [4]. Despite these and other unresolved issues, tremendous progress has been made already.

References

[1] Giaid A, Yanagisawa M, Langleben D, et al. Expression of endothelin-1 in the lungs of patients with pulmonary hypertension. N Engl J Med 1993;328: 1732–9.

[2] Voelkel NF, Cool CD, Lee SD, et al. Primary pulmonary hypertension between inflammation and cancer. Chest 1998;114:225S–30S.

[3] Humbert M, Morrell NW, Archer SL, et al. Cellular and molecular pathobiology of pulmonary arterial hypertension. J Am Coll Cardiol 2004;43:13S–24S.

[4] Michelakis ED. Spatio-temporal diversity of apoptosis within the vascular wall in pulmonary hypertension: heterogeneous BMP signalling may have therapeutic implications. Circ Res 2006;98:172–5.

[5] Shichimi M, Kato H, Marumo F, et al. Endothelin-1 as an autocrine/paracrine apoptosis survival factor for endothelial cells. Hypertension 1997;30: 1198–203.

[6] Jankov RP, Kantores C, Belcastro R, et al. Endothelin-1 inhibits apoptosis of pulmonary arterial smooth muscle in the neonatal rat. Pediatr Res 2006;60:245–51.

[7] Stewart DJ, Levy RD, Cernacek P, et al. Increased plasma endothelin-1 in pulmonary hypertension: marker or mediator of disease? Ann Intern Med 1991;114:464–9.

[8] Battistini B, Berthiaume N, Kelland NF, et al. Profile of past and current clinical trials involving endothelin receptor antagonists: the novel "-Sentan" class of drug. Exp Biol Med 2006;231:653–95.

[9] Arai H, Hori S, Aramori I, et al. Cloning and expression of a cDNA encoding an endothelin receptor. Nature 1990;348:730–2.

[10] Sakurai T, Yanagisawa M, Takuwa Y, et al. Cloning of a cDNA encoding a non-isopeptide-selective subtype of the endothelin receptor. Nature 1990;348: 732–4.

[11] Evans AM, Cobban HJ, Nixon GF. ET_A receptors are the primary mediators of myofilament calcium sensitization induced by ET-1 in rat pulmonary

artery smooth muscle: a tyrosine kinase independent pathway. Br J Pharmacol 1999;127:153–60.

[12] Black SM, Mata-Greenwood E, Dettman RW, et al. Emergence of smooth muscle cell endothelin B-mediated vasoconstriction in lambs with experimental congenital heart disease and increased blood flow. Circulation 2003;108:1646–54.

[13] Shi-Wen X, Chen Y, Denton CP, et al. Endothelin-1 promotes myofibroblast induction through the ETA receptor via a rac/phosphoinositide 3-kinase/Akt-dependent pathway and is essential for the enhanced contractile phenotype of fibrotic fibroblasts. Mol Biol Cell 2004;15:2707–19.

[14] Davie N, Haleen SJ, Upton PD, et al. ETA and ETB receptors modulate the proliferation of human pulmonary artery smooth muscle cells. Am J Respir Crit Care Med 2002;165:398–405.

[15] Bauer M, Wilkens H, Langer F, et al. Selective upregulation of endothelin B receptor gene expression in severe pulmonary hypertension. Circulation 2002; 105:1034–6.

[16] De Nucci G, Thomas R, D'Orleans-Juste P, et al. Pressor effects of circulating endothelin are limited by its removal in the pulmonary circulation and by the release of prostacyclin and endothelium-derived relaxing factor. Proc Natl Acad Sci U S A 1988;85: 9797–800.

[17] Dupuis J, Stewart DJ, Cernacek P, et al. Human pulmonary circulation is an important site for both clearance and production of endothelin-1. Circulation 1996;94:1578–84.

[18] Dupuis J, Goresky CA, Fournier A. Pulmonary clearance of circulating endothelin-1 in dogs in vivo: exclusive role of ETB receptors. J Appl Physiol 1996;81:1510–5.

[19] Clozel M. Editorial. Heart Fail Rev 2001;6:249–51.

[20] Clozel M. Effects of bosentan on cellular processes involved in pulmonary arterial hypertension: do they explain the long term benefit? Ann Med 2003; 35:605–13.

[21] Langleben D, Dupuis J, Langleben I, et al. Etiology-specific endothelin-1 clearance in human precapillary pulmonary hypertension. Chest 2006;129: 689–95.

[22] Fattinger K, Funk C, Pantze M, et al. The endothelin antagonist bosentan inhibits the canalicular bile salt export pump: a potential mechanism for hepatic adverse reactions. Clin Pharmacol Ther 2001;69: 223–31.

[23] Channick RN, Simonneau G, Sitbon O, et al. Effects of the dual endothelin-receptor antagonist bosentan in patients with pulmonary hypertension: a randomised placebo-controlled study. Lancet 2001;358: 1119–23.

[24] Rubin LJ, Badesch DB, Barst RJ, et al. Bosentan therapy for pulmonary arterial hypertension. N Engl J Med 2002;346:896–903.

[25] Galie N, Hinderliter AL, Torbicki A, et al. Effects of the oral endothelin-receptor antagonist bosentan on

echocardiographic and Doppler measures in patients with pulmonary arterial hypertension. J Am Coll Cardiol 2003;41:1380–6.

[26] Sitbon O, Badesch DB, Channick RN, et al. Effects of the dual endothelin receptor antagonist bosentan in patients with pulmonary arterial hypertension. Chest 2003;124:247–54.

[27] McLaughlin VV, Sitbon O, Badesch DB, et al. Survival with first-line bosentan in patients with primary pulmonary hypertension. Eur Respir J 2005; 25:244–9.

[28] Sitbon O, McLaughlin VV, Badesch DB, et al. Survival in patients with class III idiopathic pulmonary arterial hypertension treated with first line oral bosentan compared with an historical cohort of patients started on intravenous epoprostenol. Thorax 2005;60:1025–30.

[29] Barst RJ, Ivy D, Dingemanse J, et al. Pharmacokinetics, safety, and efficacy of bosentan in pediatric patients with pulmonary arterial hypertension. Clin Pharmacol Ther 2003;73:372–82.

[30] Sitbon O, Gressin V, Speich R, et al. Bosentan for the treatment of human immunodeficiency virus-associated pulmonary arterial hypertension. Am J Respir Crit Care Med 2004;170:1212–7.

[31] Galie N, Beghetti M, Gatzoulis MA, et al. Bosentan therapy in patients with Eisenmenger syndrome: a multicenter, double-blind, randomized, placebo-controlled study. Circulation 2006;114:48–54.

[32] Barst RJ, Rich S, Widlitz A, et al. Clinical efficacy of sitaxsentan, an oral endothelin-A receptor antagonist, in patients with pulmonary arterial hypertension. Chest 2002;121:1860–8.

[33] Barst RJ, Langleben D, Frost A, et al. Sitaxsentan therapy for pulmonary arterial hypertension. Am J Respir Crit Care Med 2004;169:441–7.

[34] Barst RJ, McGoon M, McLaughlin V, et al. Beraprost therapy for pulmonary arterial hypertension. J Am Coll Cardiol 2003;41:2119–25.

[35] Oudiz RJ, Barst RJ, Hansen JE, et al. Cardiopulmonary exercise testing and six-minute walk correlations in pulmonary arterial hypertension. Am J Cardiol 2006;97:123–6.

[36] Langleben D, Hirsch AM, Shalit E, et al. Sustained symptomatic, functional, and hemodynamic benefit with the selective endothelin-A receptor antagonist, sitaxsentan, in patients with pulmonary arterial hypertension. Chest 2004;126:1377–81.

[37] Barst RJ, Langleben D, Badesch D, et al. Treatment of pulmonary arterial hypertension with the selective

endothelin-A receptor antagonist sitaxsentan. J Am Coll Cardiol 2006;47:2049–56.

[38] Pulido T, Kurzyna M, Souza R, et al. Sitaxsentan 100 mg proves more effective than sitaxsentan 50 mg in patients with pulmonary arterial hypertension. Proc Am Thorac Soc 2006;3:A417.

[39] Benza R, Frost A, Girgis R, et al. Chronic treatment of pulmonary arterial hypertension with sitaxsentan and bosentan. Proc Am Thorac Soc 2006;3:A729.

[40] Benza R, Mehta S, Keogh A, et al. Sitaxsentan treatment for patients with pulmonary arterial hypertension failing bosentan treatment. Proc Am Thorac Soc 2005;2:A201.

[41] Galie N, Badesch DB, Oudiz R, et al. Ambrisentan therapy for pulmonary arterial hypertension. J Am Coll Cardiol 2005;46:529–35.

[42] Olschewski H, Galie N, Ghofrani HA, et al. Ambrisentan improves exercise capacity and time to clinical worsening in patients with pulmonary arterial hypertension. Proc Am Thorac Soc 2006;3: A728.

[43] Provencher S, Sitbon O, Humbert M, et al. Long-term outcome with first-line bosentan therapy in idiopathic pulmonary arterial hypertension. Eur Heart J 2006;27:589–95.

[44] Kim NH, Channick RN, Rubin LJ. Successful withdrawl of long-term epoprostenol therapy for pulmonary arterial hypertension. Chest 2003;124: 1612–5.

[45] Ivy DD, Doran A, Claussen L, et al. Weaning and discontinuation of epoprostenol in children with idiopathic pulmonary arterial hypertension receiving concomitant bosentan. Am J Cardiol 2004;93: 943–6.

[46] Suleman N, Frost AE. Transition from epoprostenol and treprostinil to the oral endothelin receptor antagonist bosentan in patients with pulmonary hypertension. Chest 2004;126:808–15.

[47] Hoeper MM, Taha N, Bekjarova A, et al. Bosentan treatment in patients with primary pulmonary hypertension receiving nonparenteral prostanoids. Eur Respir J 2003;22:330–4.

[48] Humbert M, Barst RJ, Robbins IM, et al. Combination of bosentan with epoprostenol in pulmonary arterial hypertension: BREATHE-2. Eur Respir J 2004;24:353–9.

[49] McLaughlin VV, Oudiz R, Frost A, et al. Randomized study of adding inhaled iloprost to existing bosentan in pulmonary arterial hypertension. Am J Respir Crit Care Med 2006;174:1257–63.

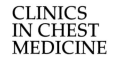

CLINICS
IN CHEST
MEDICINE

ELSEVIER
SAUNDERS

Clin Chest Med 28 (2007) 127–142

Prostanoid Therapy for Pulmonary Arterial Hypertension

Wayne L. Strauss, MD, PhD[a], Jeffrey D. Edelman, MD[b],*

[a]Division of Pulmonary and Critical Care Medicine, Department of Medicine, Oregon Health and
Sciences University, Mail Code UHN67, 3181 SW Sam Jackson Park Road, Portland, OR 97239, USA
[b]Division of Pulmonary and Critical Care Medicine, Department of Medicine, University of Washington
Medical Center, Box 356522, 1959 NE Pacific Street, Seattle, WA 98159, USA

Prostaglandins were first described by von Euler in 1933 and prostaglandin I_2 (PGI_2, prostacyclin, epoprostenol), a product of endothelial cells in all vascular tissues, was first discovered in 1976. The potential clinical roles of epoprostenol in the acute [1] and chronic [2] treatment of pulmonary arterial hypertension (PAH) were initially described in case series in the early 1980s. Epoprostenol was approved for the chronic treatment of idiopathic PAH by the U.S. Food and Drug Administration (FDA) in 1996 after a randomized, controlled trial showed improved short-term survival [3]. The availability of this agent dramatically changed the approach to treatment and prognosis for patients who have PAH. Since this time, the indications for the use of epoprostenol have expanded and structural modifications have led to the development of additional longer acting molecular analogs for clinical use (Table 1) [4]. Epoprostenol and its structural analogs are collectively termed *prostanoids*. Prostanoid agents currently being used or evaluated for treatment of PAH include epoprostenol, treprostinil, iloprost, and beraprost. Epoprostenol, treprostinil, and iloprost are currently available in the United States. The structures of these molecules are shown in Fig. 1 [5]. Ongoing areas of investigation include alternative routes of prostanoid administration and the use of prostanoids

in treating other classes of pulmonary hypertension (PH).

Epoprostenol and the arachidonic acid pathway

Epoprostenol is a member of the eicosanoid family. Eicosanoids are the 20 carbon essential fatty acids derived from arachidonic acid. This family of biologically active mediators includes the prostacyclins, thromboxanes, and leukotrienes. Eicosanoids are critical mediators of smooth muscle contraction, vasodilation and constriction, vascular permeability, platelet aggregation, and lymphocyte chemotaxis and proliferation. Metabolism of phospholipids by phospholipase A2 yields arachidonic acid. Leukotrienes are produced by metabolism of arachidonic acid through the 5-lipoxygenase pathway. Prostaglandins and thromboxanes are produced by metabolism of arachidonic acid through the cyclooxygenase pathway (Fig. 2).

Epoprostenol and pulmonary arterial hypertension pathogenesis

Vasoconstriction, cellular proliferation, and thrombosis lead to the development and progression of PAH. Pulmonary vascular endothelial cell products involved in the regulation of these processes include epoprostenol, nitric oxide, endothelin, serotonin, and thromboxane [6–8]. Since it was discovered, epoprostenol has been known to be a potent vasodilatory, cytoprotective, and antithrombotic agent. Epoprostenol inhibits platelet aggregation and thrombus formation

---

* Corresponding author.

E-mail address: edelmanj@u.washington.edu
(J.D. Edelman).

Table 1
Prostanoid agent routes of administration and half-life

Prostanoid agent	Routes of administration for PAH treatment	Half-life in circulation
Epoprostenol	Intravenous[a]	6 min [44]
Treprostinil	Subcutaneous	240 min [47]
	Intravenous	
	Inhaled[a]	
	Oral[a]	
Iloprost	Inhaled	20–30 min [62]
	Intravenous[a]	
Beraprost	Oral[b]	60 min [4]

[a] Route of administration not approved in the United States.
[b] Agent not approved for PAH treatment in the United States.

and also promotes dispersion of preexisting plate-let aggregates [9–11]. The cytoprotective effect of epoprostenol has been shown in animal models of tissue injury, including prevention of gastric ulcer formation, reduction in myocardial infarct size, and prevention of endotoxin-mediated lung injury [12–15]. The evaluation of epoprostenol in the treatment of PAH has shown several additional properties. The observation that the chronic response to treatment significantly exceeded the acute vasodilatory response suggested that epoprostenol might also be a mediator of

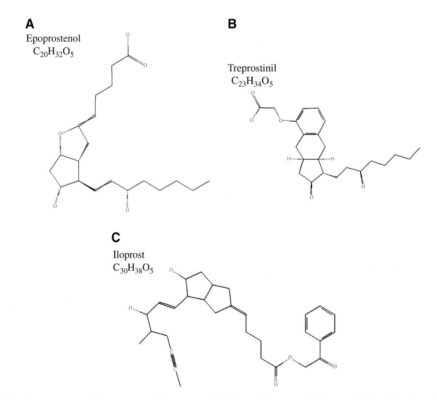

Fig. 1. Molecular structures of epoprostenol (*A*), treprostinil (*B*), and iloprost (*C*). (*From* Wishart DS, Knox C, Guo AC, et al. Drugbank: a comprehensive resource for in silico drug discovery and exploration. Nucleic Acids Res 2006; 34(Database issue):D668–72; with permission.)

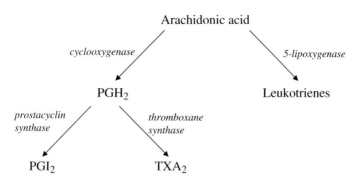

Fig. 2. Synopsis of arachidonic acid pathways leading to PGI$_2$ (epoprostenol) production.

vascular remodeling [16]. Chronic therapy with epoprostenol in PAH leads to normalization of factor VIII, von Willebrand's antigen, and ristocetin cofactor, which are markers of endothelial cell injury [17]. Chronic epoprostenol therapy also leads to increased levels of thrombomodulin and P-selectin [18]. Inhibition of endothelin-1 production by endothelial cells in vitro and improved pulmonary clearance of this molecule in response to epoprostenol have also been shown [19,20]. Lastly, epoprostenol also has a potent positive inotropic effect [21,22].

Reduced epoprostenol production and expression of its receptor have been shown to occur in PAH, whereas alteration in epoprostenol production or receptor expression can modulate PH development in animal models. Decreased urinary excretion of the epoprostenol metabolite 6-keto-prostaglandin F1α and reduced expression of prostacyclin synthase by endothelial cells suggest that epoprostenol synthesis by endothelial cells is diminished in PAH [23,24]. Urinary excretion of thromboxane A2 metabolites is increased in PAH, suggesting that an imbalance in arachidonic acid metabolism favoring thromboxane over epoprostenol production may be a cause or result of PAH [24]. Overexpression of prostacyclin synthase in transgenic mice or by direct gene transfer into mouse skeletal muscle leads to increased production of epoprostenol, as reflected by increased levels of the stable metabolite 6-ketoprostaglandin F1α, and protects against development of pulmonary hypertension in response to exposure to hypoxia or monocrotaline [25,26]. Knockout of the prostacyclin receptor in mice can lead to accentuated pulmonary hypertensive response to hypoxemia [27]. Epoprostenol has also been shown to inhibit smooth muscle proliferation and induce apoptosis of smooth muscle cells in vitro [28–31].

Clinical applications

The potential role for epoprostenol in the evaluation and treatment of PAH was identified soon after its discovery. However, nearly 2 decades elapsed before epoprostenol was approved for use by the FDA in 1996. Although this agent is clearly effective in treating PAH, its side-effect profile, risks, and inconveniences and its continuous intravenous route of delivery prompted the development of alternative agents. Epoprostenol, treprostinil, and iloprost are the three prostanoids currently approved for use in the United States; beraprost is available outside of the United States. Table 1 summarizes the routes of administration and half-life for each agent.

Available agents

Epoprostenol

Epoprostenol was first discovered in 1976. Early clinical studies suggested potential benefit of epoprostenol in cardiopulmonary bypass, peripheral vascular disease, and Raynaud's phenomenon [32]. A trial of epoprostenol in refractory left-sided congestive heart failure was terminated because of increased mortality in the treatment arm [33]. In the early 1980s, epoprostenol was first shown during invasive hemodynamic monitoring through pulmonary artery catheterization to have acute vasodilatory effects in the pulmonary circulation in seven patients who had PAH and given escalating doses of continuously infused epoprostenol (from 2 to 12 ng/kg/min) [1]. A decrease in mean pulmonary arterial pressure (MPAP) from 62 to 55 mm Hg ($P < .05$) was observed with a substantial decline in total pulmonary resistance (TPR) from 17.1 to 9.7 Wood units ($P<.005$) and increase in cardiac output from 4.22 to 6.57 L/min ($P<.01$). Three subjects remained on continuous infusion of epoprostenol for 24 to 44 hours, with sustained reduction in TPR and increased cardiac output. In this study, all subjects experienced immediate response to epoprostenol infusion, a finding not observed in subsequent studies. Long and Rubin [34] showed the acute vasodilatory effects of epoprostenol in a larger group of 100 patients.

The chronic use of infused epoprostenol was first reported in 1984 in a single patient with sustained improvements in symptoms, hemodynamics, and exercise tolerance over 13 months [2]. A subsequent nonrandomized study showed improvement in symptoms and exercise tolerance in 10 patients treated for durations ranging from 1 to 25 months [35]. A randomized pilot study comparing 11 patients treated with continuous infusion of epoprostenol with 12 patients treated with standard medical therapy showed significant hemodynamic improvement after 8 weeks of epoprostenol treatment [36]. At 8 weeks, cardiac output improved from 3.3 L/min to 3.9 L/min ($P = .020$) and pulmonary vascular resistance (PVR) decreased from 21.6 to 13.9 Wood units ($P = .039$) in the treatment group with no significant changes in the standard medical therapy group. An open-label study of 18 patients receiving continuous intravenous epoprostenol showed sustained improvement in hemodynamics (6 and 12 months) and 6-minute walk distance (6, 12, and 18 months) with improved survival compared with historical controls [37].

A landmark randomized trial compared 12 weeks of infusion of epoprostenol plus standard medical therapy with standard medical therapy alone in 81 patients, all of whom had severe PAH (primary PH based on previous National Institutes of Health [NIH] registry criteria [38]) with class III to IV symptoms [3]. The 41 patients assigned to the epoprostenol group and the 40 assigned to the conventional therapy group were well matched for baseline demographics and hemodynamic data. Eight deaths occurred in the conventional treatment group, all from disease progression, with none in the epoprostenol group, showing a mortality benefit of epoprostenol therapy ($P = .003$). Hemodynamic and exercise tolerance benefits were also observed. After this study, epoprostenol was approved for chronic intravenous use in the United States. A similar randomized, controlled trial showed improvements in hemodynamics and exercise tolerance in patients

who had scleroderma and PAH, although no survival benefit was observed [39]. Although data supporting the benefit of continuous epoprostenol in other PAH subcategories are limited, epoprostenol has been accepted as appropriate therapy for patients who have virtually all forms of advanced PAH.

The substantial mortality benefit seen with short-term (12-week) epoprostenol infusion and the widespread treatment availability of this agent have made controlled trials assessing long-term mortality impact ethically untenable. The availability of treatment with a favorable impact on short-term mortality has also limited the use of mortality as an end point in subsequent trials evaluating newer treatment agents. Thus, the assessment of long-term mortality impact for epoprostenol and newer agents is limited to comparison with historical controls or predicted mortality based on a regression equation derived from the NIH registry [38]. A single institutional series described 161 consecutive patients treated with epoprostenol for class III and IV PAH and followed up for a mean of 36.3 months [40]. Observed survival rates for patients treated with epoprostenol therapy at 1, 2, and 3 years were 87.8%, 76.3%, and 62.8%, respectively, which were significantly greater than the expected calculated survival rates of 58.9%, 46.3%, and 35.4% based on the NIH registry equation.

Another series of 178 consecutive patients treated with epoprostenol at a single institution examined long-term survival [41]. At 1, 2, 3, and 5 years, the survival rates were 85%, 70%, 63%, and 55%, respectively, compared with expected survival rates of 58%, 43%, 33%, and 28% based on the NIH registry equation. The availability of epoprostenol and subsequent newer therapies has dramatically altered the approach to timing of lung transplantation for patients who have PAH [42,43]. Patients who have a history of right heart failure or right atrial pressure of 12 mm Hg or more and those who remain class III or IV or do not experience a significant decrease in pulmonary resistance after 3 months of epoprostenol therapy are at increased risk for mortality [41]. Thus, these parameters may identify treated patients who require evaluation for lung or heart–lung transplantation.

Epoprostenol degrades spontaneously in blood to 6-ketoprostaglandin F1α and is also enzymatically degraded to 6,15-diketo-13,14-dihydro-prostaglandin F1α. Both of these inactive metabolites are excreted in the urine. Because epoprostenol has a short half-life in circulation at 37°C of approximately 6 minutes [44], it is suitable for use in assessing vasoreactivity during rapid titration. The presence of significant vasoreactivity, defined by a decrease in mean pulmonary arterial pressure of 10 mm Hg or greater to a level of 40 mm Hg or lower with no change or an increase in cardiac output, identifies patients who may respond to calcium channel blocker therapy [45]. The absence of a vasodilatory response does not preclude chronic therapy with epoprostenol or other agents. The long-term hemodynamic response to epoprostenol exceeds the acute response, and patients who do not show vasoreactivity usually respond to chronic treatment [16].

Several problems exist with epoprostenol therapy. The drug is administered through an indwelling central venous catheter exposing patients to risk for line-associated infections, sepsis, thrombosis, and air embolism. Although a short half-life in circulation (6 minutes) may be desirable for acute vasodilator testing, it exposes patients on chronic therapy to significant risk for severe rebound pulmonary hypertensive crisis if medication is discontinued for more than several minutes because of pump failure or dislodging of the central venous catheter. Epoprostenol is also unstable at room temperature and must be mixed at 8-hour intervals when used in these conditions. When kept cool using ice packs surrounding the medication cassette, infusion may be maintained for 24 hours before changing the medication cassette. The dosing of epoprostenol can be difficult, with dose escalation required to maintain response, but with the possibility of overdosing the medication and the development of symptomatic high output heart failure [46]. Distinguishing a hyperdynamic state from disease progression can be difficult without repeat right heart catheterization.

Treprostinil

Treprostinil is a stable analog of epoprostenol that does not require refrigeration. It is approved by the FDA for either continuous intravenous or subcutaneous infusion. Treprostinil has a half-life of approximately 4 hours [47]. Metabolism of treprostinil occurs predominantly in the liver and metabolites are excreted in the urine. The longer half-life of treprostinil reduces the risks associated with treatment disruption in comparison to epoprostenol. The stability of this agent also permits administration through nonparenteral routes,

thus affording the opportunity to avoid risks associated with central venous catheterization.

A multicenter randomized trial compared subcutaneous infusion of treprostinil with placebo in 470 subjects who had PAH with predominantly class III and IV symptoms [48]. Most subjects had idiopathic PAH with smaller percentages of connective tissue and congenital right-to-left shunt–associated disease represented in the study. The primary end point was change in 6-minute walk distance over baseline. The treprostinil group had a 16 m increase in walk test distance compared with the placebo group ($P = .006$). Two important observations were made during this study. Patients who had more limited functional status on entry seemed to have the greatest improvement in 6-minute walk distance, and patients able to receive a higher dose of treprostinil also experienced the greatest improvements in distance. Injection site pain is the most common dose-limiting side effect, and frequently limits subcutaneous use of the drug in clinical practice. Sustained improvement in exercise tolerance and symptoms with subcutaneous treprostinil was also reported in patients who had idiopathic PAH (n = 99) and chronic thromboembolic pulmonary hypertension (CTEPH) (n = 23), with mean follow-up of 26 months [49].

In a long-term open-label study of 860 patients who had PAH treated with subcutaneous treprostinil with follow-up of up to 4 years, 76% of patients had class III functional limitations at enrollment. Approximately half the patients had idiopathic PAH, with the rest having disease associated with congenital cardiac shunts, connective-tissue disorders, CTEPH, HIV, and portal hypertension–associated pulmonary hypertension (POPH). Of the patients in the study, 506 (59%) discontinued treprostinil. Clinical reasons for discontinuation included adverse events/injection site pain (23%), death (16%), clinical deterioration (14%), or transplantation (1%). All patients were initially on monotherapy, but bosentan or sildenafil were added in 105 and 26 patients, respectively, and 98 patients were switched to alternative prostanoid treatments. Survival rates for the cohort were 87% at 1 year and 68% at 4 years. In the subgroup of patients who had idiopathic PAH, 1- and 4-year survival rates were 91% and 72%, respectively, compared with expected survival rates from the NIH registry of 69% and 38%, respectively [50].

Because of the frequency of infusion site complications with the subcutaneous route, several trials have studied intravenous treprostinil. Although a central venous catheter is required, the longer half-life of the drug may offer improved safety profile over epoprostenol in the setting of inadvertent drug discontinuation. A study of 51 healthy volunteers given treprostinil as a continuous infusion at 10 ng/kg/min through both intravenous and subcutaneous routes showed steady-state bioequivalence with elimination half-life of 4.4 and 4.6 hours, respectively [51]. The acute hemodynamic effects of intravenous treprostinil and epoprostenol were shown to be equivalent in a nonrandomized cross-over study [52].

A second similarly designed study also showed the short-term effects of intravenous and subcutaneous treprostinil to be equivalent [52]. A 12-week, multicenter, open-label trial of intravenous treprostinil was conducted in 16 patients who had PAH that was either idiopathic, connective tissue disease–associated, or related to congenital heart disease [53]. The primary end point was distance in the 6-minute walk test, with an observed improvement of 89 m ($P = .001$). In a second 12-week open-label study, 31 patients were transitioned from intravenous epoprostenol to intravenous treprostinil for treatment of PAH [54]. The primary end point for the study was change in 6-minute walk distance. Of the 31 subjects, 27 successfully transitioned to treprostinil. No difference was seen in the distance walked at the end of the study (438 m versus 439 m). However, hemodynamic measurements suggested deterioration with small but statistically significant worsening in cardiac output and PVR after 12 weeks of treprostinil therapy.

Because of its stability, treprostinil may be administered through an aerosolized route. In an experimental model of pulmonary hypertension in sheep comparing aerosolized and intravenous treprostinil at identical doses, the aerosolized dose led to greater vasodilatory effects in the pulmonary circulation with lesser systemic vasodilatory effects [55,56]. Administration of a single 15-μg dose of nebulized treprostinil to three human subjects led to a reduction in PVR exceeding 3 hours in three patients. Two patients were treated with chronic inhaled treprostinil (15 μg four times daily) for 3 months with improvement in 6-minute walk distance and functional class [57]. A second study evaluated the additional effect of inhaled treprostinil (30 or 45 μg four times daily) in 12 patients who had PAH who remained symptomatic despite oral bosentan.

Improvements in MPAP, PVR, 6-minute walk distance, and functional class were observed [58]. Randomized, multicenter, double-blind, placebo-controlled trials evaluating the efficacy and safety of inhaled and oral treprostinil in PAH are currently underway.

Iloprost

Iloprost is stable analog of epoprostenol that can be delivered through intravenous or inhaled routes. Although intravenous use of iloprost has only been evaluated in small groups of patients, these studies suggest similar acute and intermediate-term (7 weeks) improvement in hemodynamic response and exercise tolerance compared with epoprostenol [59,60]. Despite the convenience of inhaled drug delivery, iloprost has a relatively short half-life (20–30 minutes) and requires six to nine inhalations daily through a hand-held ultrasonic or jet nebulizer device [61,62]. Typically, patients do not interrupt sleep for inhaled treatments. A study of 24 patients who had idiopathic PAH treated with inhaled iloprost for 12 months showed sustained increase in 6-minute walk distance over baseline (increase of 75 and 85 m at 3 and 12 months, respectively; $P < .05$). Moderate improvements were seen in PVR, cardiac output, and pulmonary artery mean pressures. Patients who had the greatest acute improvement in hemodynamics after a single inhalation seemed to have the largest sustained effects [63].

A 12-week multicenter, placebo-controlled study evaluated 203 patients who had functional class III and IV PAH (idiopathic, associated with collagen vascular disorders or appetite suppressants) or CTEPH. Patients in the treatment arm received 2.5- or 5.0-μg doses of iloprost six to nine times daily. A combined end point of a 10% increase in 6-minute walk distance and improvement of at least one WHO class was experienced by 16.9% of patients in the iloprost group and 4.9% in the placebo arm ($P = .007$). Iloprost treatment led to an increase of 36 m in 6-minute walk distance for the entire treatment group, with a 58-m increase noted the idiopathic PAH subgroup. Statistically significant improvements in postinhalation cardiac output and PVR were seen at 12 months compared with baseline in patients treated with iloprost, with no differences seen in the placebo arm. Fewer deaths or clinical deteriorations were observed in the iloprost group compared with the placebo group (4.9% versus 11.8%), but this difference was not statistically significant. Significant therapeutic benefit was not observed in the patients who had CTEPH [64].

An uncontrolled, observational study prospectively followed up 76 patients who had idiopathic PAH on iloprost monotherapy for up to 5 years with predefined end points of death, transplantation, and intensification of treatment with oral or intravenous agents. At 3, 12, 24, 36, 48, and 60 months, the percentage of patients not meeting an end point was 81%, 53%, 29%, 20%, and 17%, respectively. After 1 year, only 41% of patients remained on inhaled monotherapy, suggesting that patients initially treated with inhaled iloprost may require alternate or additional treatments at an early juncture [65]. Several uncontrolled studies have shown clinical improvement for patients treated with inhaled iloprost combined with the endothelin-1 receptor blocking agent bosentan or the phosphodiesterase-5 inhibitor sildenafil [66–68]. A randomized, placebo-controlled, multicenter trial is evaluating the safety and effectiveness of adding iloprost or placebo to sildenafil therapy for PAH.

Concerns exist about the interruption of inhaled iloprost therapy during sleep hours. Because many patients have relative alveolar hypoventilation and hypoxia during sleep, they may be particularly susceptible to hypoxic vasoconstriction and worsening of right heart strain when drug is absent. However, the nighttime holiday from drug may promote retention of prostacyclin receptor density on the cell surface and maintain sensitivity to prostanoids, thus mitigating the tachyphylaxis seen with continuously administered agents.

Beraprost

Because of the limitations and difficulties of continuous intravenous or subcutaneous therapy and intermittent inhaled treatment, developing a suitable oral prostanoid is desirable. Beraprost is a prostanoid stable at body temperature and gastric pH and is therefore suitable for oral dosing. A small, uncontrolled, observational study reported on response to beraprost in 12 patients who had WHO class III or IV idiopathic PAH [69]. Hemodynamic monitoring was performed at baseline and after 2 months of treatment in 10 patients who experienced a change in mean PVR from 19.3 to 14.3 Wood units and MPAP from 66 to 58 mm Hg. Long-term benefit of at least one improvement in functional class was observed in 8 patients with a mean follow-up

of 5 months. The remaining 4 patients died of progressive disease. A retrospective review of 58 patients discharged from the hospital with a new diagnosis of idiopathic PAH compared those treated with conventional therapy with those treated with beraprost [70]. Thirty-four patients discharged before 1992 were treated with conventional therapy, and the 24 patients discharged after that date were treated with oral beraprost at the highest tolerated dose (dosed 3–4 times daily at a total dose of 60–180 μg/d) in addition to conventional therapy. Twenty-seven of the 34 patients in the conventional therapy group died (mean follow-up duration of 44 months) compared with 4 of 24 patients in the beraprost group (mean follow-up duration of 20 months). The Kaplan-Meier survival curve showed a statistically significant improvement in survival ($P < .001$).

A double-blind, randomized, placebo-controlled trial of beraprost in 130 patients who had idiopathic PAH or PAH associated with collagen vascular disorders, portal hypertension, HIV, and congenital heart defects assessed change in 6-minute walk distance and hemodynamics over 12 weeks [71]. All subjects had WHO class II and III symptoms. The mean difference in walk distance change between the two groups was 25 m ($P = .036$) at 12 weeks. No significant changes were noted in hemodynamic parameters. A posthoc subgroup analysis suggested that improvement in walk distance occurred only in the patients who had primary pulmonary hypertension (idiopathic PAH or familial PAH by current definition).

A 12-month, double-blind, placebo-controlled trial evaluated beraprost (120 μg four times daily) in the treatment of patients who had idiopathic PAH or PAH associated with congenital shunts or collagen-vascular disorders [72]. The primary end point was disease progression (death, need for epoprostenol, and 25% decline in peak oxygen consumption) and secondary end points included exercise capacity (6-minute walk distance and peak VO$_2$, Borg dyspnea score), hemodynamics, symptoms of PAH, and quality of life. Fewer patients in the beraprost group experienced disease progression at 6 months (1/60 in the beraprost group and 11/56 in the control arm; $P = .002$); however, no difference in disease progression was observed at 3, 9, and 12 months. Significant improvement in 6-minute walk test distance over baseline was noted in the beraprost group at 3 and 6 months but not at 9 and 12 months. Beraprost was not approved by the FDA.

Prostanoid selection

Intravenous prostanoid therapy remains the preferred treatment for patients who have advanced PAH and WHO class IV symptoms who are at high risk for short-term mortality. Questions remain about how best to use prostanoid therapy in PAH within the context of multiple prostanoid agents, endothelin receptor antagonists, and phosphodiesterase-5 inhibitors. Given the complexity of administering and dosing currently available prostanoids, it may be advantageous to delay these therapies in certain patients, but no randomized data exist to help define the optimal time to begin treatment. Epoprostenol remains the only drug proven to improve short-term prognosis. Because of its temperature stability and potential safety margin related to longer half-life, treprostinil may be a preferable choice for certain patients requiring infused therapy, although it is not as efficacious as epoprostenol (ie, higher doses are required) and cost may become an issue. Head-to-head comparison data with epoprostenol assessing outcome equivalence, particularly in the sickest patients, are not available. Similar data limitations apply to the use of inhaled iloprost. Therefore, choosing a particular agent is based on clinical judgment and physician-to-patient discussion of known risks and benefits of the various treatment options. The option of an oral prostanoid might be helpful for patients unable to tolerate other modes of delivery. Oral treprostinil is currently being studied and oral beraprost remains available outside the United States.

Combined therapies

The availability of multiple classes of agents for treating PAH raises the question of whether combination therapy provides additional benefit. Through targeting multiple disease pathways, achieving greater response with fewer side effects may be possible. Although oral and inhaled prostanoids may be less effective than infused agents, their convenience and potentially favorable safety profile make them attractive choices for studies evaluating combination therapy with agents from other drug classes. In a single-center experience, 14 of 73 patients undergoing chronic inhaled iloprost therapy met clinical criteria for disease progression and underwent additional treatment with sildenafil [68]. For patients on inhaled iloprost monotherapy, six-minute walk distance improved from 256 to 346 m after 3 months ($P = .002$), and to 349 m after 12 months ($P = .002$) of therapy with iloprost combined with sildenafil. Hemodynamic parameters also improved. In another single-institution study, 21 consecutive patients treated with inhaled iloprost or oral beraprost with stable dosing for more than 3 months received bosentan [67]. One patient dropped out of the study because of hepatic toxicity. After 3 months of combination therapy, the mean 6-minute walk distance improved from 346 m to 404 m ($P < .001$), with continued improvements noted at further follow-up points. Patients underwent formal cardiopulmonary exercise testing at baseline and 3 months, with improvement in maximal oxygen consumption from 11.0 to 13.8 mL/min/kg ($P < .001$).

A recent randomized placebo-controlled trial involving 67 patients evaluated the addition of inhaled iloprost (5 μg six to nine times daily) versus placebo to chronic bosentan therapy. Most patients (94%) were NYHA functional class III at baseline. Most patients had idiopathic PAH (55%), with the remainder having scleroderma, other connective tissue diseases, HIV infection, repaired congenital heart disease, and anorexigen use. After 12 weeks of combination therapy, greater improvement in 6-minute walk distance was observed ($P = .051$) in the iloprost group (30 m), compared with the placebo group (4 m). Eleven of 32 patients treated with iloprost versus 2 of 33 patients treated with placebo showed improvement in NYHA functional class ($P = .002$). None of 32 patients treated with iloprost versus 5 of 33 patients treated with placebo met predefined criteria for clinical worsening ($P = .0219$). Significant difference ($P < .001$) was also noted in postinhalation MPAP in the iloprost group (−6 mm Hg from baseline) compared with the placebo group (+2 mm Hg) [73].

Limited data exist on the combination of bosentan with epoprostenol. A series of 33 patients who had PAH were started on epoprostenol therapy with 14 weeks of dose titration and then randomized 2:1 to bosentan or placebo as add-on therapy [74]. No statistically significant differences occurred in 6-minute walk distance or hemodynamic parameters between the groups. Four patients withdrew from the bosentan arm because of clinical worsening, death, and adverse advents, whereas only one patient withdrew from the placebo arm because of an adverse event.

Current questions include determining which drug combinations are beneficial and whether combination therapy should be reserved for monotherapy failures or instituted early in the disease course. Several studies evaluating the combination of prostanoid agents with other therapies are currently underway. The use of epoprostenol in combination with sildenafil for treating PAH is being assessed in an open-label study. A randomized, placebo-controlled, multicenter trial is evaluating the safety and effectiveness of adding iloprost or placebo to sildenafil therapy for PAH. Another randomized, placebo-controlled, multicenter study is assessing the addition of oral treprostinil to other approved oral PAH therapies (endothelin-receptor antagonists or phosphodiesterase-5 inhibitors).

Special considerations

Pediatric idiopathic pulmonary arterial hypertension

Approximately 10% of patients who have idiopathic PAH are younger than 21 years [75]. A retrospective study compared outcomes in children younger than 16 years (7 months to 13 years) who had idiopathic PAH and not manifest an acute vasodilator response or improve on conventional therapy. The study period from 1982 to 1995 included an interval during which epoprostenol was unavailable. Survival in the 31 patients treated with epoprostenol was 100%, 94%, 94%, and 94% at 1, 2, 3, and 4 years, respectively, versus 50%, 43%, 38%, and 38%, respectively, in 28 patients for whom epoprostenol would have been indicated but was unavailable [76].

Congenital cardiac defects

Many children and adults who have congenital heart defects, including atrial septal defects, ventricular septal defects, patent ductus arteriosus, and anomalous pulmonary venous return, develop PAH. Adults who have surgically corrected congenital heart disease have been included in many large studies evaluating prostanoids. Results for these patients have not been separately reported, and even less is known about the treatment of uncorrected disease. An uncontrolled study of epoprostenol infusion for 1 year in 20 patients who had congenital heart disease not responsive to standard therapy included 11 with uncorrected disease [77]. Although none of these patients showed an acute vasodilator response to epoprostenol, statistically significant improvement in hemodynamic and exercise parameters was noted at 1 year.

Collagen vascular disease

Patients who have collagen vascular disorders are at risk for developing PAH and fibrotic lung disease. Scleroderma both in limited and diffuse forms and mixed connective tissue disease are the collagen vascular disorders most highly associated with PAH, but all other disorders, including systemic lupus erythematosus, Sjögren's syndrome, and rheumatoid arthritis, have been associated with PAH. A recent study of 909 patients followed up in community rheumatology practices for scleroderma or mixed connective tissue disease found that 13.3% had echocardiographic evidence of undiagnosed elevated right ventricular systolic pressure [78].

Data specifically examining prostanoid treatment in patients who have connective tissue disease are available from two multicenter trials. A randomized trial of continuous intravenous infusion of epoprostenol in 111 patients who had systemic sclerosis and PAH showed improvement in the primary end point of 6-minute walk distance by 108 meters compared with those treated with placebo ($P < .001$) [39]. Of the epoprostenol patients, 21 improved one WHO class, whereas none improved in the placebo arm. A subgroup analysis of a randomized, placebo-controlled subcutaneous treprostinil trial included 90 of 470 patients who had systemic lupus erythematosus, diffuse and limited scleroderma, and mixed connective tissue disease [79]. Modest statistically significant improvements were seen in cardiac index and PVR, and a nonsignificant improvement was seen in 6-minute walk distance (25 m; $P = .055$). Randomization was not stratified by presence of connective tissue disease, and imbalances occurred in parameters between the groups, including age and distribution of WHO class. Two small pilot studies of oral beraprost and intravenous iloprost in patients who had scleroderma without known PAH showed stability or improvement in diffusion capacity of carbon monoxide [80,81]. These effects were suggested to be caused by amelioration of endothelial dysfunction and injury in patients who have systemic sclerosis and increased cardiac output from direct inotropic effects [80].

HIV

People who have HIV infection are at risk for developing PAH, but little data on treatment for these patients are available. A study evaluating acute and chronic effects of iloprost on

HIV-associated PAH showed a 31% acute decline in PVR versus baseline in eight patients. Four patients who then underwent long-term treatment showed improvement in 6-minute walk distance and PVR that failed to reach statistical significance [82]. Another study of six patients who had HIV and severe PAH treated with continuous epoprostenol infusion for 1 year showed statistically significant improvement in hemodynamic measurements and improvement in WHO class [83]. A case series of patients who had HIV-associated PAH found that treatment with highly active antiretroviral therapy and epoprostenol therapy was an independent predictor of survival [84].

Portal hypertension–associated pulmonary hypertension

Treating POPH with prostanoids has unique challenges because of the vasodilated, hyperdynamic state and low systemic blood pressure of many patients who have advanced liver disease. In 1997, Kuo and colleagues [85] reported a marked reduction in MPAP and PVR and an increase in cardiac output in four patients undergoing treatment with epoprostenol for 6 to 14 months. Subsequently, Krowka and colleagues [86] reported their experience in treating 15 patients who had POPH and MPAP of 35 mm Hg or more using intravenous epoprostenol. Acute vasodilator testing led to significant change ($P < .01$) in PVR (-34%), MPAP (-16%), and cardiac output ($+21\%$). Ten patients underwent continuous therapy (duration of 8 days to 30 months) with a 47% reduction ($P < .05$) in PVR from baseline in six patients who underwent repeat catheterization. However, 60% of patients died while undergoing treatment with long-term epoprostenol.

Successful use of intravenous prostanoids (epoprostenol or iloprost) to reduce pulmonary pressures permitting liver transplantation has been described in case reports and case series [87–95]. Larger case series were recently reported from two institutions. One study describes eight consecutive patients who had POPH with MPAP of 35 mm Hg or more treated with epoprostenol (2–8 ng/kg/min), with statistically significant decline in MPAP (43–33 mm Hg; $P = .03$) and PVR (5.1–2.4 Wood units; $P = .01$), and increase in cardiac output (6.6–10 L/min; $P = 0.02$). Six patients were listed for liver transplantation. Two patients died while awaiting transplantation and the other four underwent transplantation,

with discontinuation of PH therapy in two patients and transition from epoprostenol to oral therapy in two patients [93]. A recent abstract described 19 patients who had POPH treated with epoprostenol followed up for a median duration of 38 months, with statistically significant decreases ($P < .0001$) in MPAP (48–37 mm Hg) and PVR (8.2–3.5 Wood units) in 15 patients evaluated with follow-up right heart catheterization. Significant change in liver function was not observed. Nine (47%) patients undergoing therapy were alive at follow-up, with two patients undergoing successful liver transplantation. However, eight patients (42%) who underwent treatment died and the remaining two were lost to follow-up [95].

Epoprostenol has thus been the best-evaluated agent in the treatment of POPH. The available data show that this drug can clearly lead to hemodynamic improvement in this group of patients and may permit successful liver transplantation in patients who would otherwise have been ineligible because of their unfavorable pulmonary hemodynamics. However, in the absence of liver transplantation, the mortality rate for these patients remains high despite therapy. The major causes of death in this group have not been described. However, given the extent of hemodynamic improvement reported, progressive liver disease and its associated complications are likely major contributors to mortality, as opposed to pulmonary vascular disease. Given the high mortality despite treatment (and lack of data suggesting a mortality benefit compared with untreated patients), the strongest rationale for pursuing this invasive therapy is currently to facilitate liver transplantation.

Chronic thromboembolic pulmonary hypertension

CTEPH is characterized by proliferation of organized fibrinous clot in the pulmonary vasculature with secondary pathologic changes in small pulmonary arteries and arterioles similar to those seen in idiopathic PAH. Treatment typically consists of pulmonary endarterectomy in patients who have sufficiently central vascular disease and are believed to have an acceptable level of surgical risk. Patients who have residual disease after surgery and those who have inoperable disease are generally treated similar to those who have PAH, but few data are available to guide therapy. Small numbers of patients who have CTEPH have been included in trials of pharmacologic therapy.

A retrospective study of subcutaneous treprostinil included 99 patients who had PAH and 23 who had CTEPH [49]. At 36 months of treatment, significant improvement occurred in 6-minute walk distance from 305 to 445 m ($P = .0001$) and WHO class from 3.2 to 2.1 ($P = .001$) for the entire population (subgroup data were not reported). No difference was seen in Kaplan-Meier curves for survival. A retrospective series examined 23 patients who had CTEPH treated before beraprost was available (in Japan) and 20 who were treated with beraprost [96]. Improvement of at least one WHO class occurred in 50% of the beraprost group. Sixteen patients in the conventional therapy group died within 55 months, whereas 3 died within 44 months in the beraprost group. A prospective study of patients in the intensive care unit who had CTEPH showed that one-time inhaled iloprost at the 5-μg dose in combination with sildenafil, 50 mg orally, was a potent vasodilator in these patients and that combination therapy had significantly more effect than either drug alone [97]. A more recent study compared eight patients who had CTEPH and eight patients who had idiopathic PAH treated with oral beraprost for 6 months. Treatment resulted in improved WHO functional class (2.7–2.0, $P < .05$) and 6-minute walk distance (312–373 m, $P < .003$),without significant change in MPAP. Results were similar to those for the eight patients who had idiopathic PAH [98].

Acute respiratory distress syndrome

The acute respiratory distress syndrome (ARDS) is defined by bilateral noncardiogenic pulmonary edema with increased shunting of pulmonary blood flow resulting in poor oxygenation. Patients may develop elevated right ventricular pressures and severe oxygenation failure. Inhaled epoprostenol has been studied in these patients. A single-institution study of 16 patients who had ARDS, compared the effect of inhaled epoprostenol with that of inhaled nitric oxide [99]. Doses of both medicines were titrated for maximal oxygenation, and the drugs were given in random order. At a maximal effective mean dose of 7.5 ng/kg/min, inhaled epoprostenol was associated with an improvement in the ratio of partial pressure of arterial oxygen to inspired oxygen (Pao_2/Fio_2) of 114 to 135 mm Hg ($P < .01$) and decreased shunt fraction from 33.5% to 26% ($P < .05$), compared with nitric oxide at mean dose of 17.8 ppm, which showed an improvement in Pao_2/Fio_2 of 115 to 144 ($P < .01$) and decreased shunt fraction from 33.1% to 26.6% ($P < .05$). Similar effects were seen in a small randomized trial of inhaled epoprostenol in 14 pediatric patients who had ARDS [100]. With no outcome data supporting the widespread use of inhaled epoprostenol in ARDS, these results should be interpreted cautiously; however, inhaled epoprostenol may be a reasonable therapeutic intervention in select patients who have ARDS with critical oxygenation failure.

Cardiac surgery

Patients undergoing cardiopulmonary bypass for coronary artery grafting or valvular surgery may have preexisting elevation of PVR from longstanding heart disease and are at risk for decompensated right heart failure in the postoperative period. The right ventricle seems most sensitive to the effects of cardiopulmonary bypass and cardioplegia. Inhaled agents are attractive in this setting because they tend to have less effect on systemic blood pressure than intravenous agents. A recent study of 58 patients who had mitral stenosis and preexisting pulmonary hypertension undergoing mitral valve replacement compared treatments with inhaled epoprostenol, nitric oxide, and placebo [101]. Statistically significant decreases in MPAP and PVR were observed in the epoprostenol and nitric oxide groups compared with the placebo group. No effect on mortality was seen in this small study, but both groups on active drug had shorter durations of intubation and time in the intensive care unit.

In another uncontrolled trial of 126 patients who underwent cardiopulmonary bypass and who had postoperative pulmonary hypertension, right heart failure, or refractory hypoxemia, improvement in cardiac output from 4.6 to 5.3 L/m ($P = .037$) and fall in MPAP from 35 to 24 mm Hg ($P < .001$) were seen 6 hours after initiation of epoprostenol inhalation [102]. No difference in oxygenation was seen. Currently, inhaled epoprostenol is a potential option for patients who experience decompensated right heart failure after cardiopulmonary bypass. Potential applications for prostanoids in the immediate post–cardiopulmonary bypass period also include management of patients after pulmonary thromboendarterectomy or lung and/or heart transplantation, and for acute right heart failure in the setting of protamine reversal of heparin when coming off of cardiopulmonary bypass [103,104]. Given the uncontrolled design of the studies performed, the role of epoprostenol or other prostanoids after cardiac surgery or cardiopulmonary bypass remains investigational.

Summary

The expanding arsenal of therapies has dramatically altered the outlook for patients who have PAH. Before the discovery and development of prostanoid medications for PAH treatment, options to alter disease course and prognosis were severely limited. This class of drugs is unique in its mechanisms of action and availability through multiple routes of administration. Newer PAH therapies, including endothelin-1 receptor antagonists and phosphodiesterase-5 inhibitors, ameliorate disease through alternative pathways. Although other drugs may improve surrogates for prognosis (ie, exercise tolerance, symptoms, and hemodynamics) and survival relative to historical controls, the prostanoid class includes the only agent (epoprostenol) that has been shown to have a favorable impact on short-term survival (in patients who have idiopathic PAH). As with many conditions, available data from individual trials of single agents do not provide evidence for selection of one optimal agent. Selection of individual therapies must be based on available data, clinical judgment, and patient preference. Combination of drugs acting through different mechanisms may provide additive benefit while potentially reducing undesirable side effects from higher doses of individual agents. The role of combination therapy and the use of prostanoids to treat conditions other than PAH are areas of ongoing and future investigation.

References

[1] Rubin LJ, Groves BM, Reeves JT, et al. Prostacyclin-induced acute pulmonary vasodilation in primary pulmonary hypertension. Circulation 1982; 66(2):334–8.

[2] Higenbottam T, Wheeldon D, Wells F, et al. Long-term treatment of primary pulmonary hypertension with continuous intravenous epoprostenol (prostacyclin). Lancet 1984;1(8385):1046–7.

[3] Barst RJ, Rubin LJ, Long WA, et al. A comparison of continuous intravenous epoprostenol (prostacyclin) with conventional therapy for primary pulmonary hypertension. The Primary Pulmonary Hypertension Study Group. N Engl J Med 1996; 334(5):296–302.

[4] Melian EB, Goa KL. Beraprost: a review of its pharmacology and therapeutic efficacy in the treatment of peripheral arterial disease and pulmonary arterial hypertension. Drugs 2002;62(1):107–33.

[5] Wishart DS, Knox C, Guo AC, et al. Drugbank: a comprehensive resource for in silico drug discovery and exploration. Nucleic Acids Res 2006; 34(Database issue):D668–72.

[6] Humbert M, Morrell NW, Archer SL, et al. Cellular and molecular pathobiology of pulmonary arterial hypertension. J Am Coll Cardiol 2004; 43(12 Suppl S):13S–24S.

[7] Jeffery TK, Morrell NW. Molecular and cellular basis of pulmonary vascular remodeling in pulmonary hypertension. Prog Cardiovasc Dis 2002; 45(3):173–202.

[8] Mandegar M, Fung YC, Huang W, et al. Cellular and molecular mechanisms of pulmonary vascular remodeling: role in the development of pulmonary hypertension. Microvasc Res 2004;68(2): 75–103.

[9] Moncada S, Gryglewski R, Bunting S, et al. An enzyme isolated from arteries transforms prostaglandin endoperoxides to an unstable substance that inhibits platelet aggregation. Nature 1976; 263(5579):663–5.

[10] Ubatuba FB, Moncada S, Vane JR. The effect of prostacyclin (PGT2) on platelet behaviour. Thrombus formation in vivo and bleeding time. Thromb Haemost 1979;41(2):425–35.

[11] Szczeklik A, Gryglewski RJ, Nizankowski R, et al. Circulatory and anti-platelet effects of intravenous prostacyclin in healthy men. Pharmacol Res Commun 1978;10(6):545–56.

[12] Whittle BJ. Role of prostaglandins in the defense of the gastric mucosa. Brain Res Bull 1980;5(Suppl 1): 7–14.

[13] Ogletree ML, Lefer AM, Smith JB, et al. Studies on the protective effect of prostacyclin in acute myocardial ischemia. Eur J Pharmacol 1979;56(1–2): 95–103.

[14] Ribeiro LG, Brandon TA, Hopkins DG, et al. Prostacyclin in experimental myocardial ischemia: effects on hemodynamics, regional myocardial blood flow, infarct size and mortality. Am J Cardiol 1981;47(4):835–40.

[15] Demling RH, Smith M, Gunther R, et al. The effect of prostacyclin infusion on endotoxin-induced lung injury. Surgery 1981;89(2):257–63.

[16] McLaughlin VV, Genthner DE, Panella MM, et al. Reduction in pulmonary vascular resistance with long-term epoprostenol (prostacyclin) therapy in primary pulmonary hypertension. N Engl J Med 1998;338(5):273–7.

[17] Friedman R, Mears JG, Barst RJ. Continuous infusion of prostacyclin normalizes plasma markers of endothelial cell injury and platelet aggregation in primary pulmonary hypertension. Circulation 1997;96(9):2782–4.

[18] Sakamaki F, Kyotani S, Nagaya N, et al. Increased plasma P-selectin and decreased thrombomodulin in pulmonary arterial hypertension were improved by continuous prostacyclin therapy. Circulation 2000;102(22):2720–5.

[19] Langleben D, Barst RJ, Badesch D, et al. Continuous infusion of epoprostenol improves the net balance between pulmonary endothelin-1 clearance and release in primary pulmonary hypertension. Circulation 1999;99(25):3266–71.

[20] Giaid A, Yanagisawa M, Langleben D, et al. Expression of endothelin-1 in the lungs of patients with pulmonary hypertension. N Engl J Med 1993;328(24):1732–9.

[21] Sulica R, Dinh HV, Dunsky K, et al. The acute hemodynamic effect of IV nitroglycerin and dipyridamole in patients with pulmonary arterial hypertension: comparison with IV epoprostenol. Congest Heart Fail 2005;11(3):139–44 [quiz: 145–6].

[22] Montalescot G, Drobinski G, Meurin P, et al. Effects of prostacyclin on the pulmonary vascular tone and cardiac contractility of patients with pulmonary hypertension secondary to end-stage heart failure. Am J Cardiol 1998;82(6):749–55.

[23] Tuder RM, Cool CD, Geraci MW, et al. Prostacyclin synthase expression is decreased in lungs from patients with severe pulmonary hypertension. Am J Respir Crit Care Med 1999;159(6):1925–32.

[24] Christman BW, McPherson CD, Newman JH, et al. An imbalance between the excretion of thromboxane and prostacyclin metabolites in pulmonary hypertension. N Engl J Med 1992;327(2):70–5.

[25] Tahara N, Kai H, Niiyama H, et al. Repeated gene transfer of naked prostacyclin synthase plasmid into skeletal muscles attenuates monocrotaline-induced pulmonary hypertension and prolongs survival in rats. Hum Gene Ther 2004;15(12):1270–8.

[26] Geraci MW, Gao B, Shepherd DC, et al. Pulmonary prostacyclin synthase overexpression in transgenic mice protects against development of hypoxic pulmonary hypertension. J Clin Invest 1999;103(11):1509–15.

[27] Hoshikawa Y, Voelkel NF, Gesell TL, et al. Prostacyclin receptor-dependent modulation of pulmonary vascular remodeling. Am J Respir Crit Care Med 2001;164(2):314–8.

[28] Wharton J, Davie N, Upton PD, et al. Prostacyclin analogues differentially inhibit growth of distal and proximal human pulmonary artery smooth muscle cells. Circulation 2000;102(25):3130–6.

[29] Clapp LH, Finney P, Turcato S, et al. Differential effects of stable prostacyclin analogs on smooth muscle proliferation and cyclic AMP generation in human pulmonary artery. Am J Respir Cell Mol Biol 2002;26(2):194–201.

[30] Kothapalli D, Stewart SA, Smyth EM, et al. Prostacylin receptor activation inhibits proliferation of aortic smooth muscle cells by regulating cAMP response element-binding protein- and pocket protein-dependent cyclin a gene expression. Mol Pharmacol 2003;64(2):249–58.

[31] Li RC, Cindrova-Davies T, Skepper JN, et al. Prostacyclin induces apoptosis of vascular smooth muscle cells by a cAMP-mediated inhibition of extracellular signal-regulated kinase activity and can counteract the mitogenic activity of endothelin-1 or basic fibroblast growth factor. Circ Res 2004;94(6):759–67.

[32] Vane JR, Botting RM. Pharmacodynamic profile of prostacyclin. Am J Cardiol 1995;75(3):3A–10A.

[33] Califf RM, Adams KF, McKenna WJ, et al. A randomized controlled trial of epoprostenol therapy for severe congestive heart failure: the Flolan International Randomized Survival Trial (FIRST). Am Heart J 1997;134(1):44–54.

[34] Long WA, Rubin LJ. Prostacyclin and PGE1 treatment of pulmonary hypertension. Am Rev Respir Dis 1987;136(3):773–6.

[35] Jones DK, Higenbottam TW, Wallwork J. Treatment of primary pulmonary hypertension intravenous epoprostenol (prostacyclin). Br Heart J 1987;57(3):270–8.

[36] Rubin LJ, Mendoza J, Hood M, et al. Treatment of primary pulmonary hypertension with continuous intravenous prostacyclin (epoprostenol). Results of a randomized trial. Ann Intern Med 1990;112(7):485–91.

[37] Barst RJ, Rubin LJ, McGoon MD, et al. Survival in primary pulmonary hypertension with long-term continuous intravenous prostacyclin. Ann Intern Med 1994;121(6):409–15.

[38] D'Alonzo GE, Barst RJ, Ayres SM, et al. Survival in patients with primary pulmonary hypertension. Results from a national prospective registry. Ann Intern Med 1991;115(5):343–9.

[39] Badesch DB, Tapson VF, McGoon MD, et al. Continuous intravenous epoprostenol for pulmonary hypertension due to the scleroderma spectrum of disease. A randomized, controlled trial. Ann Intern Med 2000;132(6):425–34.

[40] McLaughlin VV, Shillington A, Rich S. Survival in primary pulmonary hypertension: the impact of epoprostenol therapy. Circulation 2002;106(12):1477–82.

[41] Sitbon O, Humbert M, Nunes H, et al. Long-term intravenous epoprostenol infusion in primary pulmonary hypertension: prognostic factors and survival. J Am Coll Cardiol 2002;40(4):780–8.

[42] Conte JV, Gaine SP, Orens JB, et al. The influence of continuous intravenous prostacyclin therapy for primary pulmonary hypertension on the timing and outcome of transplantation. J Heart Lung Transplant 1998;17(7):679–85.

[43] Edelman JD, Palevsky HI. Has prostacyclin replaced transplantation as the treatment of choice for primary pulmonary hypertension. Clinical Pulmonary Medicine 2000;7(2):90–6.

[44] Flolan (epoprostenol sodium) for Injection [package insert]. Research Triangle Park (NC): GlaxoSmithKline; 2006.

[45] Galie N, Torbicki A, Barst R, et al. Guidelines on diagnosis and treatment of pulmonary arterial hypertension. The task force on diagnosis and treatment of pulmonary arterial hypertension of the European society of cardiology. Eur Heart J 2004;25(24):2243–78.

[46] Wasserman K, Oudiz R. Overdosing with prostacyclin in primary pulmonary hypertension. J Am Coll Cardiol 2000;35(7):1995–6.

[47] Remodulin (treprostinil sodium) Injection [package insert]. Research Triangle Park (NC): Corp UT; 2006.

[48] Simonneau G, Barst RJ, Galie N, et al. Continuous subcutaneous infusion of treprostinil, a prostacyclin analogue, in patients with pulmonary arterial hypertension: a double-blind, randomized, placebo-controlled trial. Am J Respir Crit Care Med 2002;165(6):800–4.

[49] Lang I, Gomez-Sanchez M, Kneussl M, et al. Efficacy of long-term subcutaneous treprostinil sodium therapy in pulmonary hypertension. Chest 2006; 129(6):1636–43.

[50] Barst RJ, Galie N, Naeije R, et al. Long-term outcome in pulmonary arterial hypertension patients treated with treprostinil. Eur Respir J 2006;28(6):1195–203.

[51] Laliberte K, Arneson C, Jeffs R, et al. Pharmacokinetics and steady-state bioequivalence of treprostinil sodium (Remodulin) administered by the intravenous and subcutaneous route to normal volunteers. J Cardiovasc Pharmacol 2004;44(2): 209–14.

[52] McLaughlin VV, Gaine SP, Barst RJ, et al. Efficacy and safety of treprostinil: an epoprostenol analog for primary pulmonary hypertension. J Cardiovasc Pharmacol 2003;41(2):293–9.

[53] Tapson VF, Gomberg-Maitland M, McLaughlin VV, et al. Safety and efficacy of IV treprostinil for pulmonary arterial hypertension: a prospective, multicenter, open-label, 12-week trial. Chest 2006; 129(3):683–8.

[54] Gomberg-Maitland M, Tapson VF, Benza RL, et al. Transition from intravenous epoprostenol to intravenous treprostinil in pulmonary hypertension. Am J Respir Crit Care Med 2005;172(12): 1586–9.

[55] Sandifer BL, Brigham KL, Lawrence EC, et al. Potent effects of aerosol compared with intravenous treprostinil on the pulmonary circulation. J Appl Physiol 2005;99(6):2363–8.

[56] Sandifer BL, Brigham KL, Lawrence EC, et al. Effects of aerosol vs IV UT-15 on prostaglandin H2 analog-induced pulmonary hypertension in sheep. Chest 2005;128(6 Suppl):616S.

[57] Voswinckel R, Ghofrani HA, Grimminger F, et al. Inhaled treprostinil [corrected] for treatment of chronic pulmonary arterial hypertension. Ann Intern Med 2006;144(2):149–50.

[58] Channick RN, Olschewski H, Seeger W, et al. Safety and efficacy of inhaled treprostinil as add-on therapy to bosentan in pulmonary arterial hypertension. J Am Coll Cardiol 2006;48(7):1433–7.

[59] Higenbottam TW, Butt AY, Dinh-Xuan AT, et al. Treatment of pulmonary hypertension with the continuous infusion of a prostacyclin analogue, iloprost. Heart 1998;79(2):175–9.

[60] Scott JP, Higenbottam T, Wallwork J. The acute effect of the synthetic prostacyclin analogue iloprost in primary pulmonary hypertension. Br J Clin Pract 1990;44(6):231–4.

[61] Gessler T, Schmehl T, Hoeper MM, et al. Ultrasonic versus jet nebulization of iloprost in severe pulmonary hypertension. Eur Respir J 2001;17(1): 14–9.

[62] Ventavis (iloprost) Inhalation Solution [package insert]. South San Francisco (CA): Cotherix; 2006.

[63] Hoeper MM, Schwarze M, Ehlerding S, et al. Long-term treatment of primary pulmonary hypertension with aerosolized iloprost, a prostacyclin analogue. N Engl J Med 2000;342(25):1866–70.

[64] Olschewski H, Simonneau G, Galie N, et al. Inhaled iloprost for severe pulmonary hypertension. N Engl J Med 2002;347(5):322–9.

[65] Opitz CF, Wensel R, Winkler J, et al. Clinical efficacy and survival with first-line inhaled iloprost therapy in patients with idiopathic pulmonary arterial hypertension. Eur Heart J 2005;26(18): 1895–902.

[66] Seyfarth HJ, Pankau H, Hammerschmidt S, et al. Bosentan improves exercise tolerance and Tei index in patients with pulmonary hypertension and prostanoid therapy. Chest 2005;128(2):709–13.

[67] Hoeper MM, Taha N, Bekjarova A, et al. Bosentan treatment in patients with primary pulmonary hypertension receiving nonparenteral prostanoids. Eur Respir J 2003;22(2):330–4.

[68] Ghofrani HA, Rose F, Schermuly RT, et al. Oral sildenafil as long-term adjunct therapy to inhaled iloprost in severe pulmonary arterial hypertension. J Am Coll Cardiol 2003;42(1):158–64.

[69] Okano Y, Yoshioka T, Shimouchi A, et al. Orally active prostacyclin analogue in primary pulmonary hypertension. Lancet 1997;349(9062):1365.

[70] Nagaya N, Uematsu M, Okano Y, et al. Effect of orally active prostacyclin analogue on survival of outpatients with primary pulmonary hypertension. J Am Coll Cardiol 1999;34(4):1188–92.

[71] Galie N, Humbert M, Vachiery JL, et al. Effects of beraprost sodium, an oral prostacyclin analogue, in patients with pulmonary arterial hypertension: a randomized, double-blind, placebo-controlled trial. J Am Coll Cardiol 2002;39(9):1496–502.

[72] Barst RJ, McGoon M, McLaughlin V, et al. Beraprost therapy for pulmonary arterial hypertension. J Am Coll Cardiol 2003;41(12):2119–25.

[73] McLaughlin VV, Oudiz RJ, Frost A, et al. Randomized study of adding inhaled iloprost to existing bosentan in pulmonary arterial hypertension. Am J Respir Crit Care Med 2006;174(11):1257–63.

[74] Humbert M, Barst RJ, Robbins IM, et al. Combination of bosentan with epoprostenol in pulmonary arterial hypertension: BREATHE-2. Eur Respir J 2004;24(3):353–9.

[75] Rich S, Dantzker DR, Ayres SM, et al. Primary pulmonary hypertension. A national prospective study. Ann Intern Med 1987;107(2):216–23.

[76] Barst RJ, Maislin G, Fishman AP. Vasodilator therapy for primary pulmonary hypertension in children. Circulation 1999;99(9):1197–208.

[77] Rosenzweig EB, Kerstein D, Barst RJ. Long-term prostacyclin for pulmonary hypertension with associated congenital heart defects. Circulation 1999;99(14):1858–65.

[78] Wigley FM, Lima JA, Mayes M, et al. The prevalence of undiagnosed pulmonary arterial hypertension in subjects with connective tissue disease at the secondary health care level of community-based rheumatologists (the UNCOVER study). Arthritis Rheum 2005;52(7):2125–32.

[79] Oudiz RJ, Schilz RJ, Barst RJ, et al. Treprostinil, a prostacyclin analogue, in pulmonary arterial hypertension associated with connective tissue disease. Chest 2004;126(2):420–7.

[80] Matsukawa Y, Saito O, Aoki M, et al. Long-term administration of beraprost, an oral prostacyclin analogue, improves pulmonary diffusion capacity in patients with systemic sclerosis. Prostaglandins Leukot Essent Fatty Acids 2002;67(1):45–9.

[81] Caramaschi P, Biasi D, Ferrari M, et al. Long-term evaluation of lung function in patients affected by scleroderma treated with cyclic iloprost infusions. Rheumatol Int 2005;25(4):250–4.

[82] Ghofrani HA, Friese G, Discher T, et al. Inhaled iloprost is a potent acute pulmonary vasodilator in HIV-related severe pulmonary hypertension. Eur Respir J 2004;23(2):321–6.

[83] Aguilar RV, Farber HW. Epoprostenol (prostacyclin) therapy in HIV-associated pulmonary hypertension. Am J Respir Crit Care Med 2000;162(5):1846–50.

[84] Nunes H, Humbert M, Sitbon O, et al. Prognostic factors for survival in human immunodeficiency virus-associated pulmonary arterial hypertension. Am J Respir Crit Care Med 2003;167(10):1433–9.

[85] Kuo PC, Johnson LB, Plotkin JS, et al. Continuous intravenous infusion of epoprostenol for the treatment of portopulmonary hypertension. Transplantation 1997;63(4):604–6.

[86] Krowka MJ, Frantz RP, McGoon MD, et al. Improvement in pulmonary hemodynamics during intravenous epoprostenol (prostacyclin): a study of 15 patients with moderate to severe portopulmonary hypertension. Hepatology 1999;30(3):641–8.

[87] Plotkin JS, Kuo PC, Rubin LJ, et al. Successful use of chronic epoprostenol as a bridge to liver transplantation in severe portopulmonary hypertension. Transplantation 1998;65(4):457–9.

[88] Kahler CM, Graziadei I, Wiedermann CJ, et al. Successful use of continuous intravenous prostacyclin in a patient with severe portopulmonary hypertension. Wien Klin Wochenschr 2000;112(14):637–40.

[89] Tan HP, Markowitz JS, Montgomery RA, et al. Liver transplantation in patients with severe portopulmonary hypertension treated with preoperative chronic intravenous epoprostenol. Liver Transpl 2001;7(8):745–9.

[90] Minder S, Fischler M, Muellhaupt B, et al. Intravenous iloprost bridging to orthotopic liver transplantation in portopulmonary hypertension. Eur Respir J 2004;24(4):703–7.

[91] Halank M, Kolditz M, Miehlke S, et al. Combination therapy for portopulmonary hypertension with intravenous iloprost and oral bosentan. Wien Med Wochenschr 2005;155(15–16):376–80.

[92] Laving A, Khanna A, Rubin L, et al. Successful liver transplantation in a child with severe portopulmonary hypertension treated with epoprostenol. J Pediatr Gastroenterol Nutr 2005;41(4):466–8.

[93] Sussman N, Kaza V, Barshes N, et al. Successful liver transplantation following medical management of portopulmonary hypertension: a single-center series. Am J Transplant 2006;6(9):2177–82.

[94] Chinnakotla S, Ashfaq M, Davis GL, et al. Liver transplantation in patients with severe portopulmonary hypertension. Transplantation 2006;82 (1 Suppl 3):331.

[95] Fix OK, Bass NM, DeMarco T, et al. Long-term follow-up of portopulmonary hypertension treated with epoprostenol. Transplantation 2006;82(1 Suppl 3):331–2.

[96] Ono F, Nagaya N, Okumura H, et al. Effect of orally active prostacyclin analogue on survival in patients with chronic thromboembolic pulmonary hypertension without major vessel obstruction. Chest 2003;123(5):1583–8.

[97] Ghofrani HA, Wiedemann R, Rose F, et al. Combination therapy with oral sildenafil and inhaled iloprost for severe pulmonary hypertension. Ann Intern Med 2002;136(7):515–22.

[98] Vizza CD, Badagliacca R, Sciomer S, Poscia R, et al. Mid-term efficacy of beraprost, an oral prostacyclin analog, in the treatment of distal CTEPH: a case control study. Cardiology. 2006;106(3):168–73.

[99] Walmrath D, Schneider T, Schermuly R, et al. Direct comparison of inhaled nitric oxide and aerosolized prostacyclin in acute respiratory distress syndrome. Am J Respir Crit Care Med 1996;153(3):991–6.

[100] Dahlem P, van Aalderen WM, de Neef M, et al. Randomized controlled trial of aerosolized prostacyclin therapy in children with acute lung injury. Crit Care Med 2004;32(4):1055–60.

[101] Fattouch K, Sbraga F, Sampognaro R, et al. Treatment of pulmonary hypertension in patients undergoing cardiac surgery with cardiopulmonary bypass: a randomized, prospective, double-blind study. J Cardiovasc Med (Hagerstown) 2006;7(2): 119–23.

[102] De Wet CJ, Affleck DG, Jacobsohn E, et al. Inhaled prostacyclin is safe, effective, and affordable in patients with pulmonary hypertension, right heart dysfunction, and refractory hypoxemia after cardiothoracic surgery. J Thorac Cardiovasc Surg 2004;127(4):1058–67.

[103] Kramm T, Eberle B, Guth S, et al. Inhaled iloprost to control residual pulmonary hypertension following pulmonary endarterectomy. Eur J Cardiothorac Surg 2005;28(6):882–8.

[104] Ocal A, Kiris I, Erdinc M, et al. Efficiency of prostacyclin in the treatment of protamine-mediated right ventricular failure and acute pulmonary hypertension. Tohoku J Exp Med 2005;207(1):51–8.

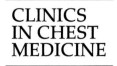

Clin Chest Med 28 (2007) 143–167

The Nitric Oxide/cGMP Signaling Pathway in Pulmonary Hypertension

James R. Klinger, MD[a,b,*]

[a]*Division of Pulmonary Sleep and Critical Care Medicine, Rhode Island Hospital,*
593 Eddy Street, Providence, RI 02903, USA
[b]*Brown Medical School, Box G-A, Providence, RI 02912, USA*

Nitric oxide (NO) is synthesized in the pulmonary vascular endothelium in response to various stimuli. Once released, it rapidly diffuses across cell membranes to reach the cytoplasm of adjacent vascular smooth muscle cells, where it binds to soluble guanylate cyclase (sGC) and increases intracellular cGMP levels. Cyclic GMP in turn phosphorylates cGMP-dependent protein kinase (PKG), which acts at several sites within the cell membrane and endoplastic reticulum to lower intracellular Ca^{2+} levels and reduce cross-linking of myosin light chain and decrease vascular tone. Although controversy exists as to the exact role that NO plays in the pathophysiology of pulmonary hypertensive diseases, numerous studies have demonstrated that pulmonary hemodynamics and functional capacity can be improved in patients with pulmonary arterial hypertension (PAH) by increasing NO delivery to the lung or slowing the metabolism of cGMP. Pharmacologic therapies that target the NO/cGMP pathway represent one of the major approaches to medical management of the patient with PAH. This article briefly reviews the background of endothelium-dependent vasorelaxation, describes the NO/cGMP/PKG pathway and its role in modulating pulmonary vascular tone and remodeling, and describes three approaches that target the NO/cGMP pathway in the treatment of patients with PAH.

This work was funded in part by American Heart Association Established Investigator Award 0240190N to the author.

* Division of Pulmonary and Critical Care Medicine, Rhode Island Hospital, 593 Eddy Street, Providence, RI 02903.

E-mail address: james_klinger@brown.edu

Endothelium-dependent vasodilation

The concept that vascular tone could be regulated by secretion of vasoactive factors from the vascular endothelium was proposed in earnest approximately 25 years ago by Furchgott and colleagues [1,2]. They found that acetylcholine caused vasodilation in isolated rabbit aorta when used at low doses. This finding was contrary to the results of other studies at that time, which showed that acetylcholine caused vasoconstriction in isolated vessels [3]. Upon further study, they discovered that accidentally rubbing the vessel segment against a foreign body during preparation for the experiment damaged the endothelial surface and rendered it insensitive to the vasodilating effect of acetylcholine. In a seminal paper published the following year [4], they were able to demonstrate that removing the endothelium from the luminal surface of aortic strips completely abolished the relaxation response to acetylcholine. Attaching a strip with intact endothelium, intimal surface to intimal surface, to the denuded strip restored the vasorelaxing effect of acetylcholine. The authors hypothesized that in response to the proper stimulus, endothelial cells released a vasodilator substance that acted on the adjacent vascular smooth muscle. This substance could not be inactivated by inhibition of the cyclo-oxygenase pathway and was not felt to be a prostaglandin. The substance was termed endothelial-derived relaxing factor (EDRF) and in additional experiments by Furchgott and by other investigators [4–6] was found to be critical for acetylcholine- and bradykinin-induced relaxation of pulmonary and systemic vessels. In 1987, EDRF was simultaneously identified as NO by two different groups of investigators [7,8].

The discovery of EDRF suggested that the circulatory system was more than a passive conduit under the control of the central nervous system and vasoactive substances secreted by distant organs. Rather, the vascular endothelium had the capacity to regulate its own blood flow by secreting vasoactive substances in response to local stimuli. The discovery of EDRF was one of the major advances of vascular biology over the last quarter century and greatly enhanced our understanding of the pathophysiology of pulmonary and other vascular diseases. In the flurry of investigations that followed the identification of EDRF, NO was found not only to modulate vascular tone but also to mediate diverse biologic functions, including inflammation, platelet aggregation, and intracellular killing. The importance of NO in biology was underscored by its recognition as "Molecule of the Year" by the journal *Science* in 1992 [9] and by the awarding of the Nobel Prize in Physiology and Medicine to Furchgott and Ignarro in 1998.

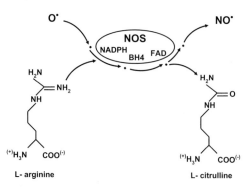

Fig. 1. Synthesis of NO by NO synthase. NO is produced when an electron from oxygen is transferred to an amino terminal nitrogen of L-arginine. Electron transfer is facilitated by the enzyme nitric oxide synthase (NOS) and uses various cofactors, including NADPH, 6(R)-5,6,7,8-tetrahydrobiopterin (BH4) and flavin adenine dinucleotide and flavin mononucleo-tide (FAD). Completion of the reaction produces NO and H_2O while converting L-arginine to L-citrulline.

The nitric oxide/cGMP signaling pathway

It is now known that NO is synthesized by the pulmonary vascular endothelium in response to various mediators, including acetylcholine, bradykinin, intracellular Ca^{2+} levels ($[Ca^{2+}]_i$), endothelin, and shear stress caused by increased flow. NO is produced by a biochemical reaction that transfers an electron from molecular oxygen through several cofactors, including reduced NADPH, 6(R)-5,6,7,8-tetrahydrobiopterin, flavin adenine dinucleotide and flavin mononucleotide to an amino terminal nitrogen of L-arginine (Fig. 1) [10]. Completion of the reaction consumes molecular oxygen and produces NO and H_2O while converting L-arginine to L-citrulline. This multistep reaction is catalyzed by a group of enzymes known as nitric oxide syntheses (NOS). Three isoforms of NOS have been described. NOS-I is a constitutively expressed enzyme referred to as neuronal endothelial NOS because of its presence in neuronal cells. Isoform II is a rapidly activated enzyme known as inducible NOS (iNOS) that is upregulated in response to inflammation and responsible for NO-mediated bacterial killing in macrophages. The third isoform, NOS-III, is found throughout the vascular endothelium and is known as endothelial NOS (eNOS). Although this enzyme is constitutively expressed, its rate of posttranscriptional processing is affected by various environmental factors, most notably shear stress and hypoxia, that significantly increase and decrease eNOS activity and production of pulmonary NO, respectively [11–13].

Newly synthesized NO in vascular endothelial cells rapidly diffuses across cellular membranes to the cytoplasm of adjacent smooth muscle cells, where it activates sGC and increases intracellular cGMP levels. Several downstream protein targets for cGMP have been identified, including cGMP gated cation channels, cGMP-dependent protein kinase (PKG), and the cyclic nucleotide phosphodiesterases (PDE) that are responsible for its degradation (Fig. 2) [14].

The most immediate effect of NO/cGMP signaling on vascular smooth muscle is a decrease in tone. Although it is possible that cGMP may act directly on cation channels on the cell surface to reduce influx of extracellular Ca^{2+}, most studies strongly implicate PKG as the mediator of cGMP-induced vasodilation. After activation by cGMP, PKG affects several regulators of cytosolic Ca^{2+} flux to decrease the concentration of $[Ca^{2+}]_i$ and thereby relax vascular smooth muscle. Among the myriad effects of activated PKG are (1) decreased Ca^{2+} entry into cells via inhibition of voltage- and receptor-operated calcium channels in the cell wall [15,16], (2) cellular hyperpolarization caused by activation of Ca^{2+} activated K^+ channels [17], (3) increased cellular extrusion of Ca^{2+} via activation of Ca^{2+}-ATPase pumps and the sodium/calcium exchanger [18,19], and (4)

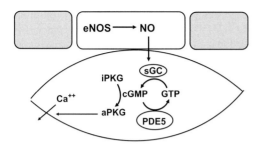

Fig. 2. NO/cGMP/PKG pathway. Highly lipid soluble NO produced in the vascular endothelium diffuses rapidly across cell membranes and activates soluble guanylyl cyclase (sGC) in the cytoplasm of the smooth muscle cell. Binding to sGC results in increased intracellular cGMP levels that activate cGMP-dependent protein kinase (PKG), which acts on various downstream targets to decrease intracellular calcium concentrations $[Ca^{++}]_i$ and thereby cause vasorelaxation.

inhibition of Ca^{2+} release from the sarcoplasmic reticulum [20]. In addition to decreasing $[Ca^{2+}]_i$, PKG may decrease smooth muscle contractile tone via calcium desensitization of the contractile elements and dephosphorylation of myosin light chains. Possible mechanisms for this effect of PKG include inhibition of myosin light chain phosphatase, inhibition of RhoA, and phosphorylation of the myosin-binding protein telokin [21,22].

Signaling through the NO/cGMP pathway also has important antimitogenic and pro-apoptotic effects on vascular smooth muscle and endothelial cells that play a pivotal role in pulmonary vascular remodeling. Activation of the NO/cGMP pathway has been shown to inhibit proliferation of bronchial smooth muscle [23] and vascular smooth muscle cells from the systemic [24–26] and pulmonary circulations [27–29] and to induce apoptosis in pulmonary vascular smooth muscle cells and endothelial cells [29–31]. Although some studies [27] found that NO donors inhibit proliferation of fetal porcine pulmonary vascular smooth muscle cells in a dose-dependent manner, other studies [32] suggest that NO has a variable effect with inhibition at high doses (10^{-3}–10^{-2} M) and a stimulatory growth effect at lower doses.

The effect of NO on endothelial cell proliferation is less clear. Transfection of sheep arterial endothelial cells with an adenoviral vector that contains the human iNOS cDNA produced 25- to 100-fold more NO than control infected cells as measured by nitrite accumulation but did not inhibit endothelial cell proliferation, viability, or apoptosis [33]. On the other hand, co-culture of

calf pulmonary artery endothelial cells with rat smooth muscle cells transfected with plasmid containing eNOS resulted in the formation of extensive capillary-like structures within 48 hours [34], suggesting that NO stimulates apoptosis and endothelial cell proliferation. This pro-angiogenic effect of NO may have beneficial effects in pulmonary vascular disease. Administration of syngeneic fibroblasts transfected with eNOS was recently shown to partially regenerate the pulmonary microcirculation and reduce pulmonary arterial pressure (PAP) and right ventricular hypertrophy in rats with monocrotaline-induced pulmonary hypertension [35].

The mechanism by which NO inhibits endothelial and smooth muscle cell proliferation is not completely understood. Most studies suggest that the antiproliferative effect of NO is mediated by cGMP [25,36–38] and downstream activation of PKG [39–41]. These conclusions stem from observations that NO inhibition of vascular smooth muscle cell growth is accompanied by an increase in intracellular cGMP levels [27], mimicked by administration of cell-permeant analogs of cGMP alone [39,40,42], potentiated by inhibition of cGMP metabolism [30,40], and blunted by inhibition of PKG [30,39,42]. Other studies have presented conflicting results regarding the role of PKG in mediating mitogenic effects of NO, however. For example, adenoviral upregulation of PKG had no effect on PDGF-induced proliferation of rat aortic vascular smooth muscle cells [41], and activation of PKG has been implicated in vascular proliferation and atherosclerotic plaque formation [43,44]. On the other hand, adenoviral upregulation of PKG has been shown to accentuate the inhibitor effect of NO on pulmonary vascular smooth muscle cell proliferation [45]. Recently, we found that inhibition of PKG completely abolished atrial natriuretic peptide-induced inhibition of pulmonary vascular smooth muscle cell proliferation [46]. Like NO, atrial natriuretic peptide increases intracellular cGMP levels via activation of guanylate cyclases. Our findings support a role for PKG in modulating cGMP-induced inhibition of pulmonary vascular smooth muscle cells.

Recent studies have shown that NO also inhibits endothelial and vascular smooth muscle cell proliferation via cGMP-independent pathways [24,47–49]. In particular, NO has been shown to change the expression and activity of cell cycle regulatory proteins [24,50]. NO also inhibits ornithine decarboxylase and polyamine synthesis [51,52]. Bauer and colleagues [51] showed that NO inhibition of ornithine decarboxylase blunts cellular proliferation via activation of p42/p44 MAPK and induction of p21(waf1/cip1). Recent data suggest that NO may also blunt vascular smooth muscle cell proliferation by direct S-nitrosation and inactivation of RhoA, identifying yet another cGMP-independent mechanism of NO-mediated antimitogenesis [53].

Part of the problem in interpreting data from studies that examine the effect of NO on cellular proliferation is the lack of uniformity in experimental conditions. In particular, the use of high passage cell cultures is complicated by the reduction or absence of PKG expression as cells approach a de-differentiated state. Under these circumstances, activation of the NO/cGMP pathway may result in greater activation of cAMP-dependent protein kinase (PKA). Several studies have shown that cGMP can inhibit vascular smooth muscle cell proliferation via activation of cAMP-dependent protein kinase (PKA) as opposed to PKG [54,55]. Another area of potential confusion is the dose of NO studied. At lower concentrations, NO has been shown to promote mitogenesis [56] and facilitate the proliferative effects of other growth factors, such as basic fibroblast growth factor [57,58]. In one study of pulmonary arterial smooth muscle cells [43], lower doses of NO augmented proliferation, whereas higher doses of NO suppressed it under the same experimental conditions. Although data from some studies are conflicting, a picture is emerging that shows NO to be capable of inhibiting and facilitating proliferation of vascular smooth muscle cells and endothelial cells depending on the concentration of NO, the stage of vascular remodeling at which NO is introduced, and the expression and activity of secondary messengers and downstream targets in the NO/cGMP pathway.

Role of the nitric oxide/cGMP pathway in modulating pulmonary vascular tone

Under normal conditions, the pulmonary circulation is a low-pressure system with a total resistance only approximately one-eighth that of the systemic circulation. Unlike the systemic circulation, in which the greatest resistance to flow is medium sized, well-muscularized arterioles under the influence of autonomic and adrenergic regulation, most of the resistance across the pulmonary vascular bed occurs at the level of peripheral precapillary vessels. The role of the NO/cGMP pathway in modulating changes in the pulmonary microcirculation under normal conditions is not completely understood, but it seems to play a vital role in regulating changes in pulmonary vascular tone at birth and in the vascular remodeling of pulmonary hypertensive diseases.

Animal studies have shown that pulmonary eNOS expression is developmentally regulated. The concentrations of eNOS and eNOS mRNA in rat lung increase during fetal life, peak shortly after birth, and then decline rapidly as the animal matures [59,60]. Although it is not yet possible to examine developmental regulation of pulmonary NOS expression in humans, similar patterns of upregulated eNOS and iNOS expression during fetal life followed by decreasing expression after birth have been reported in pigs, sheep, and baboons [61–63]. The close coordination of pulmonary NOS expression with birth suggests that the NO/cGMP pathway plays a vital role in the transition of the pulmonary circulation from a high resistance to a low resistance vascular bed during the immediate postpartum period. Animal models of fetal pulmonary hypertension are associated with decreased eNOS expression [64,65], and inhibitors of NO synthesis cause acute pulmonary vasoconstriction in the newborns of most animals [66–68]. Congenital diseases such as persistent pulmonary hypertension of the newborn and congenital diaphragmatic hernia that result in failure of the pulmonary circulation to convert to a low pressure system at birth have been associated with decreased NOS expression, decreased bioavailability of NO precursors, and reduced NO production [69,70]. Conversely, inhaled NO (iNO) has a marked vasodilator effect on the pulmonary hypertensive fetal circulation. In fact, the unique responsiveness of the newborn lung to NO has resulted in the development and approval of iNO therapy for persistent pulmonary hypertension of the newborn [71,72].

The role of the NO/cGMP pathway in regulating basal pulmonary vascular tone in adult life, however, is less clear. Immunohistochemical and in situ hybridization studies show only scant NOS expression in the peripheral resistance vessels of adult animal and human pulmonary resistance vessels [59,73–75], although other investigators have reported extensive eNOS expression throughout the human adult pulmonary circulation [76]. Inhalation of NO has little acute effect on PAP in healthy animals or humans under normoxic conditions [77–79], which suggests that under baseline conditions, pulmonary vascular tone is either unresponsive to NO or already maximally dilated by it. Support for both hypotheses has been generated by studies reporting no effect of various NOS inhibitors on resting pulmonary vascular tone and studies showing that NOS inhibition causes acute pulmonary vasoconstriction. Disagreement among these studies may be explained by differences in experimental technique, including the dose and selectivity of the NOS inhibitor used. Other factors, such as the use of crystalloid versus blood in the perfusate and the viscosity of the perfusate, also can affect results. Blood products scavenge excess NO and a higher viscosity increases endogenous NO synthesis by increasing shear stress [80]. Some of the confusion from these studies can be clarified by examining the relative effect of NOS inhibition on the pulmonary versus the systemic circulation. Using isolated lung and kidney from the same rat, Hampl and colleagues [81] found that the dose of NOS inhibitor N^{ω}-nitro-L-arginine (L-NA) needed to double perfusion pressure in the kidney had no effect on perfusion pressure in the lung. Similar findings have been demonstrated in healthy human volunteers (ie, administration of NOS inhibitors at doses sufficient to induce systemic hypertension has minimal or no effect on PAP) [82]. If endogenous NO production plays any role in maintaining basal pulmonary tone, it is likely to be minimal and significantly less than the role it plays in the systemic circulation.

On the other hand, NO has been shown to be an effective pulmonary vasodilator once pulmonary vascular tone is increased. NO blunts acute hypoxic pulmonary vasoconstriction in isolated rat lungs and human volunteers [83,84] and lowers PAP in intact sheep with thromboxane-induced pulmonary hypertension and in pigs with endotoxin-induced or embolic pulmonary hypertension [85–87] and in patients with acute lung injury [88]. In addition to acting as an acute pulmonary vasodilator, NO has been shown to decrease pulmonary vascular tone in many models of established pulmonary hypertension. Isolated lungs and pulmonary arterial rings from pulmonary hypertensive rats have a vasodilator response to NO and a vasoconstrictor response to NOS inhibition. In some studies, the vasodilator effect of NO is greater in pulmonary hypertensive lungs than in lungs and vessels obtained from control rats [89,90]. For example, Jiang and colleagues [78] found that intact rats have no pulmonary vasodilator response to iNO

under normoxic conditions but demonstrate increasingly greater vasodilation in response to NO as they develop progressive pulmonary hypertension in response to chronic hypoxia (Fig. 3). The degree of NO-induced vasodilation correlates with the degree of muscularization of the pulmonary resistance vessels [78]. These findings suggest that the pulmonary circulation becomes more responsive to the vasodilator effects of NO when pulmonary vascular tone is increased in response to acute hypoxia, administration of pulmonary vasoconstrictors, or pulmonary vascular remodeling that occurs in established pulmonary hypertension. Endogenous NO may play an increasingly important role in mitigating pulmonary vasoconstriction in diseases in which pulmonary vascular tone is increased.

Nitric oxide in the pathogenesis of pulmonary arterial hypertension

During the development of experimentally induced pulmonary hypertension, endogenous NO synthesis seems to increase. Chronic hypoxia increases expression of iNOS and eNOS in the endothelium of pulmonary resistance vessels and increases NOS activity [75,91]. As a result, levels of NO decomposition products are greater in the effluent of lungs obtained from rats with hypoxic pulmonary hypertension than in control lungs [92]. The increase in NO expression seen in these studies has been interpreted as a counterregulatory response to the development of pulmonary hypertension. If this hypothesis is correct, failure to adequately increase NO expression in response to hypertensive stimuli could contribute to the development of pulmonary vascular remodeling and sustained pulmonary hypertensive disease. In an often cited report, Giaid and colleagues [76] described diffusely positive immunostaining for eNOS throughout the pulmonary resistance vessels of lungs from patients without pulmonary hypertensive disease and near absence of eNOS expression in lungs from patients who have PAH. Decreased pulmonary endothelial expression of eNOS and increased expression of arginase II, an enzyme that decreases the bioavailability of L-arginine for NO synthesis, has also recently been reported in patients who have PAH [93]. Patients who have anorexigen-associated PAH seem to have decreased lung NO synthesis compared with patients who have idiopathic PAH (IPAH) [94], and patients who have PAH associated with

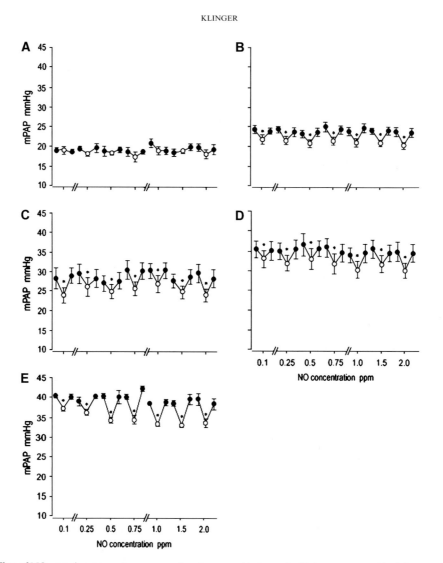

Fig. 3. Effect of NO on pulmonary artery pressure in rats exposed to hypoxia. Rats were exposed to (*A*) normoxia or (*B*) 5 days, (*C*) 10 days, (*D*) 11–20 days, and (*E*) 21–29 days of hypoxia and then anesthetized. Pulmonary catheters were inserted to measure mean pulmonary artery pressure (mPAP) during awake inhalation of room air (*closed circles*) or nitric oxide (*open circles*). Rats with more advanced hypoxic pulmonary hypertension had a greater pulmonary vasodilator response to nitric oxide. Values shown are mean ± SEM. *$P < .05$ compared with room air. ppm, parts per million. (*From* Jiang BH, Maruyama J, Yokochi A, et al. Correlation of inhaled nitric-oxide induced reduction of pulmonary artery pressure and vascular changes. Eur Respir J 2002;20(1):55; with permission.)

scleroderma have decreased levels of exhaled NO compared with controls [95].

These findings support the hypothesis that decreased endogenous expression of NO contributes to the development of PAH. The results of these studies have been challenged by other investigators, however, who have found increased expression of eNOS and iNOS in the plexiform lesions of lungs from patients who have IPAH and PAH associated with congenital left to right

shunts [96,97]. Increased pulmonary expression of eNOS also has been described in pulmonary hemangiomatosis and in smooth muscle lesions in patients who have lymphangioleiomyomatosis, which suggests that pulmonary endothelial and smooth muscle hyperplasia are associated with increased NO expression [98,99].

Studies in genetically altered mice have failed to define a clear role for NO in the pathology of pulmonary hypertensive disease. Mice with gene targeted deletion of eNOS from conception (eNOS knockout mice) have elevated PAP and increased muscularization of pulmonary arteries under baseline conditions and in response to chronic hypoxia [100–103]. Other investigators found reduced PAP and less muscularization of peripheral pulmonary vessels in eNOS knockouts exposed to chronic hypoxia compared with wild-type mice, however [104]. Discrepancies between studies such as these have not been resolved satisfactorily. Absence of eNOS expression during development may result in an abnormal pulmonary circulation with increased resistance because of inadequate development of pulmonary capillaries or insufficient inhibition of vascular growth factors. It seems that the NO/cGMP pathway modulates pulmonary vascular remodeling, but what effect it has may depend on several factors, including the local concentration of NO, the concentration of free radicals, the stage of pulmonary vascular remodeling that is present at the time that NO synthesis is altered, and likely the balance of expression of other growth factors that contribute to the underlying pulmonary hypertensive diseases.

Despite the uncertainty of the role of NO/cGMP in the development of pulmonary hypertensive diseases, there has been wide consensus that activating the NO/cGMP pathway in established pulmonary hypertension can help reduce PAP and reverse pulmonary vascular remodeling. Inhalation of exogenous NO or increasing endogenous NO production via a variety of methods, such as aerosol or cell-based gene transfer, to increase eNOS expression in the lung has been shown to lower PAP and reduce right ventricular hypertrophy and muscularization of pulmonary arteries in animal models of pulmonary hypertension [105–108].

Nitric oxide/cGMP in the treatment of pulmonary arterial hypertension

There are three general approaches to using the NO/cGMP pathway to treat PAH: (1) increase supply of exogenous NO, (2) increase production of endogenous NO, and (3) delay the metabolism of NO-induced synthesis of cGMP (Fig. 4).

Delivery of exogenous nitric oxide

Increasing delivery of exogenous NO to vascular tissue can be accomplished by administration of NO donors or inhalation of medical grade NO. NO donors, such as nitroglycerin, sodium

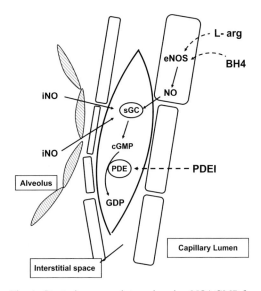

Fig. 4. Strategic approach to enhancing NO/cGMP for treatment of PAH. Ingestion of L-arginine (L-arg) or tetrahydrobiopterin (BH4) increases circulating levels of these compounds and facilitates endogenous synthesis of NO in the precapillary pulmonary vascular endothelium. NO produced by the pulmonary vascular endothelium or inhaled into the alveolus diffuses to precapillary pulmonary vascular smooth muscle, where it activates soluble guanylate cyclase (sGC) and increases intracellular cyclic GMP (cGMP) levels. Inhibition of PDE type V (PDE-V) delays metabolism of cGMP and thereby amplifies the vasodilator effect of endogenous and exogenous NO.

nitroprusside, and several long-acting oral nitrates, have been used to treat systemic hypertension and reduce right ventricular preload and left ventricular afterload for years. These agents also have been effective at dilating coronary arteries. Their ability to lower PAP in PAH is limited, however. Early vasodilator trials of nitrates in patients who had pulmonary hypertension were largely unsuccessful. Part of the reason for their failure was their lack of selectivity for the pulmonary circulation. The dose required for a significant effect on the pulmonary vascular bed usually caused systemic hypotension, which made them unsuitable for the treatment of PAH.

Inhaled NO, on the other hand, has several biochemical properties that make it ideally suited for treatment of pulmonary vascular disease. In addition to its gaseous state, NO is highly lipid soluble and able to diffuse rapidly through the alveolar epithelial basement membrane to reach adjacent precapillary pulmonary arteries, where it causes vasodilation [109]. Its high affinity for the iron moiety of hemoglobin also results in its near immediate confiscation and deactivation when it reaches the blood stream. As a result, excess NO that reaches the intravascular space is rapidly inactivated before it can be transported to the systemic circulation, which makes it a highly selective pulmonary vasodilator with virtually no downstream effects (Fig. 5) [110].

The most effective dose of iNO for dilating the pulmonary circulation has not been determined precisely and likely varies between individuals and between disease states, depending on the availability of endogenous NO, alveolar ventilation, and PDE activity. Animal studies in sheep found that the maximal pulmonary vasodilator effect occurred at 64 ppm with an ED_{50} of 39 ppm [111]. At 64 ppm, NO caused a 25% to 30% decrease in PAP. Increasing the dose of iNO to 512 ppm did not decrease PAP further [111]. Similar results were seen in small studies of patients who have adult respiratory distress syndrome [112,113]. The ED_{50} for the pulmonary vasodilator effect of iNO was 2 to 3 ppm. The ED_{50} for improvement in oxygenation was only approximately 0.1 ppm, with a worsening of oxygenation at doses above 10 ppm [112]. This occurs because at higher doses, iNO diffuses to adjacent lung units that are poorly ventilated, which causes increased blood flow to areas of low V/Q and/or intrapulmonary

shunt and worsens venous admixture. In one study of patients who had PAH [114], 10, 20, and 40 ppm reduced mPAP to the same degree, which suggested that the ED_{50} for the pulmonary vasodilator effect of iNO in PAH patients is <10 ppm.

The vasodilator effect of NO is rapid, occurs within minutes, and is short-lived, with a half-life in the order of minutes [111,112]. Clinical trials have shown that approximately 35% of patients who have PAH have an acute vasodilator response to iNO [114]. A positive vasodilator response to iNO correlates closely with patient response to prostacyclin [114] and calcium channel blockers [115–117], but without the systemic hypotension or decreased oxygenation that has been seen with the other two agents [115]. The rapid onset of action, short half-life, and selectivity of NO for the pulmonary circulation make it an ideal agent for acute vasodilator testing during right heart catheterization in patients who have PAH [116].

Inhaled NO was first administered to patients who had PAH in the early 1990s. Pepke-Zaba and colleagues [118] gave intravenous prostacyclin and iNO at 40 ppm to eight patients who had PAH. Both agents caused a significant reduction in pulmonary vascular resistance, but prostacyclin also caused a significant reduction in systemic vascular resistance that was not seen with iNO. The authors concluded that iNO acted as a selective

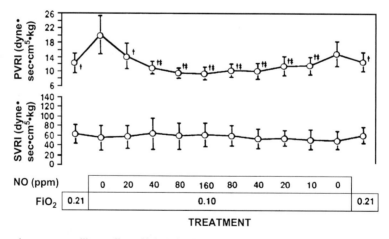

Fig. 5. Selective pulmonary vasodilator effect of inhaled NO. Changing the fraction of inspired oxygen (FiO_2) from 0.21 to 0.10 in mechanically ventilated fetal lambs causes a sudden increase in pulmonary vascular resistance index (PVRI). Addition of NO to the ventilatory circuit causes a dose-dependent decrease in PVRI with complete reversal of hypoxic pulmonary vasoconstriction at 80 ppm. The selective pulmonary vasodilator effect of NO is demonstrated by lack of any effect of NO on systemic vascular resistance index (SVRI). $n = 7$. Values shown are mean ± SD. † $P < .05$ compared with breathing FiO_2 0.10 without NO. ‡ $P < .05$ compared with breathing FiO_2 0.10 with NO 20 ppm. (*From* Roberts JD Jr, Chen TY, Kawai N, et al. Inhaled nitric oxide reverses pulmonary vasoconstriction in the hypoxic and acidotic newborn lamb. Circ Res 1993;72:249; with permission.)

pulmonary vasodilator in PAH. Shortly afterwards, iNO was shown to be effective in reducing PAP in patients in various clinical settings, including postoperative patients after mitral valve surgery [119] or heart transplantation [120] and in patients who have adult respiratory distress syndrome [88], pulmonary hypertension associated with chronic obstructive pulmonary disease [121,122], persistent pulmonary hypertension of the newborn [123–126], pulmonary hypertension associated with congenital heart defects [127], PAH associated with connective tissue disease [128,129], and pulmonary hypertension associated with pulmonary fibrosis [130,131], sarcoidosis [132] and high altitude sickness [133,134]. Patient responses to iNO vary, but on average, the mean decrease in PAP is approximately 20% [135], and approximately 35% of patients have a significant vasodilator response [114].

In the United States, iNO is approved for the treatment of acute respiratory failure in newborns, including persistent pulmonary hypertension of the newborn, but not for PAH in adult patients. Guidelines for its use in the pediatric [136] and adult [137,138] population have been published, but formal studies of the effects of long-term inhalation have not been conducted. Inhalation of NO causes an increase in serum nitrates and methemoglobin [139]. At a minimum, continuous monitoring of nitrogen dioxide (NO_2), a toxic gas that forms rapidly when NO is exposed to oxygen, is required, as is a baseline methemoglobin level and repeat level 24 hours after initiation of therapy. NO cannot be allowed to mix with oxygen until just before inhalation, and if it is used in a patient's room, exhaled gas should be vented to the outside to prevent buildup of the ambient NO concentration. The Occupational Safety and Health Administration has set an 8-hour maximum exposure level of 25 ppm for NO concentration in breathable air [140]. In general, dangerous levels of NO_2 and methemoglobin are not seen with concentrations of NO < 80 ppm and FiO_2 < 0.9 [136].

Long-term iNO is administered using concentrated NO in a portable tank delivered to the patient via nasal prongs. This technique has been shown to decrease PAP as effectively as iNO administered by full face [141]. Pulse-dose delivery devices, similar to those used for oxygen-conserving devices, deliver a pulse of NO during inspiration, which increases the efficiency of the dose delivered and decreases the amount of excess gas leaked into the atmosphere.

Chronic treatment with iNO has been shown to blunt hypoxic pulmonary hypertension in animal studies [108,142,143] and improve 6-minute walking distance (MWD) in patients who have PAH [144], but long-term experience in human subjects is limited. Channick and colleagues [145] studied eight patients who had PAH and found that iNO given by nasal prongs reduced mPAP by an average of 8 mm Hg and pulmonary vascular resistance by 22%. They created a device for providing long-term iNO via nasal cannula and treated one patient for up to 9 months with iNO at home without adverse events [145]. Before the development of other therapies for PAH, we also used long-term iNO therapy at our institution to treat patients who have PAH. Over an 8-year period, we treated six patients with iNO at home, some for as long as 2 years.

Inhaled NO has the advantage of selectively lowering pulmonary vascular resistance in areas of well-ventilated lung and has been shown to reduce shunt fraction and improve oxygenation in patients who have adult respiratory distress syndrome and during exercise in patients who have chronic obstructive pulmonary disease [88,146]. This property makes iNO ideally suited for patients who have PAH associated with severe hypoxia. Long-term iNO is complicated by the need for continuous inhalation via a pulse-dose delivery device attached to portable tanks, however, which makes long-term use onerous for patients. Severe adverse events, such as rebound pulmonary hypertension [147–149], can occur with even momentary interruption of inhaled gas. This event likely occurs as the result of a suppressive effect of chronic iNO on the activity of pulmonary vascular eNOS or sGC [150,151], although iNO does not seem to decrease eNOS expression or activity in rats [152]. Inhaled NO also has been shown to raise pulmonary capillary wedge pressure acutely in patients who have left ventricular dysfunction [153]. We experienced acute pulmonary edema in two patients with scleroderma who received iNO as part of their vasodilator trial [154]. Together, these limitations make long-term iNO use for the treatment of PAH problematic. Patients who require inhaled pulmonary vasodilator therapy to lower PAP without worsening venous admixture may be better served with intermittent inhalation of a prostacyclin analog. Long-term iNO is currently only available through a small number of clinical trials at specialized institutions.

shown to inhibit experimentally induced pulmonary vasoconstriction in isolated blood perfused rat lungs [208] and intact animals [209–212] but do not prevent monocrotaline-induced pulmonary hypertension in rats [213] and have been generally ineffective in patients who have primary pulmonary hypertension (PPH) [214]. These agents are generally weak pulmonary vasodilators but are effective bronchodilators and have positive inotropic effects that may explain some of their success in treating pulmonary hypertension associated with chronic obstructive airways disease and the postoperative period after mitral valve repair [215–219].

Because of the high concentration of PDE-V in pulmonary compared with systemic vessels, PDE-V inhibitors are more selective pulmonary vasodilators than inhibitors of PDE-I or -III. Dipyridamole, a relatively weak PDE-V inhibitor, was shown to blunt hypoxic pulmonary hypertension as early as 1977 [37] but later was found to have no effect on pulmonary hemodynamics in ten women who had PPH [220]. Use of more potent and selective inhibitors of cGMP metabolism to dilate the pulmonary circulation did not begin until the 1990s. Braner and colleagues [221] found that a selective inhibitor of cGMP metabolism decreased resting PAP and blunted experimentally induced pulmonary vasoconstriction in newborn lambs. Further studies demonstrated that specific inhibitors of PDE-V could lower PAP and blunt right ventricular overload and pulmonary vascular remodeling in rats with hypoxia and monocrotaline-induced pulmonary hypertension [222–225].

The use of PDE-V inhibitors to treat established pulmonary hypertension proceeded cautiously because of concerns for precipitating systemic vasodilation. Early studies used inhalational delivery techniques to target the pulmonary circulation [226] or used PDE-V inhibitors in combination with iNO or other NO donors [227]. By selectively increasing cGMP production in the lung, investigators hoped to increase the ratio of pulmonary-to-systemic vasodilator activity. The PDE-V inhibitor zaprinast was found to potentiate the pulmonary vasodilator effect of NO and prolong its effect [228–230]. In 1998, sildenafil was approved by the US Food and Drug Administration for the treatment of erectile dysfunction. The availability of this highly selective, potent, and orally active PDE-V inhibitor greatly intensified clinical investigation in the use of PDE-V inhibitors to treat PAH.

The first reports of the successful use of sildenafil alone to reverse pulmonary hypertension in animals and treat PAH began to appear at the turn of the century [231–238]. In 2001, Zhao and colleagues [203] gave sildenafil to ten healthy volunteers and found that it nearly abolished the acute pulmonary vasoconstrictor response to hypoxia. In the same year, Wilkens and colleagues [239] found that sildenafil lowered PAP in five patients who had PAH and potentiated the pulmonary vasodilator effect of inhaled iloprost. More importantly, no systemic effects were noted. These findings were confirmed the following year in a larger trial by Ghofrani and colleagues [240], which suggested that sildenafil could be used as an adjunct and possibly as monotherapy in PAH. Other studies found sildenafil to be at least as potent a pulmonary vasodilator as iNO in PAH [241] and PAH associated with pulmonary fibrosis [242]. In 2003, several laboratories published studies that showed that chronic treatment with sildenafil could blunt the development of pulmonary hypertension in animals [243–245], which added to the evidence that long-term use of this readily available PDE-V inhibitor may be beneficial for patients who have PAH.

Long-term studies of sildenafil to treat PAH were first reported from India in July 2002 (Table 1). One study [246] examined the effect of sildenafil on nine adults who had IPAH and five children who had operative congenital heart disease; the other study [247] examined 29 adults who had IPAH. Both studies reported improvement in NYHA class, 6-MWD, and change in peak PAP measured by echocardiography after 3 to 6 months of therapy. In one study [246] that obtained hemodynamic measurements in four selected patients, mean PAP fell from 62 mm Hg to 47 mm Hg after an average of 7 months of treatment. Similar results were reported by Michelakis and colleagues [248] the following year in five patients who had PPH. In that study, 3 months of sildenafil decreased pulmonary vascular resistance by more than 40% without affecting systemic blood pressure in five patients who had PAH. Treatment with sildenafil also reduced right ventricular mass as assessed by MRI. Less salient effects on pulmonary hemodynamics were seen in a slightly larger trial of sildenafil for PAH in England [249], but significant improvements were seen in PAP, cardiac output, and pulmonary vascular resistance, and patients had marked clinical improvement, including an average increase of 112 m in 6-MWD. Ghofrani and colleagues [250] also found significant

Table 1
Clinical trials of sildenafil for long-term treatment of pulmonary arterial hypertension

Author	Ref	Year	n	Dose	Design	Length	Subjects	mPAP (mm Hg)	6-MWD (meters)
Kothari SS	[246]	2002	14	50 mg tid	Open label	7 mo	IPAH, CSPS	−15	144
Sastry BK	[247]	2002	29	25–100 mg tid	Open label	3 mo	IPAH	−14[a]	130
Michelakis ED	[248]	2003	5	50 mg tid	Open label	3 mo	IPAH, ES	−18	128
Mikhail GW	[249]	2004	10	50 mg tid	Open label	3 mo	IPAH	−5.4	112
Ghofrani HA	[250]	2003	12	50 mg tid	Open label	6.5 mo	CTPEH	−7.7	54
Bharani A	[251]	2003	10	25 mg tid	RCT/Crossover	2 wk	IPAH, CSPS, CTEPH, ILD	−20[a]	97
Sastry BK	[252]	2004	22	25–100 mg tid	RCT/Crossover	6 wk	IPAH	−7[a]	211 s[b]
Galie N	[254]	2005	278	20–80 mg tid	RCT	12 wk	IPAH, PHCTD, CSPS	−2.1–−4.7	45–50
Wilkins MR	[256]	2005	26	50 mg tid	RCT	16 wk	IPAH, PHCTD		114
Singh TP	[253]	2006	20	50 mg tid	RCT/Crossover	6 wk	IPAH, ES	−20.5	97

Abbreviations: CTEPH, chronic thromboembolic pulmonary hypertension; CSPS, congenital pulmonary to systemic shunt; ES, Eisenmenger's syndrome; IPAH, idiopathic pulmonary arterial hypertension; MPAP, mean pulmonary arterial pressure; PHCTD, pulmonary arterial hypertension associated with connective tissue disease; RCT, randomized, controlled trial; 6-MWD, 6-minute walking distance.

[a] Change in peak right ventricular pressure as measured by two-dimensional echocardiogram.

[b] Exercise time in seconds.

improvement in pulmonary vascular resistance and 6-MWD in 12 patients who had chronic thromboembolic pulmonary hypertension.

Randomized, controlled trials of sildenafil versus placebo began with small crossover design studies in 2003. Bharani and colleagues [251] gave sildenafil, 25 mg, every 8 hours or matching placebo to ten patients with PAH who were not responding to conventional therapy. Patients received sildenafil or placebo for 2 weeks, followed by a 2-week washout period and crossover to the alternative therapy for another 2 weeks. The order in which sildenafil or placebo was taken was randomized. Patients and investigators were blinded. Although the study was small and included patients with chronic thromboembolic pulmonary hypertension and interstitial lung disease, 2 weeks of sildenafil caused significant improvements in functional class, walking distance, and peak PAP measured by echocardiogram. Similar results were obtained in two larger, double-blind crossover studies [252,253]. Sastry and colleagues [252] randomized 22 patients to sildenafil or placebo. Hemodynamics and symptoms were better after 6 weeks of sildenafil than 6 weeks of placebo. No adverse events were observed while patients were on sildenafil, but one patient had syncope and another died while taking placebo. Similar results were recently reported by Singh and colleagues [253] in ten patients who had IPAH and ten patients who had Eisenmenger's syndrome.

After these initial trials, a 12-week, double-blind, placebo-controlled multinational trial was conducted in 53 centers around the world between October 2002 and November 2003. The Sildenafil Use for Pulmonary Arterial Hypertension (SUPER) study [254] randomized 278 patients (277 received at least one dose of study drug) to receive placebo or one of three doses of sildenafil (20, 40, or 80 mg) three times daily. Subjects included patients who had IPAH or PAH associated with connective tissue disease or occurring after surgical repair of congenital systemic-to-pulmonary shunts with a 6-MWD of >100 but not more than 450 m. Patients had an equal chance of getting one of the four treatment arms. The primary outcome variable was change in 6-MWD. All three doses of sildenafil produced a significant increase in the 6-MWD compared to placebo after 4 weeks of treatment, and this difference persisted throughout the 12-week study period. The mean placebo-corrected treatment effects among 277 patients at week 12 were 38, 45, and 42 m for

patients who received 20, 40, and 80 mg of sildenafil, respectively ($P < .001$ for all three treatment arms). A significant improvement in pulmonary hemodynamics was also seen after 12 weeks of sildenafil. Whereas pulmonary vascular resistance increased an average of 49 dyne cm sec^2 in the placebo group, it fell 122, 143, and 261 dyne cm sec^2 in the 20-, 40-, and 80-mg sildenafil treatment groups, respectively ($P \leq .01$ for all three groups). The percentage of patients improving at least 1 WHO functional class during the 12-week study was 7% for placebo and 21% to 36% for patients who received sildenafil ($P \leq .005$ for all three groups). Clinical worsening, defined as hospitalization for PAH, initiation of prostacyclin or bosentan therapy, or death, developed in 10% of patients taking placebo and 4%, 3%, 7% of patients taking 20, 40, and 80 mg sildenafil, respectively ($P = NS$).

Of the 265 patients who completed the 12-week study, 259 were enrolled in an extension study with the dose of sildenafil increased to 80 mg every 8 hours. Two hundred twenty-nine patients completed at least 1 year of sildenafil monotherapy. Change in 6-MWD from the baseline in the original study was 51 m, which indicated that the beneficial effect of sildenafil on exercise capacity was maintained for at least a year at this dose.

The SUPER study not only provided strong clinical evidence that PDE-V inhibition is an effective treatment for PAH but also indicated that the degree of improvement seen and 1-year survival was at least as great as that seen in studies of endothelin receptor antagonists and intravenous prostacyclin. A large percentage of patients enrolled in the SUPER study had relatively good functional capacity at enrollment (39% were WHO class II and none were WHO class IV), however, which made it difficult to compare results with studies of other pulmonary vasodilators. No studies have compared the long-term efficacy of sildenafil or other PDE inhibitors to that of prostacyclin analogs, although one study reported improvement with sildenafil in some patients who did not respond to prostanoid therapy [255]. In the only head-to-head comparison of PDE-V inhibition with another pulmonary vasodilator, sildenafil given at a dose of 50 mg three times daily was not significantly better than bosentan, 125 mg, given twice daily [256] at improving 6-MWD or pulmonary hemodynamics in WHO class III patients with IPAH or PAH associated with connective tissue disease. There were

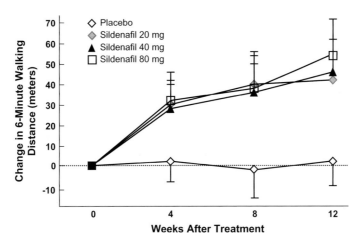

Fig. 6. Effect of increasing doses of sildenafil on 6-MWD. Mean changes from baseline, with 95% confidence intervals, in the 6-MWD are shown for the placebo and sildenafil groups over the first 12 weeks. All three doses of sildenafil (20, 40, or 80 mg of sildenafil three times daily) produced virtually identical improvement in exercise capacity. Data were collected from 266 patients with intention-to-treat analysis. $P < .001$ for the comparison of sildenafil with placebo. (*From* Galie N, Ghofrani HA, Torbicki A, et al. Sildenafil Use in Pulmonary Arterial Hypertension (SUPER) Study Group. Sildenafil citrate therapy for pulmonary arterial hypertension. N Engl J Med 2005;353(20):2153; with permission.)

significant reductions in right ventricular mass and plasma BNP levels with sildenafil that were not seen in the bosentan group, however.

The optimal dose of sildenafil has not been determined but seems to be in the range of 50 to 200 mg daily. In an early study by Chockalingam and colleagues [257], 50 mg sildenafil given twice daily improved pulmonary hemodynamics in patients who had PAH, but no additional effect was seen by raising the dose to 100 mg twice daily. In

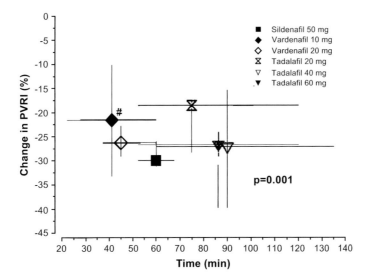

Fig. 7. Effect of different PDE inhibitors on mPAP in patients with PAH. Mean changes from baseline, with 95% confidence intervals in pulmonary vascular resistance index (PVRI) in patients with pulmonary arterial hypertension along with time of maximal response. A total of 60 patients were studied as follows: 50 mg sildenafil (*n* = 19), 10 mg vardenafil (*n* = 7), 20 mg vardenafil (*n* = 9), 20 mg tadalafil (*n* = 9), 40 mg tadalafil (*n* = 8), 60 mg tadalafil (*n* = 8). (*From* Ghofrani HA, Voswinckel R, Reichenberger F, et al. Differences in hemodynamic and oxygenation responses to three different phosphodiesterase-5 inhibitors in patients with pulmonary arterial hypertension: a randomized prospective study. J Am Coll Cardiol 2004;44(7):1494; with permission.)

the SUPER trial [254], 20 mg every 8 hours seemed to be about as effective as 40 or 80 mg over 12 weeks (Fig. 6). Patients in the extension study were treated with 80 mg three times daily for the year that they were followed. Whether not long-term treatment is effective with lower doses of sildenafil is not known. Currently, a reasonable strategy seems to be starting patients at a lower dose and increasing if no response to treatment is seen or if the patient's status deteriorates.

In addition to sildenafil, two other PDE-V inhibitors are approved for treatment of erectile dysfunction. Although neither of these agents has been approved for treatment of PAH, their longer half-life and somewhat greater selectivity and potency for PDE-V make them attractive targets for PAH. The acute pulmonary hemodynamic effects of tadalafil and vardenafil seem to be similar to those of sildenafil in patients who have PAH [258] (Fig. 7). Only sildenafil and tadalafil were shown to decrease the pulmonary-to-systemic vascular resistance ratio, however. The efficacy of long-term treatment of PAH with tadalafil and vardenafil has been examined in only a handful of small clinical trials, but both agents have been reported to be well tolerated and improve functional capacity and hemodynamics [259–261]. A multicenter, phase III, randomized, controlled trial of tadalfil versus placebo is currently in late stage clinical testing for this indication.

Summary

The NO/cGMP pathway plays an important role in mitigating pulmonary vasoconstrictive responses and vascular remodeling during the development of pulmonary hypertension. Synthesis of endogenous NO seems to increase during the development of pulmonary hypertensive disease, possibly in an attempt to compensate for elevated PAP, increased proliferation of pulmonary vascular smooth muscle, and loss of the pulmonary microvascular bed. Manipulations of the NO/cGMP pathway that increase the availability of NO in the pulmonary resistance vessels can lower PAP acutely in many patients who have established PAH and may delay or reverse remodeling of the pulmonary vascular bed. Chronic administration of iNO may not be practical for treating PAH, but increasing endogenous NO production through administration of substrate or cofactors for NOS holds promise. The development of PDE inhibitors that

selectively delay the metabolism of cGMP in pulmonary vascular smooth muscle has led to a new approach to the long-term treatment of PAH that is rapidly becoming first-line therapy for patients with WHO class II and III disease and adjunct therapy for patients treated with prostanoids or endothelin receptor antagonists. Long-term clinical studies of PDE inhibitors are needed to determine their effect on survival in PAH.

References

[1] Furchgott RF, Davidson D, Lin CI. Conditions which determine whether muscarinic agonists contract or relax rabbit aortic rings and strips. Blood Vessels 1979;16(4):213–4.

[2] Furchgott RF, Zawadzki JV. Relaxation of rabbit aortic smooth-muscle by acetylcholine. Pharmacologist 1979;21(3):271.

[3] Furchgott RF. The pharmacology of vascular smooth muscle. Pharmacol Rev 1955;7(2):183–265.

[4] Furchgott RF, Zawadzki JV. The obligatory role of endothelial cells in the relaxation of arterial smooth muscle by acetylcholine. Nature 1980;288(5789): 373–6.

[5] Chand N, Altura BM. Influence of primary prostaglandins on isolated canine renal arteries and veins. Prostaglandins Med 1981;7(1):49–62.

[6] Chand N, Altura BM. Acetylcholine and bradykinin relax intrapulmonary arteries by acting on endothelial cells: role in lung vascular diseases. Science 1981;213(4514):1376–9.

[7] Palmer RM, Ferrige AG, Moncada S. Nitric oxide release accounts for the biological activity of endothelium-derived relaxing factor. Nature 1987; 327(6122):524–6.

[8] Ignarro LJ, Buga GM, Wood KS, et al. Endothelium-derived relaxing factor produced and released from artery and vein is nitric oxide. Proc Natl Acad Sci U S A 1987;84(24):9265–9.

[9] Koshland DE. The molecule of the year. Science 1992;258(5090):1861.

[10] Marletta MA. Nitric oxide synthase structure and mechanism. J Biol Chem 1993;268(17):12231–4.

[11] McQuillan LP, Leung GK, Marsden PA, et al. Hypoxia inhibits expression of eNOS via transcriptional and posttranscriptional mechanisms. Am J Physiol 1994;267(5 Pt 2):H1921–7.

[12] Liao JK, Zulueta JJ, Yu FS, et al. Regulation of bovine endothelial constitutive nitric oxide synthase by oxygen. J Clin Invest 1995;96(6):2661–6.

[13] Davis ME, Cai H, Drummond GR, et al. Shear stress regulates endothelial nitric oxide synthase expression through c-Src by divergent signaling pathways. Circ Res 2001;89(11):1073–80.

[14] Francis SH, Blount MA, Zoraghi R, et al. Molecular properties of mammalian proteins that interact

with cGMP: protein kinases, cation channels, phosphodiesterases, and multi-drug anion transporters. Front Biosci 2005;10:2097–117.

[15] Andriantsitohaina R, Lagaud GJ, Andre A, et al. Effects of cGMP on calcium handling in ATP-stimulated rat resistance arteries. Am J Physiol 1995; 268(3 Pt 2):H1223–31.

[16] Bkaily G, Peyrow M, Yamamoto T, et al. Macroscopic Ca2+ -Na+ and K+ currents in single heart and aortic cells. Mol Cell Biochem 1988;80(1–2): 59–72.

[17] Archer SL, Huang JM, Hampl V, et al. Nitric oxide and cGMP cause vasorelaxation by activation of a charybdotoxin-sensitive K channel by cGMP-dependent protein kinase. Proc Natl Acad Sci U S A 1994;91(16):7583–7.

[18] Furukawa K, Ohshima N, Tawada-Iwata Y, et al. Cyclic GMP stimulates Na+/Ca2+ exchange in vascular smooth muscle cells in primary culture. J Biol Chem 1991;266(19):12337–41.

[19] Furukawa K, Tawada Y, Shigekawa M. Regulation of the plasma membrane Ca2+ pump by cyclic nucleotides in cultured vascular smooth muscle cells. J Biol Chem 1988;263(17):8058–65.

[20] Komalavilas P, Lincoln TM. Phosphorylation of the inositol 1,4,5-trisphosphate receptor by cyclic GMP-dependent protein kinase. J Biol Chem 1994;269(12):8701–7.

[21] Surks HK, Mochizuki N, Kasai Y, et al. Regulation of myosin phosphatase by a specific interaction with cGMP-dependent protein kinase I alpha. Science 1999;286(5444):1583–7.

[22] Sauzeau V, Le Jeune H, Cario-Toumaniantz C, et al. Cyclic GMP-dependent protein kinase signaling pathway inhibits RhoA-induced Ca2+ sensitization of contraction in vascular smooth muscle. J Biol Chem 2000;275(28):21722–9.

[23] Patel HJ, Belvisi MG, Donnelly LE, et al. Constitutive expressions of type I NOS in human airway smooth muscle cells: evidence for an antiproliferative role. FASEB J 1999;13(13):1810–6.

[24] Tanner FC, Meier P, Greutert H, et al. Nitric oxide modulates expression of cell cycle regulatory proteins: a cytostatic strategy for inhibition of human vascular smooth muscle cell proliferation. Circulation 2000;101:1982–9.

[25] Garg UC, Hassid A. Nitric oxide-generating vasodilators and 8-bromo-cyclic guanosine monophosphate inhibit mitogenesis and proliferation of cultured rat vascular smooth muscle cells. J Clin Invest 1989;83(5):1774–7.

[26] Kolpakov V, Gordon D, Kulik TJ. Nitric oxide-generating compounds inhibit total protein and collagen synthesis in cultured vascular smooth muscle cells. Circ Res 1995;76(2):305–9.

[27] Ambalavanan N, Mariani G, Bulger A, et al. Role of nitric oxide in regulating neonatal porcine pulmonary artery smooth muscle cell proliferation. Biol Neonate 1999;76(5):291–300.

[28] Jourdan KB, Evans TW, Lamb NJ, et al. Autocrine function of inducible nitric oxide synthase and cyclooxygenase-2 in proliferation of human and rat pulmonary artery smooth-muscle cells: species variation. Am J Respir Cell Mol Biol 1999;21(1): 105–10.

[29] Krick S, Platoshyn O, Sweeney M, et al. Nitric oxide induces apoptosis by activating K+ channels in pulmonary vascular smooth muscle cells. Am J Physiol Heart Circ Physiol 2002;282(1): H184–93.

[30] Pollman MJ, Yamada T, Horiuchi M, et al. Vasoactive substances regulate vascular smooth muscle cell apoptosis: countervailing influences of nitric oxide and angiotensin II. Circ Res 1996;79: 748–56.

[31] Smith JD, McLean SD, Nakayama DK. Nitric oxide causes apoptosis in pulmonary vascular smooth muscle cells. J Surg Res 1998;79:121–7.

[32] Thomae KR, Nakayama DK, Billiar TR, et al. The effect of nitric oxide on fetal pulmonary artery smooth muscle growth. J Surg Res 1995;59(3): 337–43.

[33] Tzeng E, Kim YM, Pitt BR, et al. Adenoviral transfer of the inducible nitric oxide synthase gene blocks endothelial cell apoptosis. Surgery 1997;122(2): 255–63.

[34] Zhao YD, Courtman DW, Ng DS, et al. Microvascular regeneration in established pulmonary hypertension by angiogenic gene transfer. Am J Respir Cell Mol Biol 2006;35(2):182–9.

[35] Babaei S, Stewart DJ. Overexpression of endothelial NO synthase induces angiogenesis in a co-culture model. Cardiovasc Res 2002;55(1):190–200.

[36] Dubey RK, Jackson EK, Luscher TF. Nitric oxide inhibits angiotensin II-induced migration of rat aortic smooth muscle cell: role of cyclic-nucleotides and angiotensin 1 receptors. J Clin Invest 1995; 96(1):141–9.

[37] Nakaki T, Nakayama M, Kato R. Inhibition by nitric oxide and nitric oxide-producing vasodilators of DNA synthesis in vascular smooth muscle cells. Eur J Pharmacol 1990;189(6):347–53.

[38] Rosenkrantz JG, Lynch FP, Vogel JH. Hypoxic pulmonary hypertension: its modification by dipyridamole. J Surg Res 1972;12(5):330–3.

[39] Costa RS, Assreuy J. Multiple potassium channels mediate nitric oxide-induced inhibition of rat vascular smooth muscle cell proliferation. Nitric Oxide 2005;13(2):145–51.

[40] Hamad AM, Johnson SR, Knox AJ. Antiproliferative effects of NO and ANP in cultured human airway smooth muscle. Am J Physiol 1999;277(5 Pt 1): L910–8.

[41] Boerth NJ, Dey NB, Cornwell TL, et al. Cyclic GMP-dependent protein kinase regulates vascular smooth muscle cell phenotype. J Vasc Res 1997;34(4):245–59.

[42] Yu SM, Hung LM, Lin CC. cGMP-elevating agents suppress proliferation of vascular smooth

muscle cells by inhibiting the activation of epidermal growth factor signaling pathway. Circulation 1997;95(5):1269–77.

[43] Wolfsgruber W, Feil S, Brummer S, et al. A proatherogenic role for cGMP-dependent protein kinase in vascular smooth muscle cells. Proc Natl Acad Sci U S A 2003;100(23):13519–24.

[44] Fukuo K, Inoue T, Morimoto S, et al. Nitric oxide mediates cytotoxicity and basic fibroblast growth factor release in cultured vascular smooth muscle cells: a possible mechanism of neovascularization in atherosclerotic plaques. J Clin Invest 1995; 95(2):669–76.

[45] Chiche JD, Schlutsmeyer SM, Bloch DB, et al. Adenovirus-mediated gene transfer of cGMP-dependent protein kinase increases the sensitivity of cultured vascular smooth muscle cells to the antiproliferative and pro-apoptotic effects of nitric oxide/cGMP. J Biol Chem 1998;273(51):34263–71.

[46] Klinger JR, Murray JD. Atrial natriuretic peptide inhibits murine pulmonary vascular smooth muscle cell proliferation via natriuretic peptide receptor-A. Proc Am Thor Soc 2006;3:A857.

[47] Kibbe MR, Li J, Nie S, et al. Inducible nitric oxide synthase (iNOS) expression upregulates p21 and inhibits vascular smooth muscle cell proliferation through p42/44 mitogen-activated protein kinase activation and independent of p53 and cyclic guanosine monophosphate. J Vasc Surg 2000;31(6): 1214–28.

[48] Sandirasegarane L, Charles R, Bourbon N, et al. NO regulates PDGF-induced activation of PKB but not ERK in A7r5 cells: implications for vascular growth arrest. Am J Physiol Cell Physiol 2000; 279(1):C225–35.

[49] Heller R, Polack T, Grabner R, et al. Nitric oxide inhibits proliferation of human endothelial cells via a mechanism independent of cGMP. Atherosclerosis 1999;144(1):49–57.

[50] Sarkar R, Meinberg EG, Stanley JC, et al. Nitric oxide reversibly inhibits the migration of cultured vascular smooth muscle cells. Circ Res 1996;78(2): 225–30.

[51] Bauer PM, Buga GM, Ignarro LJ. Role of p42/p44 mitogen-activated-protein kinase and p21waf1/cip1 in the regulation of vascular smooth muscle cell proliferation by nitric oxide. Proc Natl Acad Sci U S A 2001;98(22):12802–7.

[52] Ignarro LJ, Buga GM, Wei LH, et al. Role of the arginine-nitric oxide pathway in the regulation of vascular smooth muscle cell proliferation. Proc Natl Acad Sci U S A 2001;98(7):4202–8.

[53] Zuckerbraun BS, Stoyanovsky DA, Sengupta R, et al. Nitric oxide-induced inhibition of smooth muscle cell proliferation involves S-nitrosation and inactivation of RhoA. Am J Physiol Cell Physiol 2006; [Epub ahead of print].

[54] Cornwell TL, Arnold E, Boerth NJ, et al. Inhibition of smooth muscle cell growth by nitric oxide

and activation of cAMP-dependent protein kinase by cGMP. Am J Physiol 1994;267(5 Pt 1): C1405–13.

[55] D'Souza FM, Sparks RL, Chen H, et al. Mechanism of eNOS gene transfer inhibition of vascular smooth muscle cell proliferation. Am J Physiol Cell Physiol 2003;284(1):C191–9.

[56] Du M, Islam M, Lin L, et al. Promotion of proliferation of murine BALB/CT3 fibroblasts mediated by nitric oxide at lower concentrations. Biochem Mol Biol Int 1997;41:625–31.

[57] Ziche M, Parenti A, Ledda F, et al. Nitric oxide promotes proliferation and plasminogen activator production by coronary venular endothelium through endogenous bFGF. Circ Res 1997;80: 845–52.

[58] Hassid A, Arabshahi H, Bourcier T, et al. Nitric oxide selectively amplifies FGF-2-induced mitogenesis in primary rat aortic smooth muscle cells. Am J Physiol Heart Circ Physiol 1994;267:H1040–8.

[59] Kawai N, Bloch DB, Filippov G, et al. Constitutive endothelial nitric oxide synthase gene expression is regulated during lung development. Am J Physiol 1995;268(4 Pt 1):L589–95.

[60] North AJ, Star RA, Brannon TS, et al. Nitric oxide synthase type I and type III gene expression are developmentally regulated in rat lung. Am J Physiol 1994;266(6 Pt 1):L635–41.

[61] Parker TA, le Cras TD, Kinsella JP, et al. Developmental changes in endothelial nitric oxide synthase expression and activity in ovine fetal lung. Am J Physiol Lung Cell Mol Physiol 2000;278(1): L202–8.

[62] Arrigoni FI, Hislop AA, Pollock JS, et al. Birth upregulates nitric oxide synthase activity in the porcine lung. Life Sci 2002;70(14):1609–20.

[63] Shaul PW, Afshar S, Gibson LL, et al. Developmental changes in nitric oxide synthase isoform expression and nitric oxide production in fetal baboon lung. Am J Physiol Lung Cell Mol Physiol 2002;283(6):L1192–9.

[64] Shaul PW, Yuhanna IS, German Z, et al. Pulmonary endothelial NO synthase gene expression is decreased in fetal lambs with pulmonary hypertension. Am J Physiol 1997;272(5 Pt 1): L1005–12.

[65] North AJ, Moya FR, Mysore MR, et al. Pulmonary endothelial nitric oxide synthase gene expression is decreased in a rat model of congenital diaphragmatic hernia. Am J Respir Cell Mol Biol 1995;13(6):676–82.

[66] Davidson D, Eldemerdash A. Endothelium-derived relaxing factor: evidence that it regulates pulmonary vascular resistance in the isolated neonatal guinea pig lung. Pediatr Res 1991;29(6):538–42.

[67] Fineman JR, Heymann MA, Soifer SJ. N omega-nitro-L-arginine attenuates endothelium-dependent pulmonary vasodilation in lambs. Am J Physiol 1991;260(4 Pt 2):H1299–306.

[68] Nelin LD, Dawson CA. The effect of N omega-nitro-L-arginine methylester on hypoxic vasoconstriction in the neonatal pig lung. Pediatr Res 1993;34(3):349–53.

[69] Fineman JR, Wong J, Morin FC 3rd, et al. Chronic nitric oxide inhibition in utero produces persistent pulmonary hypertension in newborn lambs. J Clin Invest 1994;93(6):2675–83.

[70] Vosatka RJ, Kashyap S, Trifiletti RR. Arginine deficiency accompanies persistent pulmonary hypertension of the newborn. Biol Neonate 1994; 66(2–3):65–70.

[71] Davidson D, Barefield ES, Kattwinkel J, et al. Inhaled nitric oxide for the early treatment of persistent pulmonary hypertension of the term newborn: a randomized, double-masked, placebo-controlled, dose-response, multicenter study. The I-NO/PPHN Study Group. Pediatrics 1998;101(3 Pt 1):325–34.

[72] Roberts JD Jr, Fineman JR, Morin FC 3rd, et al. Inhaled nitric oxide and persistent pulmonary hypertension of the newborn: the Inhaled Nitric Oxide Study Group. N Engl J Med 1997;336(9): 605–10.

[73] Kobzik L, Bredt DS, Lowenstein CJ, et al. Nitric oxide synthase in human and rat lung: immunocytochemical and histochemical localization. Am J Respir Cell Mol Biol 1993;9(4):371–7.

[74] Xue C, Johns RA. Endothelial nitric oxide synthase in the lungs of patients with pulmonary hypertension. N Engl J Med 1995;333(24):1642–4.

[75] Xue C, Rengasamy A, Le Cras TD, et al. Distribution of NOS in normoxic vs. hypoxic rat lung: upregulation of NOS by chronic hypoxia. Am J Physiol 1994;267(6 Pt 1):L667–78.

[76] Giaid A, Saleh D. Reduced expression of endothelial nitric oxide synthase in the lungs of patients with pulmonary hypertension. N Engl J Med 1995; 333(4):214–21.

[77] Koizumi T, Gupta R, Banerjee M, et al. Changes in pulmonary vascular tone during exercise: effects of nitric oxide (NO) synthase inhibition, L-arginine infusion, and NO inhalation. J Clin Invest 1994; 94(6):2275–82.

[78] Jiang BH, Maruyama J, Yokochi A, et al. Correlation of inhaled nitric-oxide induced reduction of pulmonary artery pressure and vascular changes. Eur Respir J 2002;20(1):52–8.

[79] Pison U, Lopez FA, Heidelmeyer CF, et al. Inhaled nitric oxide reverses hypoxic pulmonary vasoconstriction without impairing gas exchange. J Appl Physiol 1993;74(3):1287–92.

[80] Hampl V, Herget J. Role of nitric oxide in the pathogenesis of chronic pulmonary hypertension. Physiol Rev 2000;80(4):1337–72.

[81] Hampl V, Weir EK, Archer SL. Endothelilun-derived nitric oxide is less important for basal tone regulation in the pulmonary than the renal vessels of adult rat. Journal of Vascular Medicine and Biology 1994;5:22–30.

[82] Stamler JS, Loh E, Roddy MA, et al. Nitric oxide regulates basal systemic and pulmonary vascular resistance in healthy humans. Circulation 1994;89: 2035–40.

[83] Rich GF, Roos CM, Anderson SM, et al. Inhaled nitric oxide: dose response and the effects of blood in the isolated rat lung. J Appl Physiol 1993;75(3): 1278–84.

[84] Frostell CG, Blomqvist H, Hedenstierna G, et al. Inhaled nitric oxide selectively reverses human hypoxic pulmonary vasoconstriction without causing systemic vasodilation. Anesthesiology 1993;78(3): 427–35.

[85] Fratacci MD, Frostell CG, Chen TY, et al. Inhaled nitric oxide: a selective pulmonary vasodilator of heparin-protamine vasoconstriction in sheep. Anesthesiology 1991;75(6):990–9.

[86] Weitzberg E, Rudehill A, Lundberg JM. Nitric oxide inhalation attenuates pulmonary hypertension and improves gas exchange in endotoxin shock. Eur J Pharmacol 1993;233(1):85–94.

[87] Bottiger BW, Motsch J, Dorsam J, et al. Inhaled nitric oxide selectively decreases pulmonary artery pressure and pulmonary vascular resistance following acute massive pulmonary microembolism in piglets. Chest 1996;110(4):1041–7.

[88] Rossaint R, Falke KJ, Lopez F, et al. Inhaled nitric oxide for the adult respiratory distress syndrome. N Engl J Med 1993;328(6):399–405.

[89] Wanstall JC, Hughes IE, O'Donnell SR. Evidence that nitric oxide from the endothelium attenuates inherent tone in isolated pulmonary arteries from rats with hypoxic pulmonary hypertension. Br J Pharmacol 1995;114(1):109–14.

[90] Muramatsu M, Tyler RC, Rodman DM, et al. Thapsigargin stimulates increased NO activity in hypoxic hypertensive rat lungs and pulmonary arteries. J Appl Physiol 1996;80(4):1336–44.

[91] Le Cras TD, Xue C, Rengasamy A, et al. Chronic hypoxia upregulates endothelial and inducible NO synthase gene and protein expression in rat lung. Am J Physiol 1996;270(1 Pt 1): L164–70.

[92] Isaacson TC, Hampl V, Weir EK, et al. Increased endothelium-derived NO in hypertensive pulmonary circulation of chronically hypoxic rats. J Appl Physiol 1994;76(2):933–40.

[93] Xu W, Kaneko FT, Zheng S, et al. Increased arginase II and decreased NO synthesis in endothelial cells of patients with pulmonary arterial hypertension. FASEB J 2004;18(14):1746–8.

[94] Archer SL, Djaballah K, Humbert M, et al. Nitric oxide deficiency in fenfluramine- and dexfenfluramine-induced pulmonary hypertension. Am J Respir Crit Care Med 1998;158(4):1061–7.

[95] Kharitonov SA, Cailes JB, Black CM, et al. Decreased nitric oxide in the exhaled air of patients with systemic sclerosis with pulmonary hypertension. Thorax 1997;52(12):1051–5.

[96] Mason NA, Springall DR, Burke M, et al. High expression of endothelial nitric oxide synthase in plexiform lesions of pulmonary hypertension. J Pathol 1998;185:313–8.

[97] Berger RM, Geiger R, Hess J, et al. Altered arterial expression patterns of inducible and endothelial nitric oxide synthase in pulmonary plexogenic arteriopathy caused by congenital heart disease. Am J Respir Crit Care Med 2001;163(6):1493–9.

[98] Kradin R, Matsubara O, Mark EJ. Endothelial nitric oxide synthase expression in pulmonary capillary hemangiomatosis. Exp Mol Pathol 2005; 79(3):194–7.

[99] Dweik RA, Laskowski D, Ozkan M, et al. High levels of exhaled nitric oxide (NO) and NO synthase III expression in lesional smooth muscle in lymphangio-leiomyomatosis. Am J Respir Cell Mol Biol 2001;24(4):414–8.

[100] Steudel W, Ichinose F, Huang PL, et al. Pulmonary vasoconstriction and hypertension in mice with targeted disruption of the endothelial nitric oxide synthase (NOS 3) gene. Circ Res 1997;81:34–41.

[101] Steudel W, Scherrer-Crosbie M, Bloch KD, et al. Sustained pulmonary hypertension and right ventricular hypertrophy after chronic hypoxia in mice with congenital deficiency of nitric oxide synthase 3. J Clin Invest 1998;101(11):2468–77.

[102] Fagan KA, Fouty BW, Tyler RC, et al. The pulmonary circulation of homozygous or heterozygous eNOS-null mice is hyperresponsive to mild hypoxia. J Clin Invest 1999;103(2):291–9.

[103] Fagan KA, Tyler RC, Sato K, et al. Relative contributions of endothelial, inducible, and neuronal NOS to tone in the murine pulmonary circulation. Am J Physiol 1999;277(3 Pt 1):L472–8.

[104] Quinlan TR, Li D, Laubach VE, et al. eNOS-deficient mice show reduced pulmonary vascular proliferation and remodeling to chronic hypoxia. Am J Physiol Lung Cell Mol Physiol 2000;279(4): L641–50.

[105] Budts W, Pokreisz P, Nong Z, et al. Aerosol gene transfer with inducible nitric oxide synthase reduces hypoxic pulmonary hypertension and pulmonary vascular remodeling in rats. Circulation 2000; 102(23):2880–5.

[106] Campbell AI, Kuliszewski MA, Stewart DJ. Cell-based gene transfer to the pulmonary vasculature: endothelial nitric oxide synthase overexpression inhibits monocrotaline-induced pulmonary hypertension. Am J Respir Cell Mol Biol 1999;21(5): 567–75.

[107] Kanki-Horimoto S, Horimoto H, Mieno S, et al. Implantation of mesenchymal stem cells overexpressing endothelial nitric oxide synthase improves right ventricular impairments caused by pulmonary hypertension. Circulation 2006;114(1 Suppl): I181–5.

[108] Kouyoumdjian C, Adnot S, Levame M, et al. Continuous inhalation of nitric oxide protects against development of pulmonary hypertension in chronically hypoxic rats. J Clin Invest 1994;94(2):578–84.

[109] Tod ML, O'Donnel DC, Gordon JB. Sites of inhaled NO-induced vasodilation during hypoxia and U-46619 infusion in isolated lamb lungs. Am J Physiol 1995;268(4 Pt 2):H1422–7.

[110] Rimar S, Gillis CN. Selective pulmonary vasodilation by inhaled nitric oxide is due to hemoglobin inactivation. Circulation 1993;88(6):2884–7.

[111] Dyar O, Young JD, Xiong L, et al. Dose-response relationship for inhaled nitric oxide in experimental pulmonary hypertension in sheep. Br J Anaesth 1993;71(5):702–8.

[112] Gerlach H, Rossaint R, Pappert D, et al. Time-course and dose-response of nitric oxide inhalation for systemic oxygenation and pulmonary hypertension in patients with adult respiratory distress syndrome. Eur J Clin Invest 1993;23(8): 499–502.

[113] Puybasset L, Rouby JJ, Mourgeon E, et al. Inhaled nitric oxide in acute respiratory failure: dose-response curves. Intensive Care Med 1994;20(5): 319–27.

[114] Sitbon O, Brenot F, Denjean A, et al. Inhaled nitric oxide as a screening vasodilator agent in primary pulmonary hypertension: a dose-response study and comparison with prostacyclin. Am J Respir Crit Care Med 1995;151(2 Pt 1): 384–9.

[115] Jolliet P, Bulpa P, Thorens JB, et al. Nitric oxide and prostacyclin as test agents of vasoreactivity in severe precapillary pulmonary hypertension: predictive ability and consequences on haemodynamics and gas exchange. Thorax 1997;52(4):369–72.

[116] Ricciardi MJ, Knight BP, Martinez FJ, et al. Inhaled nitric oxide in primary pulmonary hypertension: a safe and effective agent for predicting response to nifedipine. J Am Coll Cardiol 1998;32(4): 1068–73.

[117] Sitbon O, Humbert M, Jagot JL, et al. Inhaled nitric oxide as a screening agent for safely identifying responders to oral calcium-channel blockers in primary pulmonary hypertension. Eur Respir J 1998;12(2):265–70.

[118] Pepke-Zaba J, Higenbottam TW, Dinh-Xuan AT, et al. Inhaled nitric oxide as a cause of selective pulmonary vasodilatation in pulmonary hypertension. Lancet 1991;338(8776):1173–4.

[119] Girard C, Lehot JJ, Pannetier JC, et al. Inhaled nitric oxide after mitral valve replacement in patients with chronic pulmonary artery hypertension. Anesthesiology 1992;77(5):880–3.

[120] Foubert L, Latimer R, Oduro A, et al. Use of inhaled nitric oxide to reduce pulmonary hypertension after heart transplantation. J Cardiothorac Vasc Anesth 1993;7(4):506–7.

[121] Adnot S, Kouyoumdjian C, Defouilloy C, et al. Hemodynamic and gas exchange responses to infusion of acetylcholine and inhalation of nitric oxide in

patients with chronic obstructive lung disease and pulmonary hypertension. Am Rev Respir Dis 1993;148(2):310–6.

[122] Moinard J, Manier G, Pillet O, et al. Effect of inhaled nitric oxide on hemodynamics and VA/Q inequalities in patients with chronic obstructive pulmonary disease. Am J Respir Crit Care Med 1994;149(6):1482–7.

[123] Kinsella JP, Neish SR, Ivy DD, et al. Clinical responses to prolonged treatment of persistent pulmonary hypertension of the newborn with low doses of inhaled nitric oxide. J Pediatr 1993; 123(1):103–8.

[124] Abman SH, Kinsella JP, Schaffer MS, et al. Inhaled nitric oxide in the management of a premature newborn with severe respiratory distress and pulmonary hypertension. Pediatrics 1993;92(4):606–9.

[125] Allman KG, Young JD, Stevens JE, et al. Nitric oxide treatment for fulminant pulmonary hypertension. Arch Dis Child 1993;69(4):449–50.

[126] Kinsella JP, Toews WH, Henry D, et al. Selective and sustained pulmonary vasodilation with inhalational nitric oxide therapy in a child with idiopathic pulmonary hypertension. J Pediatr 1993;122(5 Pt 1):803–6.

[127] Winberg P, Lundell BP, Gustafsson LE. Effect of inhaled nitric oxide on raised pulmonary vascular resistance in children with congenital heart disease. Br Heart J 1994;71(3):282–6.

[128] Jolliet P, Thorens JB, Chevrolet JC. Pulmonary vascular reactivity in severe pulmonary hypertension associated with mixed connective tissue disease. Thorax 1995;50(1):96–7.

[129] Williamson DJ, Hayward C, Rogers P, et al. Acute hemodynamic responses to inhaled nitric oxide in patients with limited scleroderma and isolated pulmonary hypertension. Circulation 1996;94(3):477–82.

[130] Channick RN, Hoch RC, Newhart JW, et al. Improvement in pulmonary hypertension and hypoxemia during nitric oxide inhalation in a patient with end-stage pulmonary fibrosis. Am J Respir Crit Care Med 1994;149(3 Pt 1):811–4.

[131] Yoshida M, Taguchi O, Gabazza EC, et al. The effect of low-dose inhalation of nitric oxide in patients with pulmonary fibrosis. Eur Respir J 1997; 10(9):2051–4.

[132] Preston IR, Klinger JR, Landzberg MJ, et al. Vasoresponsiveness of sarcoidosis-associated pulmonary hypertension. Chest 2001;120(3):866–72.

[133] Scherrer U, Vollenweider L, Delabays A, et al. Inhaled nitric oxide for high-altitude pulmonary edema. N Engl J Med 1996;334(10):624–9.

[134] Anand IS, Prasad BA, Chugh SS, et al. Effects of inhaled nitric oxide and oxygen in high-altitude pulmonary edema. Circulation 1998;98(22):2441–5.

[135] Preston IR, Klinger JR, Houtches J, et al. Acute and chronic effects of sildenafil in patients with pulmonary arterial hypertension. Respir Med 2005;99(12):1501–10.

[136] Miller OI, Celermajer DS, Deanfield JE, et al. Guidelines for the safe administration of inhaled nitric oxide. Arch Dis Child Fetal Neonatal Ed 1994;70(1):F47–9.

[137] Zapol WM. Inhaled nitric oxide. Acta Anaesthesiol Scand Suppl 1996;109:81–3.

[138] Young JD, Dyar OJ. Delivery and monitoring of inhaled nitric oxide. Intensive Care Med 1996;22(1):77–86.

[139] Young JD, Sear JW, Valvini EM. Kinetics of methaemoglobin and serum nitrogen oxide production during inhalation of nitric oxide in volunteers. Br J Anaesth 1996;76(5):652–6.

[140] Occupational Safety and Health Administration. Regulations (Standards – 29 CFR), occupational safety and health standards. Subpart Z: toxic and hazardous substances, limits for air contaminants. 1910.1000 Table Z-1.

[141] Klein W. Hemodynamic effects of aminophylline in primary pulmonary hypertension. Wien Klin Wochenschr 1969;81(37):651–3.

[142] Roberts JD Jr, Roberts CT, Jones RC, et al. Continuous nitric oxide inhalation reduces pulmonary arterial structural changes, right ventricular hypertrophy, and growth retardation in the hypoxic newborn rat. Circ Res 1995;76(2):215–22.

[143] Horstman DJ, Frank DU, Rich GF. Prolonged inhaled NO attenuates hypoxic, but not monocrotaline-induced, pulmonary vascular remodeling in rats. Anesth Analg 1998;86(1):74–81.

[144] Parsons S, Celermajer D, Savidis E, et al. The effect of inhaled nitric oxide on 6-minute walk distance in patients with pulmonary hypertension. Chest 1998; 114(1):70S–2S.

[145] Channick RN, Newhart JW, Johnson FW, et al. Pulsed delivery of inhaled nitric oxide to patients with primary pulmonary hypertension: an ambulatory delivery system and initial clinical tests. Chest 1996;109(6):1545–9.

[146] Roger N, Barbera JA, Roca J, et al. Nitric oxide inhalation during exercise in chronic obstructive pulmonary disease. Am J Respir Crit Care Med 1997; 156(3 Pt 1):800–6.

[147] Miller OI, Tang SF, Keech A, et al. Rebound pulmonary hypertension on withdrawal from inhaled nitric oxide. Lancet 1995;346(8966):51–2.

[148] Lavoie A, Hall JB, Olson DM, et al. Life-threatening effects of discontinuing inhaled nitric oxide in severe respiratory failure. Am J Respir Crit Care Med 1996;153(6 Pt 1):1985–7.

[149] Cueto E, Lopez-Herce J, Sanchez A, et al. Life-threatening effects of discontinuing inhaled nitric oxide in children. Acta Paediatr 1997;86(12):1337–9.

[150] Scott WS, Nakayama DK. Sustained nitric oxide exposure decreases soluble guanylate cyclase mRNA and enzyme activity in pulmonary

artery smooth muscle. J Surg Res 1998;79(1):66–70.

[151] Sheehy AM, Burson MA, Black SM. Nitric oxide exposure inhibits endothelial NOS activity but not gene expression: a role for superoxide. Am J Physiol 1998;274(5 Pt 1):L833–41.

[152] Frank DU, Horstman DJ, Morris GN, et al. Regulation of the endogenous NO pathway by prolonged inhaled NO in rats. J Appl Physiol 1998;85(3):1070–8.

[153] Loh E, Stamler JS, Hare JM, et al. Cardiovascular effects of inhaled nitric oxide in patients with left ventricular dysfunction. Circulation 1994;90(6):2780–5.

[154] Preston IR, Klinger JR, Houtchens J, et al. Pulmonary edema caused by inhaled nitric oxide therapy in two patients with pulmonary hypertension associated with the CREST syndrome. Chest 2002;121(2):656–9.

[155] Pusch R, Habler O, Kleen M, et al. Inhaled sodium nitroprusside: non-selective reduction of thromboxane analogue-induced pulmonary vasoconstriction in healthy sheep. Eur J Med Res 1995;1(3):149–52.

[156] Vanderford PA, Wong J, Chang R, et al. Diethylamine/nitric oxide (NO) adduct, an NO donor, produces potent pulmonary and systemic vasodilation in intact newborn lambs. J Cardiovasc Pharmacol 1994;23(1):113–9.

[157] Hampl V, Tristani-Firouzi M, Hutsell TC, et al. Nebulized nitric oxide/nucleophile adduct reduces chronic pulmonary hypertension. Cardiovasc Res 1996;31(1):55–62.

[158] Brilli RJ, Krafte-Jacobs B, Smith DJ, et al. Aerosolization of novel nitric oxide donors selectively reduce pulmonary hypertension. Crit Care Med 1998;26(8):1390–6.

[159] Brilli RJ, Krafte-Jacobs B, Smith DJ, et al. Intratracheal instillation of a novel NO/nucleophile adduct selectively reduces pulmonary hypertension. J Appl Physiol 1997;83(6):1968–75.

[160] Lam CF, van Heerden PV, Sviri S, et al. The effects of inhalation of a novel nitric oxide donor, DETA/NO, in a patient with severe hypoxaemia due to acute respiratory distress syndrome. Anaesth Intensive Care 2002;30(4):472–6.

[161] McCaffrey MJ, Bose CL, Reiter PD, et al. Effect of L-arginine infusion on infants with persistent pulmonary hypertension of the newborn. Biol Neonate 1995;67(4):240–3.

[162] Block ER, Herrera H, Couch M. Hypoxia inhibits L-arginine uptake by pulmonary artery endothelial cells. Am J Physiol 1995;269:L574–80.

[163] Fike CD, Kaplowitz MR, Rehorst-Paea LA, et al. L-arginine increases nitric oxide production in isolated lungs of chronically hypoxic newborn pigs. J Appl Physiol 2000;88(5):1797–803.

[164] Morris CR, Morris SM Jr, Hagar W, et al. Arginine therapy: a new treatment for pulmonary hypertension in sickle cell disease? Am J Respir Crit Care Med 2003;168(1):63–9.

[165] Morris CR, Kato GJ, Poljakovic M, et al. Dysregulated arginine metabolism, hemolysis-associated pulmonary hypertension, and mortality in sickle cell disease. JAMA 2005;294(1):81–90.

[166] McNamara DB, Bedi B, Aurora H, et al. L-arginine inhibits balloon catheter-induced intimal hyperplasia. Biochem Biophys Res Commun 1993;193(1):291–6.

[167] Taguchi J, Abe J, Okazaki H, et al. L-arginine inhibits neointimal formation following balloon injury. Life Sci 1993;53(23):PL387–92.

[168] Holm AM, Andersen CB, Haunso S, et al. Effects of L-arginine on vascular smooth muscle cell proliferation and apoptosis after balloon injury. Scand Cardiovasc J 2000;34(1):28–32.

[169] Somoza B, Gonzalez C, Cachofeiro V, et al. Chronic l-arginine treatment reduces vascular smooth muscle cell hypertrophy through cell cycle modifications in spontaneously hypertensive rats. J Hypertens 2004;22(4):751–8.

[170] Tan X, Pan JQ, Li JC, et al. L-arginine inhibiting pulmonary vascular remodelling is associated with promotion of apoptosis in pulmonary arterioles smooth muscle cells in broilers. Res Vet Sci 2005;79(3):203–9.

[171] Fineman JR, Chang R, Soifer SJ. L-arginine, a precursor of EDRF in vitro, produces pulmonary vasodilation in lambs. Am J Physiol 1991;261(5 Pt 2):H1563–9.

[172] Eddahibi S, Adnot S, Carville C, et al. L-arginine restores endothelium-dependent relaxation in pulmonary circulation of chronically hypoxic rats. Am J Physiol 1992;263(2 Pt 1):L194–200.

[173] Madden JA, Keller PA, Choy JS, et al. L-arginine-related responses to pressure and vasoactive agents in monocrotaline-treated rat pulmonary arteries. J Appl Physiol 1995;79(2):589–93.

[174] Mitani Y, Maruyama K, Sakurai M. Prolonged administration of L-arginine ameliorates chronic pulmonary hypertension and pulmonary vascular remodeling in rats. Circulation 1997;96(2):689–97.

[175] Bing W, Junbao D, Jianguang Q, et al. L-arginine impacts pulmonary vascular structure in rats with an aortocaval shunt. J Surg Res 2002;108(1):20–31.

[176] Souza-Costa DC, Zerbini T, Palei AC, et al. L-arginine attenuates acute pulmonary embolism-induced increases in lung matrix metalloproteinase-2 and matrix metalloproteinase-9. Chest 2005;128(5):3705–10.

[177] Baudouin SV, Bath P, Martin JF, et al. L-arginine infusion has no effect on systemic haemodynamics in normal volunteers, or systemic and pulmonary haemodynamics in patients with elevated pulmonary vascular resistance. Br J Clin Pharmacol 1993;36(1):45–9.

[178] Surdacki A, Zmudka K, Bieron K, et al. Lack of beneficial effects of L-arginine infusion in primary pulmonary hypertension. Wien Klin Wochenschr 1994;106(16):521–6.

[179] Boger RH, Mugge A, Bode-Boger SM, et al. Differential systemic and pulmonary hemodynamic effects of L-arginine in patients with coronary artery disease or primary pulmonary hypertension. Int J Clin Pharmacol Ther 1996;34(8):323–8.

[180] Mehta S, Stewart DJ, Langleben D, et al. Short-term pulmonary vasodilation with L-arginine in pulmonary hypertension. Circulation 1995;92(6):1539–45.

[181] Nagaya N, Uematsu M, Oya H, et al. Short-term oral administration of L-arginine improves hemodynamics and exercise capacity in patients with pre-capillary pulmonary hypertension. Am J Respir Crit Care Med 2001;163(4):887–91.

[182] Lacassie HJ, Germain AM, Valdes G, et al. Management of Eisenmenger syndrome in pregnancy with sildenafil and L-arginine. Obstet Gynecol 2004;103(5 Pt 2):1118–20.

[183] Pritchard KA Jr, Shi Y, Konduri GG. Tetrahydrobiopterin in pulmonary hypertension: pulmonary hypertension in guanosine triphosphate-cyclohydrolase-deficient mice. Circulation 2005;111(16):2022–4.

[184] Alp NJ, Channon KM. Regulation of endothelial nitric oxide synthase by tetrahydrobiopterin in vascular disease. Arterioscler Thromb Vasc Biol 2004;24:413–20.

[185] Davydova MP, Postnikov AB, D'iakonov KB, et al. Involvement of tetrahydrobiopterin in local change of endothelium-dependent vasorelaxation in pulmonary hypertension. Ross Fiziol Zh Im I M Sechenova 2003;89(12):1516–22.

[186] Nandi M, Miller A, Stidwill R, et al. Pulmonary hypertension in a GTP-cyclohydrolase 1-deficient mouse. Circulation 2005;111(16):2086–90.

[187] Khoo JP, Zhao L, Alp NJ, et al. Pivotal role for endothelial tetrahydrobiopterin in pulmonary hypertension. Circulation 2005;111(16):2126–33.

[188] Matsumoto T, Kobayashi T, Kamata K. Phosphodiesterases in the vascular system. J Smooth Muscle Res 2003;39(4):67–86.

[189] Carson CC. PDE5 inhibitors: are there differences? Can J Urol 2006;13(Suppl 1):34–9.

[190] Maclean MR, Johnston ED, Mcculloch KM, et al. Phosphodiesterase isoforms in the pulmonary arterial circulation of the rat: changes in pulmonary hypertension. J Pharmacol Exp Ther 1997;283(2):619–24.

[191] Hanson KA, Ziegler JW, Rybalkin SD, et al. Chronic pulmonary hypertension increases fetal lung cGMP phosphodiesterase activity. Am J Physiol 1998;275(5 Pt 1):L931–41.

[192] Jernigan NL, Resta TC. Chronic hypoxia attenuates cGMP-dependent pulmonary vasodilation.

Am J Physiol Lung Cell Mol Physiol 2002;282:L1366–75.

[193] Murray F, Patel HH, Suda RY, et al. Expression and activity of cAMP phosphodiesterase isoforms in pulmonary artery smooth muscle cells from patients with pulmonary hypertension: role for PDE1. Am J Physiol Lung Cell Mol Physiol 2006;[Sept 15, Epub ahead of print].

[194] Corbin JD, Beasley A, Blount MA, et al. High lung PDE5: a strong basis for treating pulmonary hypertension with PDE5 inhibitors. Biochem Biophys Res Commun 2005;334(3):930–8.

[195] Murray F, MacLean MR, Pyne NJ. Increased expression of the cGMP-inhibited cAMP-specific (PDE3) and cGMP binding cGMP-specific (PDE5) phosphodiesterases in models of pulmonary hypertension. Br J Pharmacol 2002;137(8):1187–94.

[196] Black SM, Sanchez LS, Mata-Greenwood E, et al. sGC and PDE5 are elevated in lambs with increased pulmonary blood flow and pulmonary hypertension. Am J Physiol Lung Cell Mol Physiol 2001;281(5):L1051–7.

[197] Ingerman-Wojenski CM, Silver MJ. Model system to study interaction of platelets with damaged arterial wall. II: inhibition of smooth muscle cell proliferation by dipyridamole and AH-P719. Exp Mol Pathol 1988;48(1):116–34.

[198] Souness JE, Hassall GA, Parrott DP. Inhibition of pig aortic smooth muscle cell DNA synthesis by selective type III and type IV cyclic AMP phosphodiesterase inhibitors. Biochem Pharmacol 1992;44(5):857–66.

[199] Cohen AH, Hanson K, Morris K, et al. Inhibition of cyclic 3'-5'-guanosine monophosphate-specific phosphodiesterase selectively vasodilates the pulmonary circulation in chronically hypoxic rats. J Clin Invest 1996;97:172–9.

[200] Tantini B, Manes A, Fiumana E, et al. Antiproliferative effect of sildenafil on human pulmonary artery smooth muscle cells. Basic Res Cardiol 2005;100(2):131–8.

[201] Wharton J, Strange JW, Moller GM, et al. Antiproliferative effects of phosphodiesterase type 5 inhibition in human pulmonary artery cells. Am J Respir Crit Care Med 2005;172(1):105–13.

[202] Zhao L, Mason NA, Strange JW, et al. Beneficial effects of phosphodiesterase 5 inhibition in pulmonary hypertension are influenced by natriuretic peptide activity. Circulation 2003;107(2):234–7.

[203] Zhao L, Mason NA, Morrell NW, et al. Sildenafil inhibits hypoxia-induced pulmonary hypertension. Circulation 2001;104(4):424–8.

[204] Cordes L, Danneel KT, Hauch HJ, et al. Influence of chemotherapy on pulmonary hypertension with special regard to beta-hydroxypropyl theophylline. Z Kreislaufforsch 1958;47(3–4):118–32 [in German].

[205] Klein W. Primary pulmonary hypertension: aminophylline. Wien Z Inn Med 1969;50(10):499–501.

[206] Bisgard GE, Will JA. Glucagon and aminophylline as pulmonary vasodilators in the calf with hypoxic pulmonary hypertension. Chest 1977;71(2 Suppl): 263–5 [in German].

[207] Panuccio P, Viroli L, Chelucci G, et al. Effects of theophylline-ethylendiamine on chronic pulmonary arterial hypertension secondary to chronic obstructive pulmonary disease. G Ital Cardiol 1984; 14(Suppl 1):74–6.

[208] Hill NS, Rounds S. Amrinone dilates pulmonary vessels and blunts hypoxic vasoconstriction in isolated rat lungs. Proc Soc Exp Biol Med 1983; 173(2):205–12.

[209] Tanaka H, Tajimi K, Moritsune O, et al. Effects of milrinone on pulmonary vasculature in normal dogs and in dogs with pulmonary hypertension. Crit Care Med 1991;19(1):68–74.

[210] Tanaka H, Tajimi K, Matsumoto A, et al. Vasodilatory effects of milrinone on pulmonary vasculature in dogs with pulmonary hypertension due to pulmonary embolism: a comparison with those of dopamine and dobutamine. Clin Exp Pharmacol Physiol 1990;17(10):681–90.

[211] Butt AY, Dinh-Xuan AT, Pepke-Zaba J, et al. In vitro pulmonary vasorelaxant effect of the phosphodiesterase inhibitor enoximone. Angiology 1993;44(4):289–94.

[212] Chen EP, Bittner HB, Davis RD Jr, et al. Milrinone improves pulmonary hemodynamics and right ventricular function in chronic pulmonary hypertension. Ann Thorac Surg 1997;63(3): 814–21.

[213] Burch GH, Jensen LR, Pappas J, et al. Growth factor expression and effects of amrinone in monocrotaline-induced pulmonary hypertension in rats. Biochem Mol Med 1996;58(2):204–10.

[214] Rich S, Ganz R, Levy PS. Comparative actions of hydralazine, nifedipine and amrinone in primary pulmonary hypertension. Am J Cardiol 1983; 52(8):1104–7.

[215] Hess W, Arnold B, Veit S. The haemodynamic effects of amrinone in patients with mitral stenosis and pulmonary hypertension. Eur Heart J 1986; 7(9):800–7.

[216] Hachenberg T, Mollhoff T, Holst D, et al. Cardiopulmonary effects of enoximone or dobutamine and nitroglycerin on mitral valve regurgitation and pulmonary venous hypertension. J Cardiothorac Vasc Anesth 1997;11(4):453–7.

[217] Tarr TJ, Jeffrey RR, Kent AP, et al. Use of enoximone in weaning from cardiopulmonary bypass following mitral valve surgery. Cardiology 1990; 77(Suppl 3):51–7 [discussion: 62–7].

[218] Leeman M, Lejeune P, Melot C, et al. Reduction in pulmonary hypertension and in airway resistances by enoximone (MDL 17,043) in decompensated COPD. Chest 1987;91(5):662–6.

[219] Doolan LA, Jones EF, Kalman J, et al. A placebo-controlled trial verifying the efficacy of milrinone in weaning high-risk patients from cardiopulmonary bypass. J Cardiothorac Vasc Anesth 1997;11(1): 37–41.

[220] Hermiller JB, Bambach D, Thompson MJ, et al. Vasodilators and prostaglandin inhibitors in primary pulmonary hypertension. Ann Intern Med 1982;97(4):480–9.

[221] Braner DA, Fineman JR, Chang R, et al. M&B 22948, a cGMP phosphodiesterase inhibitor, is a pulmonary vasodilator in lambs. Am J Physiol 1993;264(1 Pt 2):H252–8.

[222] Takahashi T, Kanda T, Inoue M, et al. A selective type V phosphodiesterase inhibitor, E4021, protects the development of right ventricular overload and medial thickening of pulmonary arteries in a rat model of pulmonary hypertension. Life Sci 1996;59(23):PL371–7.

[223] Eddahibi S, Raffestin B, Le Monnier de Gouville AC, et al. Effect of DMPPO, a phosphodiesterase type 5 inhibitor, on hypoxic pulmonary hypertension in rats. Br J Pharmacol 1998;125(4): 681–8.

[224] Hanasato N, Oka M, Muramatsu M, et al. E-4010, a selective phosphodiesterase 5 inhibitor, attenuates hypoxic pulmonary hypertension in rats. Am J Physiol 1999;277(2 Pt 1):L225–32.

[225] Kodama K, Adachi H. Improvement of mortality by long-term E4010 treatment in monocrotaline-induced pulmonary hypertensive rats. J Pharmacol Exp Ther 1999;290(2):748–52.

[226] Ichinose F, Adrie C, Hurford WE, et al. Selective pulmonary vasodilation induced by aerosolized zaprinast. Anesthesiology 1998;88(2):410–6.

[227] Ziegler JW, Ivy DD, Wiggins JW, et al. Effects of dipyridamole and inhaled nitric oxide in pediatric patients with pulmonary hypertension. Am J Respir Crit Care Med 1998;158(5 Pt 1):1388–95.

[228] Nagamine J, Hill LL, Pearl RG. Combined therapy with zaprinast and inhaled nitric oxide abolishes hypoxic pulmonary hypertension. Crit Care Med 2000;28(7):2420–4.

[229] Thusu KG, Morin FC 3rd, Russell JA, et al. The cGMP phosphodiesterase inhibitor zaprinast enhances the effect of nitric oxide. Am J Respir Crit Care Med 1995;152(5 Pt 1):1605–10.

[230] Ichinose F, Adrie C, Hurford WE, et al. Prolonged pulmonary vasodilator action of inhaled nitric oxide by zaprinast in awake lambs. J Appl Physiol 1995;78(4):1288–95.

[231] Worwag S, Mulla H, Luyt D, et al. Dipyridamole in the treatment of a neonate with persistent pulmonary hypertension. J R Soc Med 2000;93(2): 77–8.

[232] Abrams D, Schulze-Neick I, Magee AG. Sildenafil as a selective pulmonary vasodilator in childhood primary pulmonary hypertension. Heart 2000; 84(2):E4.

[233] Weimann J, Ullrich R, Hromi J, et al. Sildenafil is a pulmonary vasodilator in awake lambs with acute pulmonary hypertension. Anesthesiology 2000; 92(6):1702–12.

[234] Prasad S, Wilkinson J, Gatzoulis MA. Sildenafil in primary pulmonary hypertension. N Engl J Med 2000;343:1342.

[235] Sayin T, Zenci M. Sildenafil in primary pulmonary hypertension: is there a subset of patients who respond favourably? Can J Cardiol 2002;18(6):676–8.

[236] Singh B, Gupta R, Punj V, et al. Sildenafil in the management of primary pulmonary hypertension. Indian Heart J 2002;54(3):297–300.

[237] Jackson G, Chambers J. Sildenafil for primary pulmonary hypertension: short and long-term symptomatic benefit. Int J Clin Pract 2002;56(5):397–8.

[238] Littera R, La Nasa G, Derchi G, et al. Long-term treatment with sildenafil in a thalassemic patient with pulmonary hypertension. Blood 2002;100(4): 1516–7.

[239] Wilkens H, Guth A, Konig J, et al. Effect of inhaled iloprost plus oral sildenafil in patients with primary pulmonary hypertension. Circulation 2001;104(11): 1218–22.

[240] Ghofrani HA, Wiedemann R, Rose F, et al. Combination therapy with oral sildenafil and inhaled iloprost for severe pulmonary hypertension. Ann Intern Med 2002;136(7):515–22.

[241] Michelakis E, Tymchak W, Lien D, et al. Oral sildenafil is an effective and specific pulmonary vasodilator in patients with pulmonary arterial hypertension: comparison with inhaled nitric oxide. Circulation 2002;105(20):2398–403.

[242] Ghofrani HA, Wiedemann R, Rose F, et al. Sildenafil for treatment of lung fibrosis and pulmonary hypertension: a randomised controlled trial. Lancet 2002;360(9337):895–900.

[243] Kang KK, Ahn GJ, Sohn YS, et al. DA-8159, a potent cGMP phosphodiesterase inhibitor, attenuates monocrotaline-induced pulmonary hypertension in rats. Arch Pharm Res 2003;26(8):612–9.

[244] Schermuly RT, Kreisselmeier KP, Ghofrani HA, et al. Chronic sildenafil treatment inhibits monocrotaline-induced pulmonary hypertension in rats. Am J Respir Crit Care Med 2004;169(1):39–45.

[245] Sebkhi A, Strange JW, Phillips SC, et al. Phosphodiesterase type 5 as a target for the treatment of hypoxia-induced pulmonary hypertension. Circulation 2003;107(25):3230–5 [Epub 2003 Jun 9].

[246] Kothari SS, Duggal B. Chronic oral sildenafil therapy in severe pulmonary artery hypertension. Indian Heart J 2002;54(4):404–9.

[247] Sastry BK, Narasimhan C, Reddy NK, et al. A study of clinical efficacy of sildenafil in patients with primary pulmonary hypertension. Indian Heart J 2002;54(4):410–4.

[248] Michelakis ED, Tymchak W, Noga M, et al. Long-term treatment with oral sildenafil is safe and improves functional capacity and hemodynamics in patients with pulmonary arterial hypertension. Circulation 2003;108(17):2066–9.

[249] Mikhail GW, Prasad SK, Li W, et al. Clinical and haemodynamic effects of sildenafil in pulmonary hypertension: acute and mid-term effects. Eur Heart J 2004;25(5):431–6.

[250] Ghofrani HA, Schermuly RT, Rose F, et al. Sildenafil for long-term treatment of nonoperable chronic thromboembolic pulmonary hypertension. Am J Respir Crit Care Med 2003;167(8): 1139–41.

[251] Bharani A, Mathew V, Sahu A, et al. The efficacy and tolerability of sildenafil in patients with moderate-to-severe pulmonary hypertension. Indian Heart J 2003;55(1):55–9.

[252] Sastry BK, Narasimhan C, Reddy NK, et al. Clinical efficacy of sildenafil in primary pulmonary hypertension: a randomized, placebo-controlled, double-blind, crossover study. J Am Coll Cardiol 2004;43(7):1149–53.

[253] Singh TP, Rohit M, Grover A, et al. A randomized, placebo-controlled, double-blind, crossover study to evaluate the efficacy of oral sildenafil therapy in severe pulmonary artery hypertension. Am Heart J 2006;151(4):851.e1–851.e5.

[254] Galie N, Ghofrani HA, Torbicki A, et al. Sildenafil Use in Pulmonary Arterial Hypertension (SUPER) Study Group: sildenafil citrate therapy for pulmonary arterial hypertension. N Engl J Med 2005; 353(20):2148–57.

[255] Kataoka M, Satoh T, Manabe T, et al. Oral sildenafil improves primary pulmonary hypertension refractory to epoprostenol. Circ J 2005;69(4): 461–5.

[256] Wilkins MR, Paul GA, Strange JW, et al. Sildenafil versus Endothelin Receptor Antagonist for Pulmonary Hypertension (SERAPH) study. Am J Respir Crit Care Med 2005;171(11):1292–7.

[257] Chockalingam A, Gnanavelu G, Venkatesan S, et al. Efficacy and optimal dose of sildenafil in primary pulmonary hypertension. Int J Cardiol 2005; 99(1):91–5.

[258] Ghofrani HA, Voswinckel R, Reichenberger F, et al. Differences in hemodynamic and oxygenation responses to three different phosphodiesterase-5 inhibitors in patients with pulmonary arterial hypertension: a randomized prospective study. J Am Coll Cardiol 2004;44(7):1488–96.

[259] Palmieri EA, Affuso F, Fazio S, et al. Tadalafil in primary pulmonary arterial hypertension. Ann Intern Med 2004;141(9):743–4.

[260] Affuso F, Palmieri EA, Di Conza P, et al. Tadalafil improves quality of life and exercise tolerance in idiopathic pulmonary arterial hypertension. Int J Cardiol 2006;108(3):429–31.

[261] Aizawa K, Hanaoka T, Kasai H, et al. Long-term vardenafil therapy improves hemodynamics in patients with pulmonary hypertension. Hypertens Res 2006;29(2):123–8.

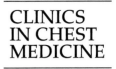

Clin Chest Med 28 (2007) 169–185

Combination Therapy and New Types of Agents for Pulmonary Arterial Hypertension

Dermot O'Callaghan, MB, MRCPI,
Sean P. Gaine, MD, PhD, FRCPI, FCCP*

Department of Respiratory Medicine, Mater Misericordiae University Hospital, University College Dublin, Eccles Street, Dublin 7, Ireland

Traditionally, the management of pulmonary arterial hypertension (PAH) has been challenging, even for experts in the field. Until the mid-1980s, the prognosis for individuals diagnosed with PAH was uniformly dismal with an expected median survival of less than 3 years from time of diagnosis [1]. In the absence of disease-modifying treatments, the only intervention shown to improve outcome was lung transplantation [2]. During the past decade, however, enormous progress has been made in the understanding of the pathophysiologic processes that characterize the disorder. The fruit of these basic scientific and clinical endeavors has been the development of several treatments that target specific cellular pathways believed to be etiologically important in PAH. On the basis of a series of randomized trials, epoprostenol, iloprost, treprostinil, bosentan, sitaxsentan, and sildenafil are licensed in the United States and Europe as monotherapy in different forms of the disease. These drugs offer not only improved symptom control but also the prospect of extended survival. Several more PAH-specific drugs are in the late stages of development and may receive regulatory approval in the near future.

The advent of novel treatments has been associated with a reduction in PAH-associated mortality, such that 5-year survival is now greater than 50% [3]. Nevertheless, despite these encouraging advances the disease remains life-threatening and most patients eventually deteriorate even on treatment. The optimal management for those who exhibit clinical decline despite targeted treatment remains a matter of considerable debate [4]. Even so, in the setting of worsening functional status and hemodynamics, the approach of combining different agents in the hope of augmenting clinical response has already been widely adopted by clinicians in many specialized centers [5–7].

This review assesses the available evidence supporting the use of drug combinations for the management of the various forms of PAH. Ongoing and forthcoming randomized trials evaluating this strategy are also highlighted. Furthermore, new types of agents to treat PAH in the future are explored.

Current therapeutic targets in pulmonary arterial hypertension

PAH comprises a group of distinct conditions characterized by proliferation and obstruction of the lung microcirculation. This process of remodelling leads to a progressive increase in pulmonary vascular resistance (PVR) and eventually right heart failure [8]. Perturbations of several physiologic parameters are recognized as important in the pathogenesis of PAH [9–11]. These include dysregulated production of vasodilators and vasoconstrictors, abnormal myocyte ion channel and growth factor receptor function, increased production of extracellular matrix, and overexpression of serotonin transporter systems.

It is now recognized that variants of PAH share similar pathophysiologic features. At the 1998 World Symposium on Primary Pulmonary

---
* Corresponding author.
E-mail address: sgaine@o2.ie (S.P. Gaine).

0272-5231/07/$ - see front matter © 2007 Elsevier Inc. All rights reserved.
doi:10.1016/j.ccm.2006.11.011

significant cost savings for patients receiving prostanoid therapy. By exploiting these molecular interrelationships it may be possible to improve overall treatment efficacy and minimize risk for toxicity by using reduced dosages of individual agents. There may now thus be a realistic alternative for patients who have intractable disease for whom lung transplantation was previously the only remaining option [48]. In the future, the therapeutic dilemma may not center on which is the most appropriate treatment for patients, but rather which combination of treatments to use and whether to commence multiple drugs together or in a stepwise fashion [43].

Clinical evidence for use of combination therapy

To date there have been few prospective trials conducted to appraise the merits of combining drugs with different modes of action for the treatment of PAH. Many investigators, however, have reported successful outcomes with this approach in animal models of pulmonary hypertension and in observational series and nonrandomized studies. Several well-designed studies are now underway or planned that should help clarify the potential benefits of various different combination strategies.

Endothelin antagonists and prostanoids

Bosentan and epoprostenol

The Bosentan Randomized Trial of Endothelin Antagonist THErapy for PAH (BREATHE-2) was the first randomized, double-blind, placebo-controlled clinical trial of combination therapy in PAH [49]. In this study, the safety and efficacy of bosentan combined with epoprostenol was compared with that of epoprostenol alone in 33 patients who had PAH that was either idiopathic or caused by underlying CTD. All enrollees had either NYHA class III or IV symptoms. Patients were randomized to receive intravenous epoprostenol for an initial 48 hours and then simultaneously assigned bosentan (titrated to 125 mg twice daily) or placebo in a 2:1 ratio. At the end of 16 weeks, the mean decrease in the total PVR was −36.3% with epoprostenol/placebo compared with −22.6% with epoprostenol/placebo ($P = .08$). A nonsignificant trend to greater improvement in several other hemodynamic parameters, including PVR, cardiac index (CI), mean pulmonary artery pressure (MPAP), and right

atrial pressure (RAP), was also observed in the combined epoprostenol/bosentan cohort. There was no difference between the groups in either functional class or 6-minute walk distance. The combination of bosentan and epoprostenol was generally well tolerated. Side effects were experienced more frequently in the combined arm, whereas those receiving prostacyclin alone experienced a more pronounced reduction in systolic blood pressure and increase in heart rate. The authors of this study contended that the lack of statistical significance in either the primary or secondary endpoints may have been accounted for by the small numbers included overall or by the uneven distribution of scleroderma patients between the groups. Three deaths occurred during or shortly after study termination in patients receiving combined therapy, although the trial was underpowered to detect differences in survival.

Bosentan and iloprost

Preliminary data are available from a placebo-controlled parallel-group multicenter investigation designed to evaluate the safety and tolerability of combination therapy with iloprost and bosentan [50]. The investigators of the STEP trial (Iloprost Inhalation Solution Safety and Pilot Efficacy Trial in combination with Bosentan for Evaluation of Pulmonary Arterial Hypertension) randomized 67 patients who had NYHA class III or IV PAH (94% and 6%, respectively) to either iloprost inhalation solution (5 μg per inhalation) or matching placebo, nebulized six times per day for 12 weeks. In total, 55% of patients had IPAH and 45% had PAH associated with CTD or congenital heart disease. Pilot efficacy data were also reported. All subjects were treated with at least 4 months of bosentan before randomization. Compliance with scheduled doses reached more than 90% in each arm. At the end of the study period, 6-minute walk distance had increased in the bosentan/iloprost group by 30 meters compared with placebo ($P < .001$). Statistically significant improvements in functional class, Borg dyspnea scores, and hemodynamics were also associated with bosentan/iloprost combination, whereas episodes of clinical deterioration occurred only among placebo-treated patients. As expected, prostanoid-related side-effects, such as facial flushing, headache, and jaw pain, occurred with greater frequency in the iloprost-treated arm. There was no significant difference in the rate of severe adverse events or clinically important laboratory abnormalities in either group, although full study details have yet to be published. No treatment-associated deaths occurred during the study period.

In light of the positive results reported in the STEP trial, the FDA approved the modification of the iloprost label in August 2005 to incorporate information regarding its use in combination with bosentan. Additional results from a 1-year open-label extension of the original investigation are expected shortly. Although primarily a safety study, the finding that combination bosentan and iloprost is associated with a significant improvement in time to clinical worsening suggests that such a strategy may in fact slow the rate of disease progression.

A phase IV study being performed in Germany is assessing the combined efficacy of the addition of bosentan in patients on maintenance iloprost. Using change in 6-minute walk distance as the primary outcome measure, the COMBI (*COM*bination of *Bosentan and Iloprost*) trial aims to evaluate 72 patients who have IPAH.

Bosentan and treprostinil

There are only scant reports available describing the use of the different formulations of treprostinil with other treatments. Several trials, however, are ongoing or are in late stages of development, which should clarify the role of this prostacyclin analog in the setting of various combinations. The FREEDOM-C study is a double-blind, placebo-controlled trial evaluating the effect of sustained-release oral treprostinil in conjunction with either an endothelin antagonist or a PDE-5 inhibitor on exercise capacity. Investigators in this international collaborative effort plan to enroll 300 patients who have various PAH-related etiologies. A further study using intravenous treprostinil as adjunctive therapy with bosentan, sildenafil, or both is also underway. Additionally, the TRIUMPH (*TR*eprostinil Sodium *I*nhalation *U*sed in the *M*anagement of *P*ulmonary Arterial *H*ypertension) study, initially established to evaluate the efficacy of nebulized treprostinil in patients already taking bosentan, has recently been updated to incorporate patients also treated with sildenafil.

Bosentan and beraprost

No large-scale study has yet been performed exclusively examining the combination of endothelin receptor antagonists and beraprost, although several reports have described the impact of bosentan as adjunct to "non-parenteral" prostanoids. In a pilot 12-week observational study, the efficacy and safety of bosentan were evaluated in 20 patients who had IPAH receiving either maximally tolerated doses of inhaled iloprost (n = 9) or oral beraprost (n = 11) [51]. Addition of bosentan resulted in substantial improvements in 6-minute walk distance (58 ± 43 m) in addition to several cardiopulmonary exercise test parameters, including maximum work rate, VO_2max, anaerobic threshold, and peak systolic blood pressure during exertion. The initial favorable effects did not seem to be sustained during follow-up, however, and formal hemodynamic evaluations by right heart catheterization were not undertaken. No significant adverse events were reported in the study period or during the 3-month extension phase.

A further nonrandomized open-label study has also reported favorable outcomes using combination bosentan/prostanoids. Improvements in the Tei index (an echocardiographic estimate of right ventricular function) and 6-minute walk distance were demonstrated among 16 patients, 13 of whom were receiving chronic beraprost or iloprost [52]. There were sustained improvements in 10 individuals after at least 1 year of follow-up without treatment-limiting side effects. Nine patients also exhibited improvement in NYHA functional class, maintained for a minimum of 6 months. It is, however, difficult to draw firm conclusions from this small feasibility study, because patients who had a range of PH etiologies (including one patient who had interstitial lung disease) were included and there was considerable heterogeneity in baseline NYHA functional classes and prostanoid doses.

Endothelin antagonists and PDE-5 inhibitors

Bosentan and sildenafil

Co-treatment with bosentan and sildenafil holds particular promise, because both treatments are orally administered, act on different intracellular targets, and are generally well tolerated. This combination was initially evaluated in a 12-week uncontrolled study of nine patients who had NYHA class III or IV IPAH despite maximum tolerated doses of bosentan [53]. After 3 months of additional sildenafil therapy, the 6-minute walk distance increased from a baseline value of 277 ± 80 m to 392 ± 61 m (P = .007), an effect that was sustained for 6 to 12 months. Statistically significant improvements in peak exercise oxygen consumption were also noted, though formal hemodynamic data were not collected. Most patients also experienced improvements in functional class. The combination was well tolerated in this small group of patients who had severe progressive PAH. A further single-center study of add-on sildenafil to chronic bosentan therapy in 18 patients reported equivocal results [7]. Concerns have been raised about the potential for regimens that contain both sildenafil and bosentan to augment the risk for liver injury, because sildenafil inhibits the enzymatic activity of CYP3A4, leading to increased plasma concentrations of bosentan. In addition, bosentan induces the CYP3A4 system, which may significantly reduce plasma levels of sildenafil, thereby reducing drug efficacy [54]. The clinical importance of these interactions remains unclear, though careful pharmacodynamic monitoring is advised in this setting.

Two industry-sponsored randomized, placebo-controlled trials are evaluating the combination of bosentan and sildenafil prospectively. The *COM*bination of *P*ulmonary *Ar*terial Hypertension *S*ildenafil *S*tudy (COMPASS) is the first ever event-driven study to be conducted in PAH, with time from baseline to first morbidity or mortality event designated as the primary endpoint. The first part of this multinational phase IV trial (COMPASS-1) is evaluating the hemodynamic effects of combination bosentan/sildenafil compared with sildenafil monotherapy, whereas COMPASS-2 is assessing morbidity and mortality in 600 patients. Another phase IV study that aims to assess the impact on exercise capacity of sildenafil at a dose of 20 mg three times daily given to patients stabilized on bosentan is due to open shortly. In addition, the *PH*osphodiesterase type-5 *I*nhibito*RT*adalafil in the Treatment in Patients with PAH (PHIRST) study, though primarily designed to test the safety and efficacy of this novel long-acting oral agent, also gauges the impact of co-treatment in a subset of patients already receiving bosentan.

PDE-5 inhibitors and prostanoids

Sildenafil and epoprostenol

An initial single-center investigation described encouraging results with the addition of long-term sildenafil in three patients who had severe PAH deteriorating despite maximum-tolerated

intravenous epoprostenol [55]. Two patients who had IPAH and one who had repaired congenital heart disease receiving 75 to 200 mg/d of sildenafil demonstrated notable improvements in hemodynamics and exercise capacity. Headache and nausea were the only therapy-related problems reported. In another study, Kuhn and colleagues [6] assessed the impact of sildenafil in a group of patients receiving maintenance epoprostenol for 2.9 ± 1.6 years. Improvements in PVR and the ratio of mean arterial pressure to MPAP ratio were recorded after administration of a single 50-mg dose of sildenafil. The combination of treatments also seemed to be more effective at augmenting CO compared with epoprostenol alone, although no statistically relevant difference was reported. There was no measurable decrease in systemic oxygen saturation, supporting previous evidence that sildenafil mediates preferential dilatation of the pulmonary arterial tree [56]. Results of an international, double-blind, phase III study evaluating the combination of epoprostenol with various doses of sildenafil over a 4-month period are expected shortly.

Sildenafil and iloprost

Several investigators have published their experiences with the addition of sildenafil in an attempt to prolong the vasorelaxant effects of iloprost (Fig. 1). In an early study involving five patients who had IPAH and associated class III or IV disease, the short-term effects of inhaled prostanoid, sildenafil, and the combination thereof were compared [57]. Nebulized iloprost resulted in significantly greater reduction in MPAP compared with sildenafil (9.4 ± 1.3 mm Hg versus

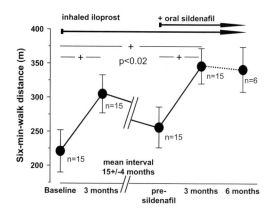

Fig. 1. Sildenafil and inhaled iloprost in PAH.

6.4 ± 1.1 mm Hg; $P < .05$); however, the combination of both drugs was superior to iloprost alone (13.8 ± 1.4 mm Hg versus 9.4 ± 1.3 mm Hg; $P < .009$). The contention that the acute vasodilatory potency of sildenafil may be synergistic to similar effects of iloprost was suggested in another study by Ghofrani and colleagues [58]. A cohort of 30 patients who had PAH, either idiopathic or caused by chronic thromboembolic disease, received inhaled NO (20–40 ppm) followed by aerosolized iloprost (2.8 μg). Patients were then randomly assigned treatment with 12.5 mg sildenafil, 50 mg sildenafil, 12.5 mg sildenafil plus 2.8 μg iloprost at 1 hour, or 50 mg sildenafil plus 2.8 μg iloprost at 1 hour. Results indicated that the combination of 50 mg oral sildenafil and inhaled iloprost had the greatest impact on hemodynamics (reduction in PVR with parallel increase in CO), followed by the combination of 12.5 mg sildenafil plus iloprost. Reduced efficacy was observed in the sildenafil and iloprost monotherapy arms, with sildenafil 12.5 mg/NO cotreatment least potent. There seemed to be no impact on arterial oxygen saturation with dual inhaled prostanoid/PDE-5 therapy.

Investigators from the same institution also studied sildenafil as adjunctive treatment in a group of PAH patients exhibiting clinical deterioration despite inhaled iloprost [59]. Deterioration was defined as subjective clinical worsening: reduced 6-minute walk distance, increasing impairment of RV function, or syncope. The entire study population (n = 14) exhibited not only initial stabilization but also a consistent improvement in 6-minute walk distance (from 256 ± 30 m to 349 ± 32 m; $P = .002$) with ameliorations sustained up to 1 year. Results also indicated favorable changes in hemodynamics and an associated improvement in modified NYHA functional class. Moreover, even after 3 months of combined therapy, baseline PVR values were further reduced with acute iloprost inhalation, suggesting an ongoing synergistic effect. Although two patients died from severe pneumonia during the study period, the investigators concluded these were not related to treatment.

These encouraging preliminary data paved the way for the VISION (*V*entavis *I*nhalation with *S*ildenafil to *I*mprove and *O*ptimize Pulmonary Arterial Hypertensio*N*) trial, currently in the recruitment stage. This international study is evaluating the outcome of approximately 180 patients who have idiopathic or familial PAH exposed to iloprost and sildenafil versus sildenafil alone,

with change in 6-minute walk distance established as the primary clinical end point. The impact of reducing the recommended number of six iloprost inhalations per day to four doses per day is also being examined.

Sildenafil and other prostanoids

Recently, treatment combinations of sildenafil with other prostacyclin analogs have begun to be explored. In an open-label pilot study, the impact of adjunctive oral sildenafil to subcutaneous treprostinil was assessed among a cohort of stable PAH patients in modified WHO functional class II to IV [60]. Investigators chose change in exercise tolerance as the primary endpoint. Treprostinil doses ranged from 35 to 90 ng/kg/min. At the end of the study period, patients demonstrated a statistically significant extension of mean treadmill times (using the Naughton-Balke protocol) from 465 ± 167 seconds at baseline to 656 ± 205 seconds after 12 weeks (42% increase; $P = .049$). Predictable vasodilator-type effects, including headache, flushing, and jaw discomfort, were reported. One patient withdrew because of onset of dyspnea and chest pain.

To date, only one study has been published evaluating PDE-5 inhibitors with oral prostacyclin analogs. Ikeda and colleagues [61] administered oral beraprost (day 1) followed by beraprost plus sildenafil (day 2) to six patients who had moderate to severe PAH and who showed greater and more prolonged reduction in MPAP and PVR compared with beraprost alone. Transient flushing affected two of six study participants as the only treatment-related adverse effect.

Other combinations

It may be possible to enhance pulmonary vasodilatation by combining NO with inhibitors of selected phosphodiesterases. This may theoretically be accomplished by increasing intracellular cGMP concentrations, not only by way of upregulation of production (NO), but also by limiting its metabolism (PDE inhibitors). Two clinical studies have been performed comparing the effects of NO and sildenafil as monotherapy and in combination [62,63]. Lepore and colleagues [62] performed hemodynamic testing in nine patients who had IPAH treated with sildenafil 50 mg alone and combined with NO and showed that cotreatment produced additive reductions in PAP and PVR, with concordant improvements in CI, compared with monotherapy. Michelakis and colleagues [63] also showed that exposure to joint sildenafil and NO resulted in a significantly greater decrease in PVR and an increase in arterial oxygen saturations in comparison with either agent alone. Sildenafil may also be used to minimize rebound pulmonary vasoconstriction after discontinuation of inhaled NO [64]. Unfortunately, inhaled NO is unlikely to emerge as a feasible maintenance therapeutic option for the foreseeable future.

Strategies for combination therapy

Over the last few years, promising data have emerged to support the potential role of combining agents with different targets to enhance therapeutic benefit. The most commonly applied combination therapy approach to date has involved the addition of a second drug when patients deteriorate (or fail to sufficiently improve) despite optimal doses of an initial therapy. Another method is to simultaneously commence two (or more) treatments at the time of diagnosis, given the likelihood of eventual monotherapy failure. Given the lack of conclusive data pertaining to combination treatment, however, the most recently published guidelines make no specific recommendation to guide clinicians on the next step to improve the status of their patients who fail monotherapy [12]. Despite this, the use of combination therapy is already widespread, with choice of regimen generally dictated by center experience, local financial constraints, and patient preferences.

A more logical approach may be the use of a goal-oriented strategy to assist timing of treatment escalation [5]. Hoeper and colleagues [5] treated 123 consecutive patients who had severe PAH over a 3-year period according to a predefined set of treatment goals. Using combinations of bosentan, sildenafil, and inhaled iloprost survival at 1, 2, and 3 years was 93.0%, 83.1%, and 79.9%, respectively; considerably better than that of a historical control group. In the subgroup of patients who had IPAH, survival was also significantly better than predicted based on the National Institutes of Health registry formula. Using the algorithm, 43.2% of patients progressed to dual treatment, and three drugs were required in 16.1%. However, fewer patients than expected progressed to intravenous prostanoids or lung transplantation.

Unfortunately, a dearth of well-designed, randomized, prospective clinical trials has so far hampered an evidence-based approach to combination therapy. Most of the studies are of a retrospective or observational nature, describing experiences with small numbers of heterogeneous patients (often from a single center) without matched control subjects characterized. Investigators have mostly chosen to investigate PAH that is idiopathic in nature or is associated with CTD or exposure to anorexigens, potentially limiting the applicability of results to other categories of pulmonary hypertension. The range of permitted baseline adjunctive "standard therapies" in studies is broad and frequently not specified, and meaningful comparison of results is further hindered by a lack of uniformity in dosing and administration schedules of investigational drugs. A range of follow-up times has been used and an array of primary and secondary endpoints as measures of efficacy used, often without supporting hemodynamic data.

Although encouraging improvements in endpoints such as exercise capacity and NYHA functional class have been reported, the short duration of these studies prevents analysis of the impact on mortality. Furthermore, despite most studies reporting no increase in adverse events, long-term safety data are lacking. The potential for drug–drug interactions that may undermine the theoretic efficacy of dual treatment cannot be discounted.

Combinations of oral/inhaled agents may occasionally facilitate dose reduction or complete discontinuation of parenterally delivered treatments, and there are reports of successful transitioning of patients from intravenous epoprostenol or subcutaneous treprostinil to more convenient therapies [65,66]. Whether the improved outcomes that seem to be the result of adjunctive therapy might have been attained by simply switching to an alternative treatment is still uncertain. It might even be argued that consideration should be given to the discontinuation of a seemingly ineffective drug when a more aggressive therapy is instituted (eg, epoprostenol). Decisions regarding such potentially hazardous treatment de-escalations should be made by expert clinicians in specialized centers, however, and attempted only in carefully selected individuals under close supervision.

As the range of drugs available for PAH increases, so do the number of potential combination options. Many of these have already been tested in studies of varying quality (Box 2). Properly designed, prospective, randomized trials, however, are required to establish which, if any, populations of PAH patients may benefit from the various combinations. Potential risks

Box 2. Combination therapy regimens evaluated in pulmonary arterial hypertension

Endothelin antagonists and prostanoids
Bosentan + epoprostenol [49]
Bosentan + iloprost [50–52]
Bosentan + beraprost [51,52]

Endothelin antagonists and PDE5 inhibitors
Bosentan + sildenafil [7,53]

PDE5 inhibitors and prostanoids
Sildenafil + epoprostenol [6,55]
Sildenafil + iloprost [57–59]
Sildenafil + beraprost [61]
Sildenafil + treprostinil [60]

associated with long-term multidrug regimens remain to be determined. The costs of treatment are already considerable, and use of more than one PAH-specific agent could necessitate significant increases in expenditures. Accordingly, most experts agree that robust and significant measures of improvement should be applied to all cases of combination therapy.

The role of pharmacogenomics [67] is likely to play an increasingly important role in therapeutic decision-making processes. This genome-wide approach is used to identify genetic polymorphisms encoding for drug metabolizing enzymes, drug transporters, and drug targets that account for inter-patient variations in drug efficacy and toxicity. Data are emerging on the use of pharmacogenomics to optimize management decisions for patients who have other pulmonary diseases, including asthma [68] and bronchogenic carcinoma [69]. Ultimately the categorization of the genetic determinants of a given patient who has PAH may permit a tailored, individualized approach dictated not by data from heterogeneous clinical trials but by analysis of unique host factors likely to influence response to therapy.

New types of agents and future therapeutic targets

Although the past decade has proved successful in clinical trials and new drug development, the next 10 years promise to be even more productive. Novel therapies will include modifications of current drugs (eg, new endothelin antagonists or prostanoids) and the targeting of entirely new pathways. The rapid increase in our understanding of the pathobiology of PAH has produced multiple potential therapeutic targets (Fig. 2). These targets are no longer concerned with vasoconstriction but rather seek to control the exuberant proliferation of each layer in

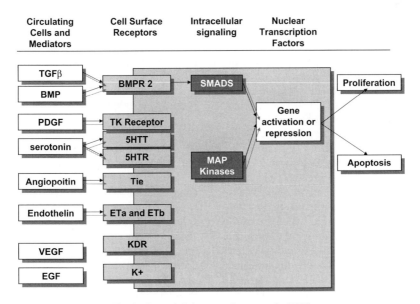

Fig. 2. Potential therapeutic targets in PAH.

vascular wall [70]. New agents include receptor antagonists (eg, serotonin), vasoactive neuropeptides (eg, vasoactive intestinal peptide), antiproliferative agents (eg, imatinib, p38 MAP kinase inhibitors, and statins) and several innovative approaches to gene therapy. Numerous investigators have already reported encouraging results using these therapies to arrest and even reverse pathologic changes in various animal models. The comparative ease with which experimentally induced pulmonary hypertension can be overcome, however, suggests that more realistic models of the disorders are probably required [71,72].

Novel therapeutic targets

Serotonin

Serotonin (5-HT) has been implicated in the pathobiology of PAH and therefore has become a potential therapeutic target. Several observations have fueled this speculation. In mice and humans, pulmonary hypertension is associated with increased 5-HT(2B) receptor expression in pulmonary arteries. Furthermore, the anorexigen dexfenfluramine, exposure to which increases the risk for pulmonary hypertension in humans, is actively metabolized to a selective 5-HT(2B) receptor agonist. Dexfenfluramine treatment potentiates hypoxia-dependent increases in pulmonary blood pressure, elastase activity, and transforming growth factor (TGF) β levels in a chronic hypoxia mouse model of pulmonary hypertension, but not in mice with genetically or pharmacologically inactive 5-HT(2B) receptors [73].

The serotonin transporter (5-HTT) is also upregulated in pulmonary hypertension, and allelic variations in the 5-HTT have been described in patients who have increased pulmonary vascular resistance, suggesting a potential role as a therapeutic target [74]. The long (L) allele is associated with augmented 5-HTT transcription and has been linked to an increased risk for developing pulmonary hypertension [75,76]. Furthermore, homozygosity for the L-allele is associated with childhood onset IPAH [77]. Increased 5-HTT expression in pulmonary artery smooth muscle cells (PA-SMCs), to a level close to that found in human IPAH, leads to PH in mice [78]. Moreover, whereas strong immunostaining for the three receptor types (ie, 5-HT1B, 5-HT2A, and 5-HT2B) and the 5-HTT was seen in remodeled pulmonary vessels from patients who had PH, only 5-HTT expression was increased in lungs and cultured PA-SMCs from patients versus control subjects.

The 5-HTT inhibitors but not the 5-HT receptor antagonists abolished 5-HT mitogenic activity and reduced the serum-induced growth response to similar levels in patients as in control subjects [11].

Although there is general agreement that serotonin is important in the pathobiology of PH, considerable controversy remains regarding how to optimally affect the serotonin axis in affected individuals. The highly selective 5-HT (2B) antagonist (PRX-08066) has demonstrated beneficial effects in experimental animal models, and phase II studies are now planned in humans. The importance of the 5-HT receptor in human PAH, however, is still a matter of speculation, and compelling evidence to support its role in constriction or proliferation in man is lacking. Another approach is also being pursued. Escitalopram, an established serotonin reuptake inhibitor used in the treatment of depression, is currently being investigated in a phase III clinical trail in France. It remains to be seen, therefore, whether manipulation of the serotonin axis will become part of our treatment portfolio in PAH.

Adrenomedullin

Adrenomedullin (AM) is a peptide with several actions that could have a therapeutic implication in PAH. Originally isolated from human pheochromocytoma tumors, AM is also known to be expressed in the heart, lung, and blood vessels. The vasodilatory actions of AM are mediated by way of cAMP- and NO-dependent mechanisms. This peptide has additional anti-inflammatory and antioxidant effects, however, and has been shown to have activity in several other biologic processes, including natriuresis, positive inotropy, inhibition of endothelial cell apoptosis, induction of angiogenesis, inhibition of cardiomyocyte apoptosis, and suppression of aldosterone production. The finding of increased AM mRNA levels and AM receptor expression in the lungs suggests a regulatory role for this mediator in the pulmonary circulation. Plasma levels of AM increase in proportion to the severity of PH and significantly correlate with mean RAP, MPAP, stroke volume, total pulmonary resistance, and the natural logarithm of plasma atrial natriuretic peptide [79]. Furthermore, intravenous administration of AM at a dose of 0.05 mcg/kg/min seems to have beneficial acute effects in PAH [80]. Inhalation of AM may also improve pulmonary hemodynamics and exercise capacity in patients who have PH. In a study of 11 patients who had IPAH, the acute hemodynamic responses to inhalation of aerosolized AM (10 mcg/kg body weight) were examined during cardiac catheterization. Treatment with AM produced a 13% decrease in MPAP and a 22% decrease in PVR, while neither systemic arterial pressure nor heart rate was altered [81]. Adrenomedullin therefore holds some promise in PAH, either by direct pharmacologic application or as peptide to be augmented in gene therapy [82].

Vasoactive intestinal peptide

Vasoactive intestinal peptide (VIP) is a neuropeptide comprised of 28 amino acids that functions primarily as a neurotransmitter but also has potent systemic and pulmonary vasodilatory actions. Specific VIP receptors (VPAC-1 and VPAC-2) activate the cAMP and cGMP second messenger systems. A deficiency of the peptide in lung tissue and serum of patients who have IPAH has been described, and corresponding receptor sites are known to be up-regulated in the disorder [83]. Inhalation of VIP decreased MPAP in eight patients who had severe IPAH (NYHA class III or IV) (Fig. 3). A metabolically stable analog (Ro 25-1553) of endogenous VIP has been shown to be highly selective of the VPAC2 receptor [84] and this agent is currently being investigated in phase III clinical trials.

Retinoids

Retinoic acid is an active metabolite of vitamin A that may play a role in modulating pulmonary vascular thickening by way of its action on smooth muscle cells. Patients who have IPAH have reduced retinoic acid levels, and retinoic acid

replacement can suppress 5-HT–induced growth in cultured human PA-SMCs in vitro [85]. Retinoic acid also induces the expression of the known cell growth suppressor, GADD45A. Furthermore, in a monocrotaline (MCT)-induced PH model in rats, all-trans retinoic acid reduced PA pressure and inhibited metalloproteinase-1 (MMP-1) mRNA overexpression and the accumulation of collagen retinoic acid [86]. It is as yet unclear whether retinoic acid therapy will prove a fruitful avenue for future therapeutic intervention.

Rho-kinase

There is emerging evidence that Rho-kinase, a potent constrictor of vascular smooth muscle, may be a potential therapeutic target in PAH. In recent work, the Rho A/Rho kinase signaling system has been shown to play a key role in the development of PH in the fawn-hooded rat [87]. In rats exposed to chronic hypoxia, acute intravenous administration of the Rho-kinase inhibitor Y-27632 results in near normalization of elevated pulmonary artery pressures but does not exhibit pulmonary vascular selectivity. The hemodynamic impact of inhaled Y-27632 was greater than that of inhaled NO, with effects lasting for at least 5 hours. Inhaled fasudil, another Rho-kinase inhibitor, causes selective MPAP reductions in fawn-hooded rats with PH that is either spontaneous or induced by MCT or chronic hypoxia [88]. Furthermore, treatment with fasudil has also been shown to improve survival in the MCT model of PH in rats [89]. There are preliminary data to suggest efficacy of this agent in humans. After 30-minute intravenous infusion in eight patients who had PAH, fasudil treatment resulted in small but significant decrements in pulmonary and systemic arterial pressures with concordant improvements in cardiac output. No significant adverse events were reported in this small study. Together these findings suggest that fasudil is worthy of pursuit as a novel therapeutic agent [90,91].

Angiopoietin-1

Activation of the TGF-β signaling system results in up-regulation of angiopoietin-1 (Ang-1), a member of the angiopoietin family of growth factors responsible for blood vessel maturation and maintenance. Significantly higher expression of Ang-1 mRNA has been demonstrated in the vasculature of patients who have PAH due to several different causes compared with normal control subjects, and increasing Ang-1 levels seem to correlate with severity of hemodynamic

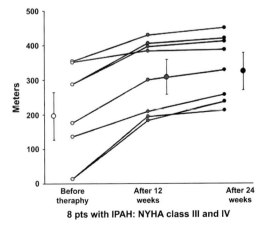

Fig. 3. The effect of inhaled VIP in PAH.

compromise. On binding to the endothelial-specific receptor Tie-2, Ang-1 seems to prevent normal vascular apoptosis by way of an inhibitory action on the BMPR-2 gene. Given that a significant proportion of familial cases of PAH have associated mutations in the TGF-β receptor pathway, these data suggest a possible pathophysiologic role for Ang-1 in disease progression [92]. Other investigators, however, have used animal models to show that administration of Ang-1 may in fact prevent the development of PAH by inhibiting endothelial cell apoptosis, thereby preventing microvessel regression and destruction [93]. These apparent contradictory actions of Ang-1 further highlight the inherent differences between human and animal models of PH and underscore the need to establish whether modulation of this mediator is likely to affect outcome in patients.

Imatinib

Several agents that specifically target growth factor signaling will soon be tested in clinical studies. Using monocrotaline-treated rats, Merklinger and colleagues [94] demonstrated that blockade of the epidermal growth factor receptors results in apoptosis of pulmonary vascular smooth muscle cells and regression of PH. Similar observations were made using animal models by Schermuly and coworkers [95] with the tyrosine kinase inhibitor imatinib, which reverses PH presumably by blocking platelet-derived growth factor signaling. Ghofrani and colleagues [96] presented the case of a patient who had severe PAH refractory to treatment with bosentan, sildenafil, and inhaled iloprost who had an impressive response to imatinib. On the basis of these data, clinical trials assessing the potential therapeutic effects of this agent in patients who have PH are ongoing. Although imatinib holds promise, formal clinical trials should be performed before physicians prescribe this drug for PAH.

Other potential targets

Several novel agents that target various pathways have shown promising results in experimental models of pulmonary hypertension. For example, p38 mitogen-activated protein kinase activity has been shown to play a key role in the pathogenesis of several inflammatory disorders. In an MCT-induced model of PAH, inhibition of this pathway using FR167653 attenuates the expression of inflammatory cytokines and prevents progression of PH [97].

The cofactor tetrahydrobiopterin (BH4) is an important regulator of nitric oxide synthase (NOS) function. The enzyme GTP-cyclohydrolase 1 (GTP-CH1) catalyzes the first step in the de novo production of tetrahydrobiopterin (BH4). The hyperphenylalaninemic mutant mouse (hph-1) displays a 90% reduction in GTP-CH1 activity and therefore deficient BH4 biosynthesis. This animal develops PH even under normoxic conditions and demonstrates increased susceptibility to hypoxia-induced PH [98]. Targeted transgenic overexpression of GTP-cyclohydrolase I (GCH), however, augments BH4 synthesis in the endothelium and prevents hypoxia-induced PH [99]. These early reports suggest that endothelial BH4 is potentially a novel therapeutic target for the future.

The 3-hydroxy-3-methylglutaryl CoA (HMG-CoA) reductase inhibitor simvastatin attenuates PH and associated smooth muscle neointimal proliferation in pneumonectomized rats injected with MCT [100,101]. These results, although encouraging, emphasize the difficulty with the current animal models of PAH. Even though formal clinical trials of statins in PAH have not yet been reported, many patients who have PAH already receive these drugs to treat hypercholesterolemia. Moreover, there is no evidence thus far that the dramatic results described in animal models can be replicated in humans. Nevertheless, statins may yet have a role in combination with other agents in early PAH.

Gene therapy

The prospects for gene therapy for pulmonary hypertension are encouraging for several reasons. First, there are several deficiencies of key vasodilating, antiproliferative agents (eg, PGI2, NO) described that could lend themselves to enzyme replacement. Similarly, overproduction of vasoconstrictive and proliferative peptides such as endothelin may be amenable to inhibition with gene therapy. Second, because the entire venous return passes through the lung it is possible to use remote sites for gene transfer rather than direct application to this organ. For similar reasons the pulmonary circulation lends itself to the use of stem cells administered intravenously that could be targeted at the vast pulmonary vascular endothelial bed. Finally, the gene responsible for the familial form of the disease (FPAH) and a significant percentage of sporadic cases has been identified (ie, BMPR-2) and could be a target for replacement therapy. Several interesting approaches to gene therapy in PAH have been undertaken in animal models, and currently a human trial is at an advanced stage of planning.

Targets and approaches to gene therapy in pulmonary hypertension

Several novel approaches to gene transfer in pulmonary hypertension have been considered. Prostacyclin is a potent vasodilator that also inhibits platelet adhesion and cell growth. In one study the effects of the human prostaglandin I_2 (prostacyclin) synthase (PGIS) gene were investigated in an MCT-induced rat model of pulmonary hypertension. Intratracheal transfer of the PGIS gene augmented pulmonary prostacyclin synthesis, improved pulmonary hemodynamics, and improved survival in MCT-exposed rats [102]. The effects of PGIS gene transfer into skeletal muscle using the naked DNA method were also investigated in MCT-induced PH. A single injection of rat PGIS cDNA-encoding plasmid into thigh muscle 3 days after bupivacaine pretreatment transiently increased muscle PGIS protein expression and muscle and serum levels of a stable prostacyclin metabolite (6-keto-prostaglandin F1). Furthermore, prostacyclin selectively increased lung cAMP levels as compared with liver and kidney. Repeated PGIS gene transfer every week lowered RV systolic pressure and ameliorated RV and pulmonary artery remodeling in these animals and conferred significant improvement in survival rate [103].

Another group explored whether transfer of the PGIS gene into the liver could also ameliorate MCT-induced PH in rats. Up-regulated PGIS gene expression was noted in the hepatocytes of the prostacyclin synthase group. ET-1 levels in the lung were also markedly lower in the PGIS group, and the survival ratio was significantly increased in the gene therapy group in comparison with the control group [104].

Although replacing an important deficiency such as PGIS makes intuitive sense, it is also possible to use gene therapy to disrupt the synthesis of substances that are counterproductive. Survivin, an inhibitor of apoptosis that is overexpressed in cancer cells, has been detected in the pulmonary arteries from animal models and from patients who have pulmonary hypertension. In this regard, gene therapy with an adenovirus carrying a dominant-negative survivin mutant reversed established MCT-induced PAH in rats [105].

Cell-based gene transfer

Bone marrow-derived endothelial progenitor cells (EPCs) normally function to repair and regenerate blood vessels. Stewart and colleagues used an MCT rat model of PH to show that EPCs are capable of engrafting and repairing MCT-damaged lungs, raising the prospect of a potential regenerative therapy [106]. EPCs cultured for 7 to 10 days and fluorescently labeled were engrafted at the level of the distal pulmonary arterioles and incorporated into the endothelial lining in the MCT-injured lung. These investigators demonstrated that EPCs transduced with human endothelial NO-synthase (eNOS) exhibited significant reversal of established disease at day 35 and improved survival in established PAH, suggesting an ability to engraft and repair the MCT-damaged lung, thereby restoring microvasculature structure and function. The regeneration of lung vascular endothelium by injection of progenitor cells may therefore represent a novel treatment paradigm for management of PAH [106]. A human study evaluating patients who have advanced disease has recently been approved in Montreal, Canada. Investigators will assess the safety and feasibility of EPC-based gene transfer using eNOS in 18 PAH patients who have NYHA class IV symptoms.

Summary

The past decade has witnessed enormous progress in our understanding of the pathobiology of pulmonary hypertension. These advancements in basic scientific and clinical endeavor have seen the development and approval of several treatments that target specific cellular pathways. These drugs offer not only symptom control but also the prospect of improved survival. Combination therapy is under investigation and seems promising. Numerous new potential therapeutic targets have also been identified, and several investigational agents have shown encouraging results in experimental models of pulmonary hypertension [95,100,107]. The success using compounds to treat PH induced in animals is often not replicated in humans [108], however, suggesting the need for more relevant models of the disease. In this regard, work using transgenic mice may be a more accurate representation of PH in humans [71,72].

The next decade promises to be even more productive than the previous with the prospect of further significant advances in management of this disease.

References

[1] Rubin LJ. Primary pulmonary hypertension. N Engl J Med 1997;336(2):111–7.

[2] Gaine SP, Rubin LJ. Primary pulmonary hypertension. Lancet 1998;352(9129):719–25.

[3] Sitbon O, Humbert M, Nunes H, et al. Long-term intravenous epoprostenol infusion in primary pulmonary hypertension: prognostic factors and survival. J Am Coll Cardiol 2002;40(4):780–8.

[4] Galie N, Seeger W, Naeije R, et al. Comparative analysis of clinical trials and evidence-based treatment algorithm in pulmonary arterial hypertension. J Am Coll Cardiol 2004;43(12 Suppl S): 81S–8S.

[5] Hoeper MM, Markevych I, Spiekerkoetter E, et al. Goal-oriented treatment and combination therapy for pulmonary arterial hypertension. Eur Respir J 2005;26(5):858–63.

[6] Kuhn KP, Wickersham NE, Robbins IM, et al. Acute effects of sildenafil in patients with primary pulmonary hypertension receiving epoprostenol. Exp Lung Res 2004;30(2):135–45.

[7] Mathai SC, Fisher MR, Housten-Harris T, et al. The addition of sildenafil to bosentan therapy in the treatment of pulmonary arterial hypertension. Chest 2005;128(4):161S–2S.

[8] Gaine S. Pulmonary hypertension. JAMA 2000; 284(24):3160–8.

[9] Yuan JX, Aldinger AM, Juhaszova M, et al. Dysfunctional voltage-gated K+ channels in pulmonary artery smooth muscle cells of patients with primary pulmonary hypertension. Circulation 1998;98(14):1400–6.

[10] Christman BW, McPherson CD, Newman JH, et al. An imbalance between the excretion of thromboxane and prostacyclin metabolites in pulmonary hypertension. N Engl J Med 1992;327(2):70–5.

[11] Marcos E, Fadel E, Sanchez O, et al. Serotonin-induced smooth muscle hyperplasia in various forms of human pulmonary hypertension. Circ Res 2004;94(9):1263–70.

[12] Rubin LJ. Diagnosis and management of pulmonary arterial hypertension: ACCP evidence-based clinical practice guidelines. Chest 2004;126(1 Suppl): 7S–10S.

[13] Humbert M, Sitbon O, Simonneau G. Treatment of pulmonary arterial hypertension. N Engl J Med 2004;351(14):1425–36.

[14] Tuder RM, Cool CD, Geraci MW, et al. Prostacyclin synthase expression is decreased in lungs from patients with severe pulmonary hypertension. Am J Respir Crit Care Med 1999;159(6):1925–32.

[15] Barst RJ, Rubin LJ, Long WA, et al. A comparison of continuous intravenous epoprostenol (prostacyclin) with conventional therapy for primary pulmonary hypertension. The Primary Pulmonary Hypertension Study Group. N Engl J Med 1996; 334(5):296–302.

[16] Badesch DB, Tapson VF, McGoon MD, et al. Continuous intravenous epoprostenol for pulmonary hypertension due to the scleroderma spectrum of disease. A randomized, controlled trial. Ann Intern Med 2000;132(6):425–34.

[17] Olschewski H, Simonneau G, Galie N, et al. Inhaled iloprost for severe pulmonary hypertension. N Engl J Med 2002;347(5):322–9.

[18] Simonneau G, Barst RJ, Galie N, et al. Continuous subcutaneous infusion of treprostinil, a prostacyclin analogue, in patients with pulmonary arterial hypertension: a double-blind, randomized, placebo-controlled trial. Am J Respir Crit Care Med 2002; 165(6):800–4.

[19] Gomberg-Maitland M, Tapson VF, Benza RL, et al. Transition from intravenous epoprostenol to intravenous treprostinil in pulmonary hypertension. Am J Respir Crit Care Med 2005;172(12): 1586–9.

[20] Barst RJ, McGoon M, McLaughlin V, et al. Beraprost therapy for pulmonary arterial hypertension. J Am Coll Cardiol 2003;41(12):2119–25.

[21] Giaid A, Yanagisawa M, Langleben D, et al. Expression of endothelin-1 in the lungs of patients with pulmonary hypertension. N Engl J Med 1993;328(24):1732–9.

[22] O'Callaghan D, Gaine SP. Bosentan: a novel agent for the treatment of pulmonary arterial hypertension. Int J Clin Pract 2004;58(1):69–73.

[23] Channick RN, Simonneau G, Sitbon O, et al. Effects of the dual endothelin-receptor antagonist bosentan in patients with pulmonary hypertension: a randomised placebo-controlled study. Lancet 2001;358(9288):1119–23.

[24] Rubin LJ, Badesch DB, Barst RJ, et al. Bosentan therapy for pulmonary arterial hypertension. N Engl J Med 2002;346(12):896–903.

[25] O'Callaghan DS, Gaine SP. Sitaxsentan: an endothelin-A receptor antagonist for the treatment of pulmonary arterial hypertension. Int J Clin Pract 2006;60(4):475–81.

[26] Galie N, Badesch D, Oudiz R, et al. Ambrisentan therapy for pulmonary arterial hypertension. J Am Coll Cardiol 2005;46(3):529–35.

[27] Barst RJ, Langleben D, Badesch D, et al. Treatment of pulmonary arterial hypertension with the selective endothelin-A receptor antagonist sitaxsentan. J Am Coll Cardiol 2006;47(10): 2049–56.

[28] Badesch D, Galie N, Langleben D, et al. Sitaxsentan improves time to clinical worsening in patients with pulmonary arterial hypertension. Chest 2005; 128(4):160S–1S.

[29] McLaughlin VV, Sitbon O, Badesch DB, et al. Survival with first-line bosentan in patients with primary pulmonary hypertension. Eur Respir J 2005; 25(2):244–9.

[30] Barst RJ, Langleben D, Frost A, et al. Sitaxsentan therapy for pulmonary arterial hypertension. Am J Respir Crit Care Med 2004;169(4):441–7.

[31] Wilkins MR. Selective or nonselective endothelin receptor blockade in pulmonary arterial hypertension. Am J Respir Crit Care Med 2004;169(4): 433–4.

[32] Wharton J, Strange JW, Moller GM, et al. Antiproliferative effects of phosphodiesterase type 5 inhibition in human pulmonary artery cells. Am J Respir Crit Care Med 2005;172(1): 105–13.

[33] Ladha F, Bonnet S, Eaton F, et al. Sildenafil improves alveolar growth and pulmonary hypertension in hyperoxia-induced lung injury. Am J Respir Crit Care Med 2005;172(6):750–6.

[34] Richalet JP, Gratadour P, Robach P, et al. Sildenafil inhibits altitude-induced hypoxemia and pulmonary hypertension. Am J Respir Crit Care Med 2005;171(3):275–81.

[35] Machado RF, Martyr S, Kato GJ, et al. Sildenafil therapy in patients with sickle cell disease and pulmonary hypertension. Br J Haematol 2005;130(3): 445–53.

[36] Galie N, Ghofrani HA, Torbicki A, et al. Sildenafil citrate therapy for pulmonary arterial hypertension. N Engl J Med 2005;353(20):2148–57.

[37] Humbert M, Sitbon O, Simonneau G. Novel therapeutic perspectives in pulmonary arterial hypertension. Eur Respir J 2003;22(2):193–4.

[38] Badesch DB, Abman SH, Ahearn GS, et al. Medical therapy for pulmonary arterial hypertension: ACCP evidence-based clinical practice guidelines. Chest 2004;126(1 Suppl):35S–62S.

[39] Farber HW, Loscalzo J. Pulmonary arterial hypertension. N Engl J Med 2004;351(16):1655–65.

[40] Rubin LJ, Galie N. Pulmonary arterial hypertension: a look to the future. J Am Coll Cardiol 2004;43(12 Suppl S):89S–90S.

[41] Barst RJ, Rubin LJ, McGoon MD, et al. Survival in primary pulmonary hypertension with long-term continuous intravenous prostacyclin. Ann Intern Med 1994;121(6):409–15.

[42] D'Alonzo GE, Barst RJ, Ayres SM, et al. Survival in patients with primary pulmonary hypertension. Results from a national prospective registry. Ann Intern Med 1991;115(5):343–9.

[43] McLaughlin VV, Hoeper MM. Pulmonary arterial hypertension: the race for the most effective treatment. Am J Respir Crit Care Med 2005;171(11): 1199–201.

[44] Hoeper MM, Spiekerkoetter E, Westerkamp V, et al. Intravenous iloprost for treatment failure of aerosolised iloprost in pulmonary arterial hypertension. Eur Respir J 2002;20(2):339–43.

[45] Rabe KF, Tenor H, Dent G, et al. Identification of PDE isozymes in human pulmonary artery and effect of selective PDE inhibitors. Am J Physiol 1994; 266(5 Pt 1):L536–43.

[46] Beavo JA. Cyclic nucleotide phosphodiesterases: functional implications of multiple isoforms. Physiol Rev 1995;75(4):725–48.

[47] Ono F, Nagaya N, Kyotani S, et al. Hemodynamic and hormonal effects of beraprost sodium, an orally active prostacyclin analogue, in patients with secondary precapillary pulmonary hypertension. Circ J 2003;67(5):375–8.

[48] Rich S, McLaughlin VV. Lung transplantation for pulmonary hypertension: patient selection and maintenance therapy while awaiting transplantation. Semin Thorac Cardiovasc Surg 1998;10(2): 135–8.

[49] Humbert M, Barst RJ, Robbins IM, et al. Combination of bosentan with epoprostenol in pulmonary arterial hypertension: BREATHE-2. Eur Respir J 2004;24(3):353–9.

[50] McLaughlin VV, Oudiz R, Frost A, et al. A randomized, double-blind, placebo-controlled study of iloprost inhalation as add-on therapy to bosentan in pulmonary arterial hypertension. Chest 2005;128(4):160S.

[51] Hoeper MM, Taha N, Bekjarova A, et al. Bosentan treatment in patients with primary pulmonary hypertension receiving nonparenteral prostanoids. Eur Respir J 2003;22(2):330–4.

[52] Seyfarth HJ, Pankau H, Hammerschmidt S, et al. Bosentan improves exercise tolerance and Tei index in patients with pulmonary hypertension and prostanoid therapy. Chest 2005;128(2):709–13.

[53] Hoeper MM, Faulenbach C, Golpon H, et al. Combination therapy with bosentan and sildenafil in idiopathic pulmonary arterial hypertension. Eur Respir J 2004;24(6):1007–10.

[54] Paul GA, Gibbs JS, Boobis AR, et al. Bosentan decreases the plasma concentration of sildenafil when coprescribed in pulmonary hypertension. Br J Clin Pharmacol 2005;60(1):107–12.

[55] Stiebellehner L, Petkov V, Vonbank K, et al. Long-term treatment with oral sildenafil in addition to continuous IV epoprostenol in patients with pulmonary arterial hypertension. Chest 2003;123(4): 1293–5.

[56] Ghofrani HA, Wiedemann R, Rose F, et al. Sildenafil for treatment of lung fibrosis and pulmonary hypertension: a randomised controlled trial. Lancet 2002;360(9337):895–900.

[57] Wilkens H, Guth A, Konig J, et al. Effect of inhaled iloprost plus oral sildenafil in patients with primary pulmonary hypertension. Circulation 2001;104(11): 1218–22.

[58] Ghofrani HA, Wiedemann R, Rose F, et al. Combination therapy with oral sildenafil and inhaled iloprost for severe pulmonary hypertension. Ann Intern Med 2002;136(7):515–22.

[59] Ghofrani HA, Rose F, Schermuly RT, et al. Oral sildenafil as long-term adjunct therapy to inhaled iloprost in severe pulmonary arterial hypertension. J Am Coll Cardiol 2003;42(1):158–64.

[60] Gomberg-Maitland M, McLaughlin V, Gulati M, et al. Efficacy and safety of sildenafil added to treprostinil in pulmonary hypertension. Am J Cardiol 2005;96(9):1334–6.

[61] Ikeda D, Tsujino I, Ohira H, et al. Addition of oral sildenafil to beraprost is a safe and effective therapeutic option for patients with pulmonary hypertension. J Cardiovasc Pharmacol 2005;45(4):286–9.

[62] Lepore JJ, Maroo A, Pereira NL, et al. Effect of sildenafil on the acute pulmonary vasodilator response to inhaled nitric oxide in adults with primary pulmonary hypertension. Am J Cardiol 2002;90(6):677–80.

[63] Michelakis E, Tymchak W, Lien D, et al. Oral sildenafil is an effective and specific pulmonary vasodilator in patients with pulmonary arterial hypertension: comparison with inhaled nitric oxide. Circulation 2002;105(20):2398–403.

[64] Atz AM, Wessel DL. Sildenafil ameliorates effects of inhaled nitric oxide withdrawal. Anesthesiology 1999;91(1):307–10.

[65] Suleman N, Frost AE. Transition from epoprostenol and treprostinil to the oral endothelin receptor antagonist bosentan in patients with pulmonary hypertension. Chest 2004;126(3):808–15.

[66] Sitbon O, Humbert M, Ioos V, et al. Transition from intravenous epoprostenol to oral bosentan in pulmonary arterial hypertension. Am J Respir Crit Care Med 2004;169:176s.

[67] Sadee W, Dai Z. Pharmacogenetics/genomics and personalized medicine. Hum Mol Genet 2005; 14(Spec No. 2):R207–14.

[68] Wechsler ME, Israel E. How pharmacogenomics will play a role in the management of asthma. Am J Respir Crit Care Med 2005;172(1):12–8.

[69] Rosell R, Crino L, Danenberg K, et al. Targeted therapy in combination with gemcitabine in non-small cell lung cancer. Semin Oncol 2003; 30(4 Suppl 10):19–25.

[70] Adnot S. Lessons learned from cancer may help in the treatment of pulmonary hypertension. J Clin Invest 2005;115(6):1461–3.

[71] Merklinger SL, Wagner RA, Spiekerkoetter E, et al. Increased fibulin-5 and elastin in S100A4/Mts1 mice with pulmonary hypertension. Circ Res 2005;97(6):596–604.

[72] Lawrie A, Spiekerkoetter E, Martinez EC, et al. Interdependent serotonin transporter and receptor pathways regulate S100A4/Mts1, a gene associated with pulmonary vascular disease. Circ Res 2005; 97(3):227–35.

[73] Launay JM, Herve P, Peoc'h K, et al. Function of the serotonin 5-hydroxytryptamine 2B receptor in pulmonary hypertension. Nat Med 2002;8(10): 1129–35.

[74] Guignabert C, Raffestin B, Benferhat R, et al. Serotonin transporter inhibition prevents and reverses monocrotaline-induced pulmonary hypertension in rats. Circulation 2005;111(21):2812–9.

[75] Eddahibi S, Humbert M, Fadel E, et al. Serotonin transporter overexpression is responsible for pulmonary artery smooth muscle hyperplasia in primary pulmonary hypertension. J Clin Invest 2001; 108(8):1141–50.

[76] Eddahibi S, Chaouat A, Morrell N, et al. Polymorphism of the serotonin transporter gene and pulmonary hypertension in chronic obstructive pulmonary disease. Circulation 2003;108(15): 1839–44.

[77] Vachharajani A, Saunders S. Allelic variation in the serotonin transporter (5HTT) gene contributes to idiopathic pulmonary hypertension in children. Biochem Biophys Res Commun 2005;334(2): 376–9.

[78] Guignabert C, Izikki M, Tu LI, et al. Transgenic mice overexpressing the 5-hydroxytryptamine transporter gene in smooth muscle develop pulmonary hypertension. Circ Res 2006;98(10):1323–30.

[79] Kakishita M, Nishikimi T, Okano Y, et al. Increased plasma levels of adrenomedullin in patients with pulmonary hypertension. Clin Sci (Lond) 1999;96(1):33–9.

[80] Nagaya N, Nishikimi T, Uematsu M, et al. Haemodynamic and hormonal effects of adrenomedullin in patients with pulmonary hypertension. Heart 2000;84(6):653–8.

[81] Nagaya N, Kyotani S, Uematsu M, et al. Effects of adrenomedullin inhalation on hemodynamics and exercise capacity in patients with idiopathic pulmonary arterial hypertension. Circulation 2004; 109(3):351–6.

[82] Nagaya N, Kangawa K. Adrenomedullin in the treatment of pulmonary hypertension. Peptides 2004;25(11):2013–8.

[83] Petkov V, Mosgoeller W, Ziesche R, et al. Vasoactive intestinal peptide as a new drug for treatment of primary pulmonary hypertension. J Clin Invest 2003;111(9):1339–46.

[84] Schmidt DT, Ruhlmann E, Waldeck B, et al. The effect of the vasoactive intestinal polypeptide agonist Ro 25-1553 on induced tone in isolated human airways and pulmonary artery. Naunyn Schmiedebergs Arch Pharmacol 2001;364(4):314–20.

[85] Preston IR, Tang G, Tilan JU, et al. Retinoids and pulmonary hypertension. Circulation 2005;111(6): 782–90.

[86] Qin Y, Zhou A, Ben X, et al. All-trans retinoic acid in pulmonary vascular structural remodeling in rats with pulmonary hypertension induced by monocrotaline. Chin Med J (Engl) 2001;114(5):462–5.

[87] Nagaoka T, Gebb SA, Karoor V, et al. Involvement of RhoA/Rho kinase signaling in pulmonary hypertension of the fawn-hooded rat. J Appl Physiol 2006;100(3):996–1002.

[88] Nagaoka T, Fagan KA, Gebb SA, et al. Inhaled Rho kinase inhibitors are potent and selective vasodilators in rat pulmonary hypertension. Am J Respir Crit Care Med 2005;171(5): 494–9.

[89] Abe K, Shimokawa H, Morikawa K, et al. Long-term treatment with a Rho-kinase inhibitor improves monocrotaline-induced fatal pulmonary hypertension in rats. Circ Res 2004; 94(3):385–93.

[90] Ishikura K, Yamada N, Ito M, et al. Beneficial acute effects of rho-kinase inhibitor in patients with pulmonary arterial hypertension. Circ J 2006;70(2):174–8.

[91] Fukumoto Y, Matoba T, Ito A, et al. Acute vasodilator effects of a Rho-kinase inhibitor, fasudil, in patients with severe pulmonary hypertension. Heart 2005;91(3):391–2.

[92] Du L, Sullivan CC, Chu D, et al. Signaling molecules in nonfamilial pulmonary hypertension. N Engl J Med 2003;348(6):500–9.

[93] Zhao YD, Campbell AI, Robb M, et al. Protective role of angiopoietin-1 in experimental pulmonary hypertension. Circ Res 2003;92(9):984–91.

[94] Merklinger SL, Jones PL, Martinez EC, et al. Epidermal growth factor receptor blockade mediates smooth muscle cell apoptosis and improves survival in rats with pulmonary hypertension. Circulation 2005;112(3):423–31.

[95] Schermuly RT, Dony E, Ghofrani HA, et al. Reversal of experimental pulmonary hypertension by PDGF inhibition. J Clin Invest 2005;115(10): 2811–21.

[96] Ghofrani HA, Seeger W, Grimminger F. Imatinib for the treatment of pulmonary arterial hypertension. N Engl J Med 2005;353(13):1412–3.

[97] Lu J, Shimpo H, Shimamoto A, et al. Specific inhibition of p38 mitogen-activated protein kinase with FR167653 attenuates vascular proliferation in monocrotaline-induced pulmonary hypertension in rats. J Thorac Cardiovasc Surg 2004;128(6): 850–9.

[98] Nandi M, Miller A, Stidwill R, et al. Pulmonary hypertension in a GTP-cyclohydrolase 1-deficient mouse. Circulation 2005;111(16):2086–90.

[99] Khoo JP, Zhao L, Alp NJ, et al. Pivotal role for endothelial tetrahydrobiopterin in pulmonary hypertension. Circulation 2005;111(16):2126–33.

[100] Nishimura T, Vaszar LT, Faul JL, et al. Simvastatin rescues rats from fatal pulmonary hypertension by inducing apoptosis of neointimal smooth muscle cells. Circulation 2003;108(13):1640–5.

[101] Nishimura T, Faul JL, Berry GJ, et al. Simvastatin attenuates smooth muscle neointimal proliferation and pulmonary hypertension in rats. Am J Respir Crit Care Med 2002;166(10):1403–8.

[102] Nagaya N, Yokoyama C, Kyotani S, et al. Gene transfer of human prostacyclin synthase ameliorates monocrotaline-induced pulmonary hypertension in rats. Circulation 2000;102(16):2005–10.

[103] Tahara N, Kai H, Niiyama H, et al. Repeated gene transfer of naked prostacyclin synthase plasmid into skeletal muscles attenuates monocrotaline-induced pulmonary hypertension and prolongs survival in rats. Hum Gene Ther 2004;15(12):1270–8.

[104] Suhara H, Sawa Y, Fukushima N, et al. Gene transfer of human prostacyclin synthase into the liver is effective for the treatment of pulmonary hypertension in rats. J Thorac Cardiovasc Surg 2002; 123(5):855–61.

[105] McMurtry MS, Archer SL, Altieri DC, et al. Gene therapy targeting survivin selectively induces pulmonary vascular apoptosis and reverses pulmonary arterial hypertension. J Clin Invest 2005;115(6): 1479–91.

[106] Zhao YD, Courtman DW, Deng Y, et al. Rescue of monocrotaline-induced pulmonary arterial hypertension using bone marrow-derived endothelial-like progenitor cells: efficacy of combined cell and eNOS gene therapy in established disease. Circ Res 2005;96(4):442–50.

[107] Hu H, Sung A, Zhao G, et al. Simvastatin enhances bone morphogenetic protein receptor type II expression. Biochem Biophys Res Commun 2006; 339(1):59–64.

[108] Opitz CF, Wensel R, Winkler J, et al. Clinical efficacy and survival with first-line inhaled iloprost therapy in patients with idiopathic pulmonary arterial hypertension. Eur Heart J 2005;26(18): 1895–902.

ELSEVIER
SAUNDERS

Clin Chest Med 28 (2007) 187–202

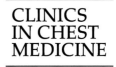
CLINICS
IN CHEST
MEDICINE

Surgical Therapies for Pulmonary Arterial Hypertension

Jeffrey S. Sager, MD, MSCE[a],*, Vivek N. Ahya, MD[b]

[a]Lung Transplantation Program, Pulmonary, Allergy and Critical Care Division, University of Pennsylvania Medical
Center, 828 West Gates Building, 3600 Spruce Street, Philadelphia, PA 19104, USA
[b]Lung Transplantation Program, Pulmonary, Allergy and Critical Care Division, University of Pennsylvania Medical
Center, 832 West Gates Building, 3400 Spruce Street, Philadelphia, PA 19104, USA

Surgical therapies for the treatment of pulmonary arterial hypertension (PAH) typically are reserved for patients who are deemed to be refractory to medical therapy and have evidence of progressive right-sided heart failure. Atrial septostomy (AS), a primarily palliative procedure, may stave off hemodynamic collapse from right-sided heart failure long enough to permit a more definitive surgical treatment such as lung or combined heart-lung transplantation.

It is imperative that chronic thromboembolic pulmonary hypertension (CTEPH) be distinguished from PAH related to other etiologies, because the treatment of choice in select symptomatic candidates is pulmonary thromboendarterectomy and not transplantation [1]. This procedure can restore near-normal cardiopulmonary function after surgery. A detailed review of the epidemiology, diagnosis, and treatment of CTEPH appears elsewhere in this volume. This article reviews the indications, risks, and potential benefits of AS and thoracic transplantation for the treatment of PAH.

Atrial septostomy

Pulmonary arterial hypertension encompasses a heterogeneous group of disorders with similar histologic and pathophysiologic abnormalities. Idiopathic pulmonary hypertension (IPAH), familial PAH, and PAH associated with connective tissue diseases, portal hypertension, HIV infection, drugs and toxins, or congenital left-to-right

shunts make up most of the categories of PAH. PAH is a progressive arteriopathy. The devastating consequences are the result of increasing right ventricular afterload, straining right ventricular function and eventually leading to right ventricular failure, hemodynamic collapse, and death. In fact, 50% of deaths reported in the National Institutes of Health (NIH) pulmonary hypertension registry resulted from right ventricular failure [2]. In the last 15 years, the introduction and widespread use of pulmonary vasodilators such as prostanoids, endothelin receptor antagonists, and phosphodiesterase type 5 inhibitors have improved functional outcomes, quality of life (QOL), and survival in patients who have PAH [3–6]. Despite these new therapies, a significant number of patients eventually develop progressive disease. Patients who have end-stage PAH typically experience limited exercise capacity, severe dyspnea on exertion, syncope, and other clinical signs of cor pulmonale such as refractory ascites and severe edema. AS attempts to relieve these symptoms by creating a shunt or relief valve in the interatrial septum, permitting decompression of the right heart (through the right atrium) into the left atrium. Relieving right ventricular strain also may enhance cardiac output; in select patients awaiting lung transplantation, this beneficial effect may prolong survival long enough to find suitable donor organs [7].

The rationale for using AS in PAH is supported by the observation that patients who have IPAH and who have a patent foramen ovale have a longer survival than those without one [8,9]. Similarly, patients who have Eisenmenger syndrome have significantly longer survival than patients who have IPAH or PAH related to other

---

* Corresponding author.
E-mail address: sagerj@uphs.upenn.edu (J.S. Sager).

causes [10–12]. The right-to-left shunting seems to protect right ventricular systolic function despite sustained systemic level pulmonary artery pressures. Austen and colleagues [13] demonstrated in dogs that an interatrial shunt decompressed the right ventricle and improved systemic blood flow with exercise. A recent study of prognostic factors in IPAH by Kawut and colleagues [14] demonstrated that a higher cardiac index and right ventricular ejection fraction were associated with improved survival. AS attempts to improve both of these indices.

Despite the potential benefits of AS, this procedure is associated with considerable risk. Appropriate patient selection and timing of AS remains uncertain. Most recommendations are gleaned from small series or case reports [7,15–24]. A recent review summarized the outcomes from four published case series of at least 10 or more patients. The immediate procedure-related mortality was 13% (7/55 patients). The risk of death was greatest in patients who had very advanced pulmonary hypertension, severe right heart failure, and resting hypoxemia [25]. Conclusions from these limited case reports suggest that only select patients who have symptoms of severe PAH such as recurrent syncope, persistent right heart failure, and marked functional incapacity (New York Heart Association class III or IV) should be considered candidates for the procedure. Recently, a report from Hong Kong described a patient who had severe IPAH who benefited from treatment with a combination of medical therapy (oral sildenafil) and AS [26]. The patient had a sustained clinical response 8 months following AS while receiving chronic sildenafil therapy, as demonstrated by a significant improvement in the 6-minute-walk test (6 MWT) distance, resolution of ascites, and reduction in pulmonary artery pressures (estimated by echocardiography). Further studies are needed to determine the efficacy and safety of combination therapy. In particular, there is concern that the right-to-left shunt created by the AS may expose the vasoactive agents to the systemic circulation and result in life-threatening systemic hypotension [27].

Procedure

Most cases of AS reported in the literature are performed using the percutaneous route [19–21]. AS requires transseptal catheterization to create an interatrial communication large enough to relieve right heart strain, improve left-sided filling, and increase cardiac output. This goal, however, must be balanced against the risk that creating too large a shunt significantly decreases systemic arterial oxygen saturation and reduces systemic oxygen delivery despite improvements in cardiac output. Even with an appropriately sized right-to-left shunt, systemic arterial oxygen saturation should be expected to decline by 5% to 10% [28].

AS can be performed by blade septostomy with or without balloon dilation or by graded static balloon dilation [7,18,20,21,29–31]. The results of graded balloon dilation AS are similar to those of blade balloon AS [17,32]. Both procedures require a transseptal puncture using either a Brockenborough needle (Medtronics, Minneapolis, MN,) or a perforating radiofrequency energy system [33–35]. Use of conventional fluoroscopic landmarks as geographic guides to locate the site of septal puncture can be problematic because patients who have severe pulmonary hypertension have marked right atrial enlargement and leftward displacement of the interatrial septum. Needle puncture requires mechanical force that may cause additional stretching and distortion of the atrial septum, increasing the potential for damage to the surrounding tissue. Even experienced centers have reported a 1.2% incidence of pericardial tamponade associated with inadvertent left atrial puncture [36]. Use of radiofrequency has the theoretic advantage of allowing more precise control of the size of the septal perforation because the thermal effects on adjacent tissue are minimal. This technique also does not stimulate nerve or muscle cells, thereby reducing pain and risk of cardiac arrhythmias [35].

Direct visualization of the atrial septum using transesophageal or intracavitary echocardiography (ICE) may reduce procedure-related complications [23,37–40]. Transthoracic echocardiography, however, may not provide adequate imaging of atrial structures [41–45]. Figs. 1 through 3 demonstrate the use of the ICE catheter during AS using a transseptal needle puncture with graded balloon dilation.

Hemodynamic effects

The immediate postprocedure increase in cardiac index ranges from 15% to 58%. Reports of improvements in pulmonary arterial pressure and pulmonary vascular resistance measurements as well as in functional capacity are variable, with several studies reporting statistically significant

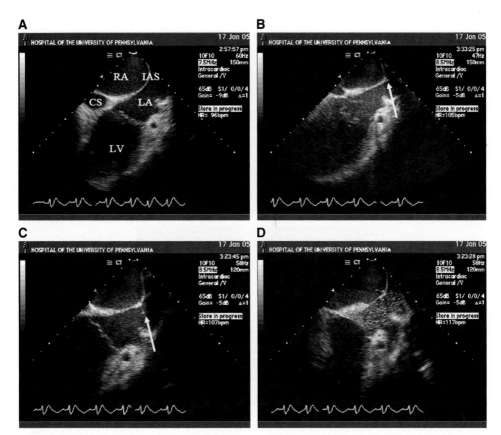

Fig. 1. (*A*) Intracardiac echocardiographic image with the catheter in the mid right atrium, with the transducer rotated clockwise toward the interatrial septum. CS, coronary sinus; LA, left atrium; IAS, interatrial septum; LV, left ventricle; RA, right atrium. (*B*) Intracardiac echocardiographic image with the intracardiac echocardiography catheter in the mid right atrium, with the transducer rotated clockwise toward the interatrial septum. Note the tenting of the fossa ovalis (*arrow*) before transseptal puncture. (*C*) Intracardiac echocardiographic image with the intracavitary echocardiography catheter in the mid right atrium, with the transducer rotated clockwise toward the interatrial septum. Note the tenting of the Brockenbrough needle (*arrow*) as it crosses into the left atrium. (*D*) Intracardiac echocardiographic image with the intracardiac echocardiography catheter in the mid right atrium, with the transducer rotated clockwise toward the interatrial septum. Injection of contrast after transseptal crossing confirms left atrial access. Note microbubbles seen in the left atrium. (Images courtesy of Howard Hermann, MD, Philadelphia, PA.)

benefit; however, the magnitude of the changes often are small and thus may not be clinically significant [19,21,46].

An excellent review published in a previous edition of *Clinics in Chest Medicine* [47] of 64 patients undergoing AS for IPAH demonstrated that mean right atrial pressure decreased by 3 mm Hg, cardiac index increased by 0.7 L/min/m^2, and net systemic oxygen transport increased despite reduction in systemic arterial oxygen saturation. Significant changes to mean pulmonary artery pressure or mean systemic artery pressure immediately postprocedure were not seen. Although the

immediate hemodynamic effects seem to be small, these assessments were performed at rest; thus, additional benefit with exercise cannot be excluded. In fact, animal models suggest that the benefits of AS may be greatest during exercise. For example, dogs with right ventricular hypertension and an atrial septal defect are able to increase left ventricular output dramatically without a significant increment in right ventricular end diastolic pressure These findings are in stark contrast to observations made in dogs without an atrial septal defect [13]. Reports of decrease in New York Heart Association (NYHA) functional

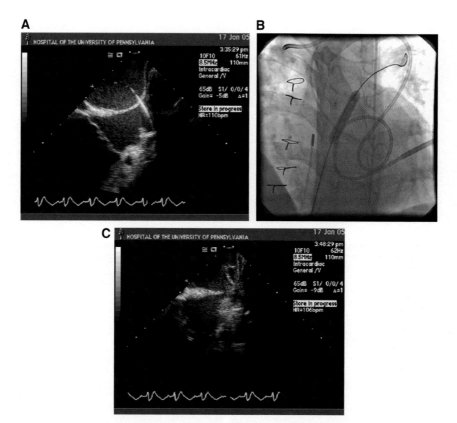

Fig. 2. (*A*) Intracardiac echocardiographic image with the catheter in the mid right atrium, with the transducer rotated clockwise toward the interatrial septum. The guide wire is seen crossing the transseptal puncture. (*B*) Fluoroscopic image of the septostomy balloon at peak inflation. (*C*) Intracardiac echocardiographic image with the intracardiac echocardiography catheter in the mid right atrium, with the transducer rotated clockwise toward the interatrial septum. The balloon is seen crossing the transseptal puncture before maximum inflation. (Images courtesy of Howard Hermann, MD, Philadelphia, PA.)

class and improved 6 MWT distance after AS indicate that the beneficial effects of this procedure may not be appreciated fully by testing obtained while the patient is at rest [21].

Long-term outcomes

Studies of the long-term impact of AS are limited. In one report of 54 patients who underwent AS, the median survival of the group was 19.5 months (range, 2–96 months) [47]. Although sustained hemodynamic benefits for 2 or more years have been documented [46], long-term survival seems to be limited by progressive disease [28]. Whether AS truly confers a survival advantage is not known. Studies reporting survival benefit compared results with historical controls obtained from the NIH registry and may no longer be relevant in the modern era of pharmacologic therapy [21]. At

present, AS should be considered only when all medical therapies have failed and patients do not have resting hypoxemia. The role of this procedure is primarily palliative or as a bridge to thoracic transplantation. Exceptions to this recommendation may be made in regions of the world where pharmacologic therapies are too expensive or are not readily available.

No longitudinal QOL data are available for patients undergoing AS. A cross-sectional study of patients who had IPAH performed at the University of Pennsylvania Medical Center indicated that greater 6-minute-walk distance and lower NYHA functional class correlated with better health-related QOL scores; however, specific hemodynamic parameters did not correlate with QOL [48]. Notably, none of these patients underwent AS, and the overall impact of AS on QOL remains unknown.

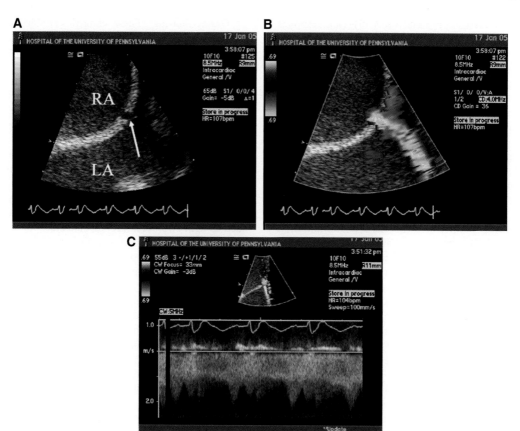

Fig. 3. (*A*) Intracardiac echocardiographic image with the intracardiac echocardiography catheter in the mid right atrium, with the transducer rotated clockwise toward the interatrial septum. After balloon atrial septostomy, the creation of a 4-mm septostomy is seen by two-dimensional imaging (*arrow*). LA, left atrium; RA, right atrium. (*B*) Intracardiac echocardiographic image with the intracardiac echocardiography catheter in the mid right atrium, with the transducer rotated clockwise toward the interatrial septum. Color Doppler flow confirms a continuous right-to-left shunt. (*C*) Continuous-wave Doppler interrogation of the septostomy demonstrates right-to-left shunting throughout the cardiac cycle. (Images courtesy of Howard Hermann, MD, Philadelphia, PA.)

Lung and heart-lung transplantation

Thoracic transplantation offers the possibility of longer survival and improved QOL in patients suffering from end-stage PAH [49]. Although advances in surgical techniques and the introduction of potent immunosuppressive agents has made short- and intermediate-term survival a reality, the transplant recipient remains vulnerable to multiple complications that threaten survival and QOL. The 2006 International Society for Heart and Lung Transplantation (ISHLT) registry reported survival rates of 78% after 1 year, 49% after 5 years, and 25% at 10 years for all lung transplant recipients who received organs between January 1994 and June 2004 [50]. Although patients who had IPAH had the highest perioperative mortality, 5-

and 10-year survival rates are similar to those of patients receiving transplants for other diseases. These humbling survival statistics show that transplantation remains risky and is justified only as the option of last resort.

Effective medical therapies during the past decade have reduced the number of patients receiving transplantation for advanced PAH. In fact, recent reports indicate that IPAH accounted for only 3.9% of all lung transplantations; in 1990 IPAH accounted for 10% of all such procedures [50,51].

Patient referral

The decision to list and offer transplantation to a patient who has PAH depends on several factors including the patient's primary diagnosis (eg,

IPAH versus congenital heart disease), response to medical therapy, functional status, predicted survival, and expected wait times for donor organs. In 1991, the NIH pulmonary hypertension registry reported a median survival of 2.8 years for patients who had IPAH [2]. Since then, effective treatment with pulmonary vasodilators has dramatically improved survival [52–54]. For example, at one transplantation center, epoprostenol treatment of patients who had IPAH on the lung transplant waiting list led to significant improvement in functional status, so that transplantation was deferred in 70% of the cohort [55].

The response to epoprostenol therapy can be assessed as early as 3 months after its initiation [56]. Patients who remain at NYHA class 3 or 4 after 3 months of therapy with intravenous epoprostenol have a 2-year survival rate of 46%; patients whose status improves to NYHA class 1 or 2 have a 2-year survival rate of 93%. Thus short-term response to epoprostenol therapy has significant prognostic implications, and patients who have poor functional status and do not respond to this treatment should be strongly encouraged to undergo evaluation for thoracic transplantation [56]. It is unclear whether other recently introduced pulmonary hypertension therapies, either alone or in combination, will have an additional beneficial effect on patient survival and further reduce the need for transplantation [57–63].

Historically, waiting times in excess of 2 years for donor lungs were common. Organ allocation was determined solely by the amount of time accrued on the waiting list, prompting early referral of patients who had IPAH, who often were not sick enough for transplantation at the time of referral but possibly might need a transplant during the anticipated 1- to 2-year wait. Unfortunately, this strategy of early referral increased the overall number of patients awaiting transplantation and consequently was disadvantageous to patients who had rapidly progressive disease and could not survive the prolonged delay until transplantation. An attempt to address this inequity was made in 2005 with the introduction of a new lung allocation policy in the United States. This policy prioritizes patients by medical urgency and likelihood of benefiting from the transplant procedure rather than simply by time accrued on the waiting list [64].

Under the new system, a lung allocation score (LAS) is calculated for each transplantation candidate based on clinical factors determined to be significant after retrospective multivariate analysis of data collected by the United Network of Organ Sharing. These clinical variables are used to calculate predicted 1-year survival with and without transplantation and net benefit from transplantation. Factors used to predict death on the waiting list for all patients (including those who have PAH) include diagnosis, forced vital capacity, age, body mass index, diabetes, NHYA functional class, 6 MWT distance, ventilator use, and need for supplemental oxygen at rest. Factors used to predict 1-year survival after transplantation are forced vital capacity, age, creatinine, NYHA functional class, and diagnosis. Notably, pulmonary artery pressures as well as important predictors of mortality in patients who have PAH such as right atrial pressure, cardiac index, history of medical treatment failure, and clinical symptoms (syncope, hemoptysis) are not included in the waiting list survival calculation. For these reasons, the new lung allocation system may not calculate medical urgency accurately for patients who have PAH. The accuracy of the calculations of survival after transplantation and net benefit of transplantation is debatable also. This measurement is based on predicted 1-year survival after transplantation. Although 1-year survival is poorer in PAH than in other conditions, because of increased perioperative complications, 5- and 10-year survival rates are similar to those for other disease groups. Because the LAS relies on data for 1-year survival, the true benefit of transplantation may be underestimated, placing patients who have PAH at an allocation disadvantage [50]. Fortunately, the new LAS system has a mechanism for the transplant physician to appeal for a higher LAS score. In addition, there is a mandate to continue data collection so that future calculations may predict prognosis with greater precision.

Prognostication remains difficult for Patients who have Eisenmenger syndrome, and thus the decision of whether to proceed to transplantation is challenging. In general, these patients seem to have a better prognosis than patients who have IPAH and a similar severity of PAH [10]. The risk-to-benefit analysis of lung transplantation in this population is not clear. These patients have lower right atrial pressures and higher cardiac indices than a comparable group of patients who have IPAH. The right-to-left shunt probably exerts a protective effect by offloading the right ventricle, permitting it to adapt more slowly [12]. Nevertheless, a dilated right ventricle, elevated right atrial pressure, and reduced cardiac index in patients who have Eisenmenger syndrome is associated with high mortality [65,66]. These patients should be considered for evaluation for lung (with or without cardiac repair) or heart-lung transplantation. Limited data suggest that heart-lung transplantation confers the greatest survival advantage to patients who have Eisenmenger syndrome caused by ventricular septal defects and other complex congenital heart diseases [67].

There are no clear guidelines regarding the appropriate timing of referral for patients who have PAH related to other diseases. Survival rates vary among the different disease processes, and decisions about transplantation must be individualized.

Selection criteria

The numerous potential life-threatening complications associated with thoracic transplantation require the application of stringent selection criteria to potential candidates to increase the likelihood of a successful outcome [60]. In general, the ideal patient should have reduced short-term survival without transplantation and be ambulatory and free of clinically significant extrathoracic organ damage. A recent update of candidate selection criteria in a consensus statement from the ISHLT outlines general indications as well as absolute and relative contraindications for transplantation [60]. Isolated right-heart dysfunction secondary to severe PAH is not a contraindication to lung transplantation because dramatic post-transplantation reduction in right ventricular afterload can lead to rapid recovery of right ventricular function (Figs. 4 and 5) [68].

Older recipients have poorer outcomes after lung transplantation [50]. In recognition of this finding, earlier consensus guidelines [69] suggested an upper age limits of 55 years for heart-lung transplantation, 60 years for bilateral lung transplantation, and 65 years for single-lung transplantation. Although a survey of lung transplantation practices in the United States indicated that many centers follow these age cutoffs, a recent update of these guidelines did not endorse an upper age limit as an absolute contraindication [60,70].

Patients who have scleroderma, especially the calcinosis, Raynaud's phenomena, esophageal dysmotility, sclerodactyly, and telangiectasia (CREST) syndrome, often have severe PAH. Although thoracic transplantation should be considered for these patients, esophageal dysmotility and gastroesophageal reflux disease pose important and strong relative contraindications. A number of studies now indicate that silent

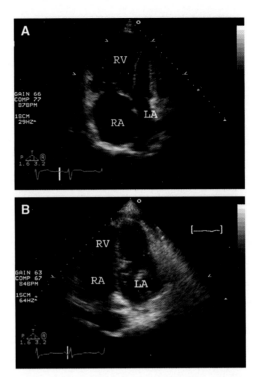

Fig. 4. (*A*) Pretransplantation four-chamber echocardiographic view in a patient who has idiopathic pulmonary arterial hypertension. Note the dilated right atrium (RA) and right ventricle (RV) with the underfilled left atrium (LA). (*B*) Six-month posttransplantation four-chamber echocardiographic view in the same patient. Note the recovery of the right atrium (RA) and right ventricle (RV) to normal size and the improved filling of the left heart chambers. LA, left atrium. (Images courtesy of Martin G. Keane, MD, Philadelphia, PA.)

aspiration of gastric contents is detrimental to graft function and may be an important risk factor for accelerated graft failure [71].

Routine health maintenance examinations, including Pap smear, mammography, and colon cancer screening, should be performed according to age-appropriate guidelines for the general population in all patients being referred for consideration of thoracic organ transplantation.

Choice of procedure

Three transplant options exist for patients who have pulmonary hypertension: single-lung transplantation, bilateral lung transplantation, and combined heart-lung transplantation. Unfortunately, there are no randomized clinical trials to indicate which procedure is optimal. Right ventricular dysfunction associated with severe

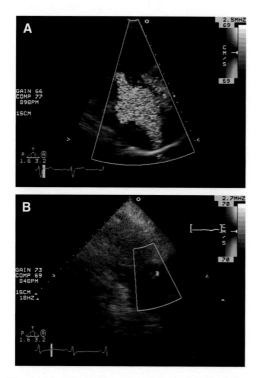

Fig. 5. (A) Pretransplantation right ventricular inflow tract with Doppler study demonstrating severe tricuspid regurgitation. (B) Posttransplantation echocardiographic view of the same patient's right ventricular inflow tract demonstrating trivial tricuspid regurgitation. (Images courtesy of Martin G. Keane, MD, Philadelphia, PA.)

pulmonary hypertension led to initial recommendations supporting combined heart-lung transplantation as the procedure of choice. Data supporting this procedure over isolated lung transplantation are conflicting, however [72–75]. It has been shown that isolated right ventricular dysfunction can recover quickly after lung transplantation, and because thoracic organs are in short supply, lung transplantation has emerged as the recommended procedure for most patients who have PAH. Combined heart-lung transplantation now is reserved primarily for patients who have complex and surgically irreparable congenital heart disease [68,76].

Although, both single- and double-lung transplant procedures have been performed successfully in patients who have severe pulmonary hypertension, a recent survey of North American transplant centers indicated that 88% strongly prefer bilateral lung transplantation in patients who have IPAH [70]. This preference is fueled by concerns that after single-lung transplantation

the marked difference in pulmonary vascular resistance between the allograft and native lung will direct most of the cardiac output toward the freshly implanted allograft, thereby magnifying the risk of reperfusion edema and primary graft dysfunction [76]. Despite these concerns, survival data published in the most recent ISHLT registry report demonstrate no significant difference in survival between single-lung transplantation and bilateral lung transplantation for PAH [50]. Advocates of single-lung transplantation argue that this procedure takes less time than the bilateral procedure; thus the potentially deleterious effects of prolonged ischemic and cardiopulmonary bypass times can be reduced.

Overall, heart-lung, single-lung, and bilateral lung transplantation all have been successfully used in the management of pulmonary hypertension. Each procedure is characterized by unique advantages and disadvantages, and no single procedure has proved clearly superior. In the absence of new information, the patient's diagnosis and severity of illness, institutional experience, and availability of donor organs will be the primary factors determining the preferred surgical procedure for a particular patient who has PAH.

Outcomes

One-year survival after lung transplantation for IPAH is approximately 66%, significantly lower than that associated with transplantation in other patient populations (ie, for emphysema, cystic fibrosis) [50]. Perioperative mortality is particularly high and results from surgical complexity, the requirement for cardiopulmonary bypass with consequent risk of bleeding, increased incidence of hemodynamic instability caused in part by underlying cardiac impairment, and early graft dysfunction [77]. The 5-year survival, however, is 47%, comparable with that of other disease groups. The 10-year survival after transplantation of patients who have PAH is, in fact, better than that of patients undergoing transplantation for chronic obstructive pulmonary disease or idiopathic pulmonary fibrosis [50].

Posttransplantation improvements in hemodynamic parameters and functional status are critical to achieving the primary goal of lung transplantation: improvement in QOL. For patients who have pulmonary vascular disease, both single-lung and bilateral lung transplantation result in immediate and sustained improvements in pulmonary vascular resistance and pulmonary arterial pressure [78]. This improvement is accompanied by an immediate increase in cardiac output and more gradual remodeling of the right ventricle, with a decrease in ventricular wall thickness [79–81].

Most patients who undergo lung transplantation have sufficient improvement in exercise capacity within 1 year of the procedure to permit resumption of an active lifestyle. Recently identified pretransplantation risk factors for poor posttransplantation functional capacity include recipient female gender, high recipient body mass index, and poor functional capacity. Bilateral lung transplantation was associated with improved functional capacity [82]. Studies comparing results of cardiopulmonary exercise testing before and after single-, bilateral, and heart-lung transplantation for various disease groups, including pulmonary vascular disease, have shown dramatic improvement in exercise tolerance after transplantation. Peak exercise capacity, although considerably enhanced, remains suboptimal when compared with normal volunteers. Cardiopulmonary exercise testing measurements typically show a reduced anaerobic threshold and maximum oxygen consumption despite the absence of significant cardiac or ventilatory limitations [83–87]. These findings suggest that abnormal peripheral oxygen use at the level of the skeletal muscle, possibly resulting from calcineurin inhibitor–induced impairment in mitochondrial function, may contribute to peak exercise limitations [88–91].

Specific data comparing QOL before and after lung transplantation for PAH are lacking. QOL surveys assessing physical, social, and psychologic functioning in the general lung transplantation population reveal significant short- and intermediate-term improvements. Long-term QOL benefit is more variable and depends on the presence and number of comorbidities and, in particular, on the degree to which graft function is compromised by the development of chronic rejection [92–95].

Postoperative complications

Although lung transplantation offers the possibility of improved survival and QOL for patients who have advanced lung disease, the plethora of possible complications after transplantation threatens these objectives. These complications may be technical, mediated by allograft-specific or independent immune responses, or the consequence of immunosuppression.

Mild, transient edema is a nearly universal feature of the freshly transplanted lung allograft. It is thought to be the consequence of increased microvascular permeability associated with ischemia-reperfusion injury to the allograft, although surgical trauma and lymphatic disruption also may be important contributing factors. Severe reperfusion lung injury or primary graft dysfunction (PGD) occurs in approximately 12% to 22% of lung transplant recipients [96–99]. Donor female sex, African American donor ethnicity, and recipient diagnosis of IPAH are associated risk factors for the development of PGD [99]. Additionally, prolonged ischemic time is likely to be an important risk factor, although this has not been uniformly observed [100,101].

The diagnosis of PGD is based on the development of widespread radiographic infiltrates and markedly impaired oxygenation within 72 hours of transplantation in the absence of other causes of early graft dysfunction. Histopathologic examination of lung tissue from patients who have PGD reveals prevailing patterns of diffuse alveolar damage [102]. Treatment typically is supportive, relying on lung-protective mechanical ventilation strategies.

PGD has a significant impact on mortality, duration of mechanical ventilation, and hospital length of stay after lung transplantation. The 2006 ISHLT registry report indicated that PGD is the most common cause of death within the first month after lung transplantation [50]. Survivors of PGD have a protracted recovery with impaired physical function up to 1 year after transplantation [103].

Anastomotic complications after lung transplantation may occur at the site of bronchial, pulmonary arterial, and venous anastomotic sites. Dehiscence of the bronchial anastomosis once was a leading cause of perioperative mortality, but refinements in surgical techniques, tissue preservation, and immunosuppression have reduced dramatically the incidence of major dehiscence. Focal dehiscence is still encountered in 1% to 6% of recipients [104–106]; fortunately, these wounds usually heal without surgical intervention. It is hypothesized that disruption of the donor bronchial blood supply during explantation increases the risk of ischemic injury to the bronchial mucosa and contributes to the risk of developing dehiscence or other airway complications [107,108].

The most common airway complication is the development of bronchial anastomotic narrowing. It typically develops within several weeks of transplantation and has been reported to occur in 12% to 24% of lung recipients. Anastomotic strictures typically present with focal wheezing on the involved side, recurrent bouts of pneumonia or purulent bronchitis, and reduced spirometry measurements. Direct bronchoscopic visualization of the anastomosis is required for diagnosis and treatment. Techniques used to address anastomotic narrowing include balloon dilatation, electrocautery or laser débridement of excessive granulation tissue, transbronchial needle injection of corticosteroids, endobronchial stent placement, and, rarely, brachytherapy [104,109–111].

Lung transplant recipients are at considerable risk of lung injury mediated by alloreactive T cells. This process, termed "acute rejection," occurs in 55% to 75% of transplant recipients within the first year after transplantation, despite the administration of potent immunosuppressive agents [112]. Symptoms of acute rejection, such as fever, chills, malaise, and increasing dyspnea, may be absent or nonspecific. Physical examination can be normal or may reveal signs of a pleural effusion and crackles on auscultation. Declining spirometric measurements and resting- or exercise-induced hypoxemia may be seen. The standard for diagnosis depends on histopathologic evaluation of lung tissue, usually obtained by performing transbronchial lung biopsies. The presence of acute rejection can be confirmed by evidence of perivascular lymphocytic infiltrates that in advanced stages may extend into the alveolar septum [113]. Treatment involves augmentation of immunosuppression, usually by administering pulse dose corticosteroids. Recurrent or refractory acute rejection episodes may be treated with T-cell depleting antibodies or unconventional immunomodulatory strategies such as photopheresis or total lymphoid irradiation [114].

Chronic rejection is the major obstacle to long-term survival after lung transplantation. It is present in up to two thirds of all long-term survivors [115–117]. The histologic manifestation of chronic rejection, bronchiolitis obliterans, is characterized by inflammation and fibrosis of the bronchiolar walls ultimately progressing to obliteration of the airway lumen. Acute rejection, particularly when recurrent or severe, is the most common identified risk factor for chronic rejection. Alloimmune-independent risk factors also have been reported, although less consistently. These include cytomegalovirus and other respiratory viral infections and gastroesophageal reflux

disease [118,119]. Because the sensitivity of transbronchial biopsy for the detection of bronchiolitis obliterans is low, a clinical surrogate based on spirometric criteria was defined and termed the "bronchiolitis obliterans syndrome" (BOS) [120]. The incidence of BOS is greatest within the first 2 years after transplantation, but the risk remains persistent beyond this time [115]. The onset of BOS typically is insidious but may be abrupt in aggressive cases. Dyspnea, cough, and recurrent bouts of purulent tracheobronchitis, with recovery of *Pseudomonas aeruginosa* from sputum cultures, are highly characteristic features. Although chest radiographs usually are unremarkable, high-resolution CT of the chest reveals air trapping on expiratory images in most patients and evidence of bronchiectasis in some [121–123]. No effective treatment has been proven for BOS, but promising studies suggest that the immunomodulatory properties of the macrolide antibiotic azithromycin may be beneficial [124,125]. Retransplantation remains a treatment option for select patients.

Infection rates among lung transplant recipients seem to be higher than in other solid-organ transplant populations and probably are related to the higher levels of administered immunosuppression and the unique exposure of the lung allograft to the external environment [126]. Bacterial infections of the lower respiratory tract predominate and seem to have a bimodal distribution with reported incidence of 16% in the early posttransplantation period [127]. These infections re-emerge as important late complications after transplantation, particularly in patients who develop chronic rejection. Gram-negative pathogens, especially *Pseudomonas aeruginosa*, are most frequently isolated in association with both early and late infectious events [128–131].

Cytomegalovirus is the most common viral pathogen encountered in the posttransplantation period. Although antiviral therapy has dramatically reduced direct mortality from cytomegalovirus infection, this virus continues to cause frequent, troubling infections, is associated with an increased risk of bacterial and fungal superinfections, and has been implicated as a risk factor for the development of chronic rejection [132,133]. Recent studies suggest that other respiratory viral pathogens such as respiratory syncytial virus, parainfluenza virus, and adenovirus also may be associated with progressive graft dysfunction and chronic rejection [134].

Although a number of opportunistic and endemic fungal pathogens have been reported to cause pulmonary infections in lung transplant recipients, *Aspergillus* species are by far the most frequent and lethal pathogens encountered. Approximately 5% of lung recipients develop *Aspergillus* infections of the airway [135]. The devitalized cartilage and foreign suture material of the fresh bronchial anastomosis create a favorable environment for localized fungal infection at the anastomotic site. A more diffuse ulcerative tracheobronchitis is seen occasionally after severe ischemic injury to the bronchial mucosa [136]. *Aspergillus* infections of the airway typically occur in the first 6 months after transplantation and usually respond to appropriate antifungal therapy, although, rarely, progression to invasive pneumonia or fatal erosion into an adjacent pulmonary artery have been reported [135,137,138].

Invasive aspergillosis is the most serious and devastating form of *Aspergillus* infection. An overall incidence rate of 5% has been calculated from pooled studies [126]. Most cases occur within the first year after transplantation. Despite treatment with antifungal agents, mortality approaches 60% [135].

Long-term use of immunosuppressive agents may create or exacerbate pre-existing medical problems such as osteoporosis, renal insufficiency, hypertension, hypercholesterolemia, gastroparesis, and reflux disease [126]. Immunosuppression also increases the risk of neoplastic complications. For example, 2% to 8% of lung recipients develop posttransplantation lymphoproliferative disorder [139,140], a spectrum of abnormal B-cell proliferative responses ranging from benign polyclonal hyperplasia to malignant lymphomas triggered by unchecked Epstein-Barr virus proliferation in the immunosuppressed transplant recipient [141].

Summary

Transplantation remains an effective therapy for patients suffering from end-stage disease caused by PAH. The major hurdles that the transplant community faces are the shortage of donor organs and the development of chronic rejection (ie, BOS). The physician caring for the lung recipient must be vigilant for the numerous posttransplantation complications that may arise. A recent volume of *The Clinics in Chest Medicine* [142] reviews an in-depth discussion of some of the issues raised in this article. Many PAH recipients of lung transplants have an excellent QOL with nearly complete restoration of activities of daily living and other activities.

References

[1] Hoeper MM, Mayer E, Simonneau G, et al. Chronic thromboembolic pulmonary hypertension. Circulation 2006;113(16):2011–20.

[2] D'Alonzo GE, Barst RJ, Ayres SM, et al. Survival in patients with primary pulmonary hypertension. Results from a national prospective registry. Ann Intern Med 1991;115(5):343–9.

[3] Galie N, Ghofrani HA, Torbicki A, et al. Sildenafil citrate therapy for pulmonary arterial hypertension. N Engl J Med 2005;353(20):2148–57.

[4] Rubin LJ, Badesch DB, Barst RJ, et al. Bosentan therapy for pulmonary arterial hypertension. N Engl J Med 2002;346(12):896–903.

[5] Simonneau G, Barst RJ, Galie N, et al. Continuous subcutaneous infusion of treprostinil, a prostacyclin analogue, in patients with pulmonary arterial hypertension: a double-blind, randomized, placebo-controlled trial. Am J Respir Crit Care Med 2002;165(6):800–4.

[6] Barst RJ, Rubin LJ, McGoon MD, et al. Survival in primary pulmonary hypertension with long-term continuous intravenous prostacyclin. Ann Intern Med 1994;121(6):409–15.

[7] Rothman A, Sklansky MS, Lucas VW, et al. Atrial septostomy as a bridge to lung transplantation in patients with severe pulmonary hypertension. Am J Cardiol 1999;84(6):682–6.

[8] Rozkovec A, Montanes P, Oakley CM. Factors that influence the outcome of primary pulmonary hypertension. Br Heart J 1986;55(5):449–58.

[9] Glanville AR, Burke CM, Theodore J, et al. Primary pulmonary hypertension. Length of survival in patients referred for heart-lung transplantation. Chest 1987;91(5):675–81.

[10] Hopkins WE, Ochoa LL, Richardson GW, et al. Comparison of the hemodynamics and survival of adults with severe primary pulmonary hypertension or Eisenmenger syndrome. J Heart Lung Transplant 1996;15(1 Pt 1):100–5.

[11] Hopkins WE. The remarkable right ventricle of patients with Eisenmenger syndrome. Coron Artery Dis 2005;16(1):19–25.

[12] Hopkins WE, Waggoner AD. Severe pulmonary hypertension without right ventricular failure: the unique hearts of patients with Eisenmenger syndrome. Am J Cardiol 2002;89(1):34–8.

[13] Austen WG, Morrow AG, Berry WB. Experimental studies of the surgical treatment of primary pulmonary hypertension. J Thorac Cardiovasc Surg 1964;48:448–55.

[14] Kawut SM, Horn EM, Berekashvili KK, et al. New predictors of outcome in idiopathic pulmonary arterial hypertension. Am J Cardiol 2005;95(2):199–203.

[15] Collins TJ, Moore JW, Kirby WC. Atrial septostomy for pulmonary hypertension. Am Heart J 1988;116(3):873–4.

[16] Fulwani M, Nabar A, Iyer R, et al. Palliative blade-balloon atrial septostomy in primary pulmonary hypertension. Indian Heart J 1997;49(2):185–6.

[17] Hausknecht MJ, Sims RE, Nihill MR, et al. Successful palliation of primary pulmonary hypertension by atrial septostomy. Am J Cardiol 1990; 65(15):1045–6.

[18] Kerstein D, Levy PS, Hsu DT, et al. Blade balloon atrial septostomy in patients with severe primary pulmonary hypertension. Circulation 1995;91(7): 2028–35.

[19] Nihill MR, O'Laughlin MP, Mullins CE. Effects of atrial septostomy in patients with terminal cor pulmonale due to pulmonary vascular disease. Cathet Cardiovasc Diagn 1991;24(3):166–72.

[20] Rich S, Dodin E, McLaughlin VV. Usefulness of atrial septostomy as a treatment for primary pulmonary hypertension and guidelines for its application. Am J Cardiol 1997;80(3):369–71.

[21] Sandoval J, Gaspar J, Pulido T, et al. Graded balloon dilation atrial septostomy in severe primary pulmonary hypertension. A therapeutic alternative for patients nonresponsive to vasodilator treatment. J Am Coll Cardiol 1998;32(2):297–304.

[22] Thanopoulos BD, Georgakopoulos D, Tsaousis GS, et al. Percutaneous balloon dilatation of the atrial septum: immediate and midterm results. Heart 1996;76(6):502–6.

[23] Unger P, Stoupel E, Vachiery JL, et al. Atrial septostomy under transesophageal guidance in a patient with primary pulmonary hypertension and absent right superior vena cava. Intensive Care Med 1996;22(12):1410–1.

[24] Micheletti A, Hislop AA, Lammers A, et al. Role of atrial septostomy in the treatment of children with pulmonary arterial hypertension. Heart 2006;92(7): 969–72.

[25] Doyle RL, McCrory D, Channick RN, et al. Surgical treatments/interventions for pulmonary arterial hypertension: ACCP evidence-based clinical practice guidelines. Chest 2004;126(1 Suppl): 63S–71S.

[26] Chau EM, Fan KY, Chow WH. Combined atrial septostomy and oral sildenafil for severe right ventricular failure due to primary pulmonary hypertension. Hong Kong Med J 2004;10(4):281–4.

[27] Laine JF, Slama M, Petitpretz P, et al. Danger of vasodilator therapy for pulmonary hypertension in patent foramen ovale. Chest 1986;89(6):894–5.

[28] Barst RJ. Role of atrial septostomy in the treatment of pulmonary vascular disease. Thorax 2000;55(2): 95–6.

[29] Reichenberger F, Pepke-Zaba J, McNeil K, et al. Atrial septostomy in the treatment of severe pulmonary arterial hypertension. Thorax 2003;58(9): 797–800.

[30] Ali Khan MA, Bricker JT, Mullins CE, et al. Blade atrial septostomy: experience with the first 50 procedures. Cathet Cardiovasc Diagn 1991;23(4): 257–62.

[31] Allcock RJ, O'Sullivan JJ, Corris PA. Atrial septostomy for pulmonary arterial hypertension. Heart 2003;89(11):1344–7.

[32] Rothman A, Beltran D, Kriett JM, et al. Graded balloon dilation atrial septostomy as a bridge to lung transplantation in pulmonary hypertension. Am Heart J 1993;125(6):1763–6.

[33] Bunch TJ, Asirvatham SJ, Friedman PA, et al. Outcomes after cardiac perforation during radiofrequency ablation of the atrium. J Cardiovasc Electrophysiol 2005;16(11):1172–9.

[34] Sherman W, Lee P, Hartley A, et al. Transatrial septal catheterization using a new radiofrequency probe. Catheter Cardiovasc Interv 2005;66(1):14–7.

[35] Sakata Y, Feldman T. Transcatheter creation of atrial septal perforation using a radiofrequency transseptal system: novel approach as an alternative to transseptal needle puncture. Catheter Cardiovasc Interv 2005;64(3):327–32.

[36] Roelke M, Smith AJ, Palacios IF. The technique and safety of transseptal left heart catheterization: the Massachusetts General Hospital experience with 1,279 procedures. Cathet Cardiovasc Diagn 1994;32(4):332–9.

[37] Kipel G, Arnon R, Ritter SB. Transesophageal echocardiographic guidance of balloon atrial septostomy. J Am Soc Echocardiogr 1991;4(6):631–5.

[38] Bidoggia H, Maciel JP, Alvarez JA. Transseptal left heart catheterization: usefulness of the intracavitary electrocardiogram in the localization of the fossa ovalis. Cathet Cardiovasc Diagn 1991;24(3): 221–5.

[39] Oztunc F, Saltik IL, Batmaz G, et al. Balloon atrial septostomy under echocardiographic guidance. Case report. Turk J Pediatr 1998;40(3):437–40.

[40] Moscucci M, Dairywala IT, Chetcuti S, et al. Balloon atrial septostomy in end-stage pulmonary hypertension guided by a novel intracardiac echocardiographic transducer. Catheter Cardiovasc Interv 2001;52(4):530–4.

[41] Cafri C, de la Guardia B, Barasch E, et al. Transseptal puncture guided by intracardiac echocardiography during percutaneous transvenous mitral commissurotomy in patients with distorted anatomy of the fossa ovalis. Catheter Cardiovasc Interv 2000;50(4):463–7.

[42] Zanchetta M, Rigatelli G, Pedon L, et al. Role of intracardiac echocardiography in atrial septal abnormalities. J Interv Cardiol 2003;16(1):63–77.

[43] Zanchetta M, Rigatelli G, Pedon L, et al. Intracardiac echocardiography: gross anatomy and magnetic resonance correlations and validations. Int J Cardiovasc Imaging 2005;21(4):391–401.

[44] Zanchetta M, Rigatelli G, Pedon L, et al. Transcatheter atrial septal defect closure assisted by

intracardiac echocardiography: 3-year follow-up. J Interv Cardiol 2004;17(2):95–8.

[45] Boccalandro F, Baptista E, Muench A, et al. Comparison of intracardiac echocardiography versus transesophageal echocardiography guidance for percutaneous transcatheter closure of atrial septal defect. Am J Cardiol 2004;93(4):437–40.

[46] Kothari SS, Yusuf A, Juneja R, et al. Graded balloon atrial septostomy in severe pulmonary hypertension. Indian Heart J 2002;54(2):164–9.

[47] Sandoval J, Rothman A, Pulido T. Atrial septostomy for pulmonary hypertension. Clin Chest Med 2001;22(3):547–60.

[48] Taichman DB, Shin J, Hud L, et al. Health-related quality of life in patients with pulmonary arterial hypertension. Respir Res 2005;6:92.

[49] Arcasoy SM, Kotloff RM. Lung transplantation. N Engl J Med 1999;340(14):1081–91.

[50] Trulock EP, Edwards LB, Taylor DO, et al. Registry of the International Society for Heart and Lung Transplantation: twenty-third official adult lung and heart-lung transplantation report—2006. J Heart Lung Transplant 2006;25(8):880–92.

[51] Trulock EP, Edwards LB, Taylor DO, et al. Registry of the International Society for Heart and Lung Transplantation: twenty-second official adult lung and heart-lung transplant report—2005. J Heart Lung Transplant 2005;24(8):956–67.

[52] McLaughlin VV, Shillington A, Rich S. Survival in primary pulmonary hypertension: the impact of epoprostenol therapy. Circulation 2002;106(12): 1477–82.

[53] Shapiro SM, Oudiz RJ, Cao T, et al. Primary pulmonary hypertension: improved long-term effects and survival with continuous intravenous epoprostenol infusion. J Am Coll Cardiol 1997;30(2):343–9.

[54] Kuhn KP, Byrne DW, Arbogast PG, et al. Outcome in 91 consecutive patients with pulmonary arterial hypertension receiving epoprostenol. Am J Respir Crit Care Med 2003;167(4):580–6.

[55] Conte JV, Gaine SP, Orens JB, et al. The influence of continuous intravenous prostacyclin therapy for primary pulmonary hypertension on the timing and outcome of transplantation. J Heart Lung Transplant 1998;17(7):679–85.

[56] Sitbon O, Humbert M, Nunes H, et al. Long-term intravenous epoprostenol infusion in primary pulmonary hypertension: prognostic factors and survival. J Am Coll Cardiol 2002;40(4):780–8

[57] Minai OA, Arroliga AC. Long-term results after addition of sildenafil in idiopathic PAH patients on bosentan. South Med J 2006;99(8):880–3.

[58] McLaughlin VV, Oudiz RJ, Frost A, et al. Randomized study of adding inhaled iloprost to existing bosentan in pulmonary arterial hypertension. Am J Respir Crit Care Med 2006;174(11):1257–63.

[59] Lunze K, Gilbert N, Mebus S, et al. First experience with an oral combination therapy using bosentan and sildenafil for pulmonary arterial

hypertension. Eur J Clin Invest 2006;36(Suppl 3): 32–8.

[60] Orens JB, Estenne M, Arcasoy S, et al. International guidelines for the selection of lung transplant candidates: 2006 update—a consensus report from the Pulmonary Scientific Council of the International Society for Heart and Lung Transplantation. J Heart Lung Transplant 2006;25(7):745–55.

[61] Barst RJ, Langleben D, Badesch D, et al. Treatment of pulmonary arterial hypertension with the selective endothelin-A receptor antagonist sitaxsentan. J Am Coll Cardiol 2006;47(10):2049–56.

[62] Olschewski H, Simonneau G, Galie N, et al. Inhaled iloprost for severe pulmonary hypertension. N Engl J Med 2002;347(5):322–9.

[63] Hoeper MM, Galie N, Simonneau G, et al. New treatments for pulmonary arterial hypertension. Am J Respir Crit Care Med 2002;165(9):1209–16.

[64] Egan TM, Murray S, Bustami RT, et al. Development of the new lung allocation system in the United States. Am J Transplant 2006;6(5 Pt 2): 1212–27.

[65] Daliento L, Somerville J, Presbitero P, et al. Eisenmenger syndrome. Factors relating to deterioration and death. Eur Heart J 1998;19(12):1845–55.

[66] Oya H, Nagaya N, Uematsu M, et al. Poor prognosis and related factors in adults with Eisenmenger syndrome. Am Heart J 2002;143(4):739–44.

[67] Waddell TK, Bennett L, Kennedy R, et al. Heart-lung or lung transplantation for Eisenmenger syndrome. J Heart Lung Transplant 2002;21(7):731–7.

[68] Kasimir MT, Seebacher G, Jaksch P, et al. Reverse cardiac remodelling in patients with primary pulmonary hypertension after isolated lung transplantation. Eur J Cardiothorac Surg 2004;26(4):776–81.

[69] Maurer JR, Frost AE, Estenne M, et al. International guidelines for the selection of lung transplant candidates. The International Society for Heart and Lung Transplantation, the American Thoracic Society, the American Society of Transplant Physicians, the European Respiratory Society. J Heart Lung Transplant 1998;17(7):703–9.

[70] Levine SM. A survey of clinical practice of lung transplantation in North America. Chest 2004; 125(4):1224–38.

[71] Hadjiliadis D, Duane Davis R, Steele MP, et al. Gastroesophageal reflux disease in lung transplant recipients. Clin Transpl 2003;17(4):363–8.

[72] Franke UF, Wahlers T, Wittwer T, et al. Heart-lung transplantation is the method of choice in the treatment of patients with end-stage pulmonary hypertension. Transplant Proc 2002;34(6): 2181–2.

[73] Ueno T, Smith JA, Snell GI, et al. Bilateral sequential single lung transplantation for pulmonary hypertension and Eisenmenger's syndrome. Ann Thorac Surg 2000;69(2):381–7.

[74] Chapelier A, Vouhe P, Macchiarini P, et al. Comparative outcome of heart-lung and lung

transplantation for pulmonary hypertension. J Thorac Cardiovasc Surg 1993;106(2):299–307.

[75] Whyte RI, Robbins RC, Altinger J, et al. Heart-lung transplantation for primary pulmonary hypertension. Ann Thorac Surg 1999;67(4):937–41 [discussion: 941–2].

[76] Bando K, Armitage JM, Paradis IL, et al. Indications for and results of single, bilateral, and heart-lung transplantation for pulmonary hypertension. J Thorac Cardiovasc Surg 1994;108(6):1056–65.

[77] Klepetko W, Mayer E, Sandoval J, et al. Interventional and surgical modalities of treatment for pulmonary arterial hypertension. J Am Coll Cardiol 2004;43(12 Suppl S):73S–80S.

[78] Gammie JS, Keenan RJ, Pham SM, et al. Single-versus double-lung transplantation for pulmonary hypertension. J Thorac Cardiovasc Surg 1998; 115(2):397–402 [discussion: 402–3].

[79] Moulton MJ, Creswell LL, Ungacta FF, et al. Magnetic resonance imaging provides evidence for remodeling of the right ventricle after single-lung transplantation for pulmonary hypertension. Circulation 1996;94(9 Suppl):II312–9.

[80] Pasque MK, Trulock EP, Cooper JD, et al. Single lung transplantation for pulmonary hypertension. Single institution experience in 34 patients. Circulation 1995;92(8):2252–8.

[81] Mendeloff EN, Meyers BF, Sundt TM, et al. Lung transplantation for pulmonary vascular disease. Ann Thorac Surg 2002;73(1):209–17 [discussion: 217–9].

[82] Sager JS, Kotloff RM, Ahya VN, et al. Association of clinical risk factors with functional status following lung transplantation. Am J Transplant 2006; 6(9):2191–201.

[83] Orens JB, Becker FS, Lynch JP III, et al. Cardiopulmonary exercise testing following allogeneic lung transplantation for different underlying disease states. Chest 1995;107(1):144–9.

[84] Schwaiblmair M, Reichenspurner H, Muller C, et al. Cardiopulmonary exercise testing before and after lung and heart-lung transplantation. Am J Respir Crit Care Med 1999;159(4 Pt 1): 1277–83.

[85] Theodore J, Morris AJ, Burke CM, et al. Cardiopulmonary function at maximum tolerable constant work rate exercise following human heart-lung transplantation. Chest 1987;92(3):433–9.

[86] Oelberg DA, Systrom DM, Markowitz DH, et al. Exercise performance in cystic fibrosis before and after bilateral lung transplantation. J Heart Lung Transplant 1998;17(11):1104–12.

[87] Levy RD, Ernst P, Levine SM, et al. Exercise performance after lung transplantation. J Heart Lung Transplant 1993;12(1 Pt 1):27–33.

[88] McKenna MJ, Fraser SF, Li JL, et al. Impaired muscle Ca2+ and K+ regulation contribute to poor exercise performance post-lung transplantation. J Appl Physiol 2003;95(4):1606–16.

[89] Tirdel GB, Girgis R, Fishman RS, et al. Metabolic myopathy as a cause of the exercise limitation in lung transplant recipients. J Heart Lung Transplant 1998;17(12):1231–7.

[90] Mercier JG, Hokanson JF, Brooks GA. Effects of cyclosporine A on skeletal muscle mitochondrial respiration and endurance time in rats. Am J Respir Crit Care Med 1995;151(5):1532–6.

[91] Evans AB, Al-Himyary AJ, Hrovat MI, et al. Abnormal skeletal muscle oxidative capacity after lung transplantation by 31P-MRS. Am J Respir Crit Care Med 1997;155(2):615–21.

[92] TenVergert EM, Essink-Bot ML, Geertsma A, et al. The effect of lung transplantation on health-related quality of life: a longitudinal study. Chest 1998;113(2):358–64.

[93] MacNaughton KL, Rodrigue JR, Cicale M, et al. Health-related quality of life and symptom frequency before and after lung transplantation. Clin Transpl 1998;12(4):320–3.

[94] Vermeulen KM, Ouwens JP, van der Bij W, et al. Long-term quality of life in patients surviving at least 55 months after lung transplantation. Gen Hosp Psychiatry 2003;25(2):95–102.

[95] Lanuza DM, Lefaiver C, McCabe M, et al. Prospective study of functional status and quality of life before and after lung transplantation. Chest 2000;118(1):115–22.

[96] de Perrot M, Liu M, Waddell TK, et al. Ischemia-reperfusion-induced lung injury. Am J Respir Crit Care Med 2003;167(4):490–511.

[97] Christie JD, Carby M, Bag R, et al. Report of the ISHLT Working Group on Primary Lung Graft Dysfunction part II: definition. A consensus statement of the International Society for Heart and Lung Transplantation. J Heart Lung Transplant 2005;24(10):1454–9.

[98] Christie JD, Van Raemdonck D, de Perrot M, et al. Report of the ISHLT Working Group on Primary Lung Graft Dysfunction part I: introduction and methods. J Heart Lung Transplant 2005;24(10): 1451–3.

[99] Christie JD, Kotloff RM, Pochettino A, et al. Clinical risk factors for primary graft failure following lung transplantation. Chest 2003;124(4): 1232–41.

[100] Thabut G, Mal H, Cerrina J, et al. Graft ischemic time and outcome of lung transplantation: a multi-center analysis. Am J Respir Crit Care Med 2005; 171(7):786–91.

[101] Christie JD. Lung allograft ischemic time: crossing the threshold. Am J Respir Crit Care Med 2005; 171(7):673–4.

[102] Christie JD, Bavaria JE, Palevsky HI, et al. Primary graft failure following lung transplantation. Chest 1998;114(1):51–60.

[103] Christie JD, Sager JS, Kimmel SE, et al. Impact of primary graft failure on outcomes following lung transplantation. Chest 2005;127(1):161–5.

[104] Mughal MM, Gildea TR, Murthy S, et al. Short-term deployment of self-expanding metallic stents facilitates healing of bronchial dehiscence. Am J Respir Crit Care Med 2005;172(6):768–71.

[105] Schmid RA, Boehler A, Speich R, et al. Bronchial anastomotic complications following lung transplantation: still a major cause of morbidity? Eur Respir J 1997;10(12):2872–5.

[106] Schroder C, Scholl F, Daon E, et al. A modified bronchial anastomosis technique for lung transplantation. Ann Thorac Surg 2003;75(6): 1697–704.

[107] Barman SA, Ardell JL, Parker JC, et al. Pulmonary and systemic blood flow contributions to upper airways in canine lung. Am J Physiol 1988;255(5 Pt 2): H1130–5.

[108] Herrera JM, McNeil KD, Higgins RS, et al. Airway complications after lung transplantation: treatment and long-term outcome. Ann Thorac Surg 2001; 71(3):989–93 [discussion: 993–4].

[109] Seymour CW, Krimsky WS, Sager J, et al. Trans-bronchial needle injection: a systematic review of a new diagnostic and therapeutic paradigm. Respiration 2006;73(1):78–89.

[110] Chhajed PN, Malouf MA, Tamm M, et al. Interventional bronchoscopy for the management of airway complications following lung transplantation. Chest 2001;120(6):1894–9.

[111] Chhajed PN, Malouf MA, Tamm M, et al. Ultra-flex stents for the management of airway complications in lung transplant recipients. Respirology 2003;8(1):59–64.

[112] Hopkins PM, Aboyoun CL, Chhajed PN, et al. Prospective analysis of 1,235 transbronchial lung biopsies in lung transplant recipients. J Heart Lung Transplant 2002;21(10):1062–7.

[113] Yousem SA, Berry GJ, Cagle PT, et al. Revision of the 1990 working formulation for the classification of pulmonary allograft rejection: Lung Rejection Study Group. J Heart Lung Transplant 1996; 15(1 Pt 1):1–15.

[114] Whelan TP, Hertz MI. Allograft rejection after lung transplantation. Clin Chest Med 2005;26(4): 599–612, vi.

[115] Bando K, Paradis IL, Similo S, et al. Obliterative bronchiolitis after lung and heart-lung transplantation. An analysis of risk factors and management. J Thorac Cardiovasc Surg 1995;110(1):4–13 [discussion: 13–4].

[116] Boehler A, Estenne M. Obliterative bronchiolitis after lung transplantation. Curr Opin Pulm Med 2000;6(2):133–9.

[117] Sundaresan S, Trulock EP, Mohanakumar T, et al. Prevalence and outcome of bronchiolitis obliterans syndrome after lung transplantation. Washington University Lung Transplant Group. Ann Thorac Surg 1995;60(5):1341–6 [discussion: 1346–7].

[118] Kroshus TJ, Kshettry VR, Savik K, et al. Risk factors for the development of bronchiolitis obliterans syndrome after lung transplantation. J Thorac Cardiovasc Surg 1997;114(2):195–202.

[119] Nicod LP. Mechanisms of airway obliteration after lung transplantation. Proc Am Thorac Soc 2006; 3(5):444–9.

[120] Estenne M, Maurer JR, Boehler A, et al. Bronchiolitis obliterans syndrome 2001: an update of the diagnostic criteria. J Heart Lung Transplant 2002; 21(3):297–310.

[121] Bankier AA, Van Muylem A, Knoop C, et al. Bronchiolitis obliterans syndrome in heart-lung transplant recipients: diagnosis with expiratory CT. Radiology 2001;218(2):533–9.

[122] Lee ES, Gotway MB, Reddy GP, et al. Early bronchiolitis obliterans following lung transplantation: accuracy of expiratory thin-section CT for diagnosis. Radiology 2000;216(2):472–7.

[123] Leung AN, Fisher K, Valentine V, et al. Bronchiolitis obliterans after lung transplantation: detection using expiratory HRCT. Chest 1998;113(2): 365–70.

[124] Gerhardt SG, McDyer JF, Girgis RE, et al. Maintenance azithromycin therapy for bronchiolitis obliterans syndrome: results of a pilot study. Am J Respir Crit Care Med 2003;168(1):121–5.

[125] Yates B, Murphy DM, Forrest IA, et al. Azithromycin reverses airflow obstruction in established bronchiolitis obliterans syndrome. Am J Respir Crit Care Med 2005;172(6):772–5.

[126] Kotloff RM, Ahya VN. Medical complications of lung transplantation. Eur Respir J 2004;23(2): 334–42.

[127] Weill D, Dey GC, Hicks RA, et al. A positive donor gram stain does not predict outcome following lung transplantation. J Heart Lung Transplant 2002; 21(5):555–8.

[128] Horvath J, Dummer S, Loyd J, et al. Infection in the transplanted and native lung after single lung transplantation. Chest 1993;104(3):681–5.

[129] Kramer MR, Marshall SE, Starnes VA, et al. Infectious complications in heart-lung transplantation. Analysis of 200 episodes. Arch Intern Med 1993; 153(17):2010–6.

[130] Maurer JR, Tullis DE, Grossman RF, et al. Infectious complications following isolated lung transplantation. Chest 1992;101(4):1056–9.

[131] Gasink LB, Blumberg EA. Bacterial and mycobacterial pneumonia in transplant recipients. Clin Chest Med 2005;26(4):647–59, vii.

[132] Boehler A, Estenne M. Post-transplant bronchiolitis obliterans. Eur Respir J 2003;22(6):1007–18.

[133] Zamora MR. Cytomegalovirus and lung transplantation. Am J Transplant 2004;4(8):1219–26.

[134] Khalifah AP, Hachem RR, Chakinala MM, et al. Respiratory viral infections are a distinct risk for bronchiolitis obliterans syndrome and death. Am J Respir Crit Care Med 2004;170(2):181–7.

[135] Mehrad B, Paciocco G, Martinez FJ, et al. Spectrum of Aspergillus infection in lung transplant

recipients: case series and review of the literature. Chest 2001;119(1):169–75.

[136] Birsan T, Taghavi S, Klepetko W. Treatment of aspergillus-related ulcerative tracheobronchitis in lung transplant recipients. J Heart Lung Transplant 1998;17(4):437–8.

[137] Cahill BC, Hibbs JR, Savik K, et al. Aspergillus airway colonization and invasive disease after lung transplantation. Chest 1997;112(5): 1160–4.

[138] Kessler R, Massard G, Warter A, et al. Bronchial-pulmonary artery fistula after unilateral lung transplantation: a case report. J Heart Lung Transplant 1997;16(6):674–7.

[139] Levine SM, Angel L, Anzueto A, et al. A low incidence of posttransplant lymphoproliferative disorder in 109 lung transplant recipients. Chest 1999; 116(5):1273–7.

[140] Reams BD, McAdams HP, Howell DN, et al. Posttransplant lymphoproliferative disorder: incidence, presentation, and response to treatment in lung transplant recipients. Chest 2003;124(4):1242–9.

[141] Loren AW, Porter DL, Stadtmauer EA, et al. Posttransplant lymphoproliferative disorder: a review. Bone Marrow Transplant 2003;31(3):145–55.

[142] Kotloff RM, Ahya VN. Pulmonary considerations in organ and hematopoietic stem cell transplantation. Clin Chest Med 2005;26(4):517–739.

ELSEVIER
SAUNDERS

Clin Chest Med 28 (2007) 203–218

CLINICS
IN CHEST
MEDICINE

Portopulmonary Hypertension

Jason M. Golbin, DO, MS[a], Michael J. Krowka, MD[a,b],*

[a]Division of Pulmonary and Critical Care Medicine, Mayo Clinic College of Medicine,
200 First Street SW, Rochester, MN 55905, USA
[b]Division of Gastroenterology and Hepatology, Mayo Clinic College of Medicine,
200 First Street SW, Rochester, MN 55905, USA

"Portal venous hypertension coexisted with pulmonary arterial hypertension. These observations suggested two questions: What was the origin of the pulmonary vascular changes? Was there a possible relationship between these pulmonary vascular lesions and abnormalities in the portal venous system?" [1]

As a result of the success of orthotopic liver transplantation (LT), there has been increasing interest in the diagnosis and therapeutic options for the pulmonary vascular complications of hepatic disease. These pulmonary vascular complications range from the hepatopulmonary syndrome (HPS), which is characterized by intrapulmonary vascular dilatations, to portopulmonary hypertension (POPH), which is characterized by an elevated pulmonary vascular resistance as a consequence of obstruction to pulmonary arterial blood flow. This review will concentrate on POPH.

Diagnostic criteria

POPH is likely best defined as pulmonary artery hypertension (PAH) associated with portal hypertension, whether or not that portal hypertension is secondary to underlying liver disease [2]. The diagnosis of POPH is traditionally based on hemodynamic data from right heart catheterization (RHC). Diagnostic hemodynamic criteria include increased mean pulmonary artery pressure (mPAP) higher than 25 mmHg at rest, normal

pulmonary artery occlusion pressure (PAOP) less than 15 mmHg, and an increased pulmonary vascular resistance (PVR) greater than 240 dynes/s/cm^{-5}. PVR is calculated in dynes/s/cm^{-5} as PVR = [(mPAP – PAOP) ÷ Cardiac Output] × 80. The diagnostic level of PVR greater than 240 dynes/s/cm^{-5} was agreed upon by a 2004 consensus panel, even though some patients with PVR values between 120 and 240 dynes/s/cm^{-5} may have a constellation of findings consistent with POPH [2].

POPH was first described in 1951 by Mantz and Craige [3]. They described a case of a 53-year-old female who was seen for hoarseness. Imaging revealed esophageal abnormalities consistent with varicosities. On surgical exploration, the pulmonary artery was found to be greatly enlarged and had "pulsations simulating that of the aorta." In addition, a large peri-esophageal plexus of veins was discovered. During the case, the patient remained hypotensive and the chest was closed. The patient expired a few days later. Autopsy revealed a large portacaval shunt, with an extremely narrowed portal vein. Microscopic examination of the lungs revealed embolization of numerous terminal arteries and arterioles with old blood clots, which showed endothelial proliferation. Intimal thickening was seen in the medium and large pulmonary arteries.

Since this first report, numerous case reports validated this initial finding. More recently, the number of new POPH citations in PubMed have been increasing with each passing year. There were 11 citations in 2002, 14 in 2003, 17 in 2004, 28 in 2005, and 2006 is on pace to surpass 30. In addition, because of the significant implications for appropriate candidacy for LT, the disease continues to receive increased attention [4].

---

* Corresponding author. Division of Pulmonary and Critical Care Medicine, Mayo Clinic College of Medicine, 200 First Street SW, Rochester, MN 55905.
E-mail address: krowka.michael@mayo.edu (M.J. Krowka).

Before 1998, POPH was grouped with a number of other etiologies of "secondary" PAH. The updated Venice 2003 classification system now classifies POPH as a subset of pulmonary arterial hypertension, a group that includes idiopathic PAH as well as other etiologies, such as collagen vascular disease and HIV [5]. The classification system can be seen in Table 1 [5].

Many diseases and systemic conditions may involve both the portal and pulmonary circulations. These include antiphospholipid/anticardio-lipin antibodies, mixed connective tissue disease, schistosomiasis, sarcoidosis, systemic lupus erythematosus (SLE), microangiopathic hemolytic anemia, and HIV [6]. However, these conditions usually do not demonstrate the hemodynamic criteria that define POPH on right heart catheterization.

Although cirrhotic liver disease is the most common cause of portal hypertension, a small minority of patients have another etiology for their disease [7]. These include biliary atresia, extrahepatic portal vein obstruction, noncirrhotic portal fibrosis, noncirrhotic portal hypertension in SLE, and idiopathic portal fibrosis [6]. This suggests that it is the portal hypertension, not the underlying liver disease, which is the underlying etiology of POPH.

To properly interpret the hemodynamic changes associated with POPH, it is important to recall the hemodynamic changes commonly observed in patients with liver disease. Approximately 30% to 50% of patients with cirrhosis display a hyperdynamic circulation characterized by a high cardiac output (CO), a low systemic vascular resistance (SVR), and a low PVR [8]. In

Table 1
Revised clinical classification of pulmonary hypertension (Venice 2003)

1. Pulmonary arterial hypertension (PAH)
    1.1. Idiopathic (IPAH)
    1.2. Familial (FPAH)
    1.3. Associated with (APAH):
        1.3.1. Collagen vascular disease
        1.3.2. Congential systemic-to-pulmonary shunts
        1.3.3. Portal hypertension
        1.3.4. HIV infection
        1.3.5. Drugs and toxins
        1.3.6. Other (thyroid disorders, glycogen storage disease, Gaucher disease, hereditary hemorrhagic telangiectasia, hemoglobinopathies, myeloproliferative disorders, splenectomy)
    1.4. Associated with significant venous or capillary involvement
        1.4.1. Pulmonary veno-occlusive disease (PVOD)
        1.4.2. Pulmonary capillary hemangiomatosis (PCH)
    1.5. Persistent pulmonary hypertension of the newborn
2. Pulmonary hypertension with left heart disease
    2.1. Left-sided atrial or ventricular heart disease
    2.2. Left-sided valvular heart disease
3. Pulmonary hypertension associated with lung diseases and/or hypoxemia
    3.1. Chronic obstructive pulmonary disease
    3.2. Interstitial lung disease
    3.3. Sleep-disordered breathing
    3.4. Alveolar hypoventilation disorders
    3.5. Chronic exposure to high altitude
    3.6. Developmental abnormalities
4. Pulmonary hypertension due to chronic thrombotic and/or embolic disease
    4.1. Thromboembolic obstruction of proximal pulmonary arteries
    4.2. Thromboembolic obstruction of distal pulmonary arteries
    4.3. Nonthrombotic pulmonary embolism (tumor, parasites, foreign material)
5. Miscellaneous
    Sarcoidosis, histiocytosis X, lymphangiomatosis, compression of pulmonary vessels (adenopathy, tumor, fibrosing mediastinitis)

Reprinted from Simmonneau G, Galie N, Rubin LJ, et al. Clinical classification of pulmonary hypertension. J Am Coll Cardiol 2004;43(12Suppl S):10S; with permission.

these patients, pulmonary artery pressures may be elevated because of the increase in CO and blood volume. However, it is important to note that in this case the PVR will be low or normal.

This is in contrast to POPH, in which the PVR is increased, as are pulmonary artery pressures. In POPH, CO may be initially elevated secondary to liver disease, but it often decreases as the severity of the PAH progresses. Compared with idiopathic PAH, patients with POPH usually have a higher cardiac output [9]. Both conditions, however, are characterized by an elevated PVR, thus distinguishing them from patients who have liver disease without PAH [10]. These hemodynamic distinctions play an important role in the consideration of LT, for the elevation in PVR seen in POPH patients may have a deleterious effect on the outcome of surgery.

Current thinking has proposed a modification to the traditionally accepted hemodynamic criteria of POPH [11]. Some patients with underlying liver disease may be found to have an elevated PAOP on RHC, secondary to their high flow state with excess circulating volume. By the traditional criteria, even if their PVR is elevated, they would not have fulfilled each criterion for the diagnosis of POPH. A modified POPH criterion has since been proposed that uses the Transpulmonary Gradient (TPG) to properly address the patient who possesses both an increased PAOP as well as an increased PVR. The TPG = mPAP − PAOP, and a TPG higher than 12 mmHG is abnormal. An abnormal TPG reflects obstruction to flow, a key characteristic that distinguishes the increased mPAP associated with POPH (with increased PVR) from other causes of increased mPAP (high flow with excess volume) [4]. This has not yet been fully accepted by the POPH community, but represents a proposed modification that merits further study.

A classification of severity of POPH was proposed in 2004 [2]. Mild disease has an mPAP of 25 to 34 mmHg, moderate disease ranges from 35 to 44 mmHg, and severe disease has an mPAP 45 mmHg or higher. This staging system was designed to correlate with the increased mortality seen with LT in patients who are classified as moderate-to-severe [6,12].

POPH represents a completely different disease entity from hepatopulmonary syndrome (HPS), another pulmonary vascular complication of hepatic disease. HPS is defined as an arterial oxygenation defect (alveolar-arterial oxygen gradient >20 mmHg) induced by intrapulmonary vascular dilatations associated with hepatic disease [13]. Major clinical differences between HPS and POPH can be seen in Table 2.

Epidemiology and prevalence

The prevalence of POPH in patients with liver disease is not well defined. The first retrospective autopsy studies showed that the prevalence of PAH ranged from 0.25% to 0.73% in populations with portal hypertension or cirrhosis, as compared with 0.13% of those without either abnormality [14–16]. More recent work using hemodynamic studies have estimated the prevalence of POPH to be between 2% and 5% [6]. In addition, the prevalence in patients undergoing LT is likely higher, with one study showing a prevalence of 8.5% [17]. These studies, plus others, demonstrated the relationship between portal hypertension and PAH, and helped lead to the reclassification of POPH as a form of secondary PAH, as previously discussed. Conversely, the prevalence of portal hypertension in patients with PAH is approximately 10% [18].

Identification of POPH is made an average of 4 to 7 years after the diagnosis of portal hypertension [19]. However, it is not unheard of for the diagnosis of POPH to be made before the diagnosis of portal hypertension [6].

The mean age of presentation for POPH is in the fifth decade of life, as compared with the fourth decade for idiopathic PAH [8,20]. A review from 1998 showed the average age of patients with POPH to be 49 ± 13 years, slightly older than previous reports. The sex ratio was 1.1:1 (male:female), which does correlate with previous reports [8,14].

Pathology and histology

Histopathologically, the pulmonary vasculature of POPH is indistinguishable from that of other forms of PAH. POPH is characterized by vasoconstrictive, proliferative, and obliterative changes in the pulmonary vascular bed. Plexiform arteriopathy, medial hypertrophy, intimal fibrosis, adventitial proliferation, and fibrinoid necrosis of small arteries may be seen [14,15,21]. Thrombus with recanalization may be present, which likely are not the result of emboli, as no systemic sources of clot are usually found [22]. These thrombotic lesions are believed to result from in situ clot formation caused by the combination of endothelial cell injury, platelet aggregation, and a hypercoaguable state, and not by direct coagulation

Table 2
Distinction between hepatopulmonary syndrome (HPS) and portopulmonary hypertension (PPHTN)

	HPS	PPHTN
Symptomatology	Progressive dyspnea	Progressive dyspnea Chest pain Syncope
Clinical examination	Cyanosis Finger clubbing Spider angiomas (?)	No cyanosis RV heave Pronounced P2 component
ECG findings	None	RBBB Rightward axis RV hypertrophy
Arterial blood gas levels	Moderate-to-severe hypoxemia	No/mild hypoxemia
Chest radiography	Normal	Cardiomegaly Hilar enlargement
CEE	Always positive; left atrial opacification for $>$3–6 cardiac cycles after right atrial opacification	Usually negative; however, positive for $<$3 cardiac cycles (if atrial septal defect or patent foramen ovale exists)
^{99m}TcMAA shunting index	$\geq$6%	$<$6%
Pulmonary haemodynamics	Normal/low PVR	Elevated PVR Normal mPAOP
Pulmonary angiography	Normal/"spongy" appearance (type I) Discrete arteriovenous communications (type II)	Large main pulmonary arteries Distal arterial pruning
OLT	Even indicated in severe stages	Only indicated in mild-to-moderate stages

Abbreviations: CEE, contrast-enhanced echocardiography; mPAOP, mean pulmonary artery occlusion pressure; OLT, orthotopic liver transplantation; PVR, pulmonary vascular resistance; RBBB, right bundle-branch block; RV, right ventricle; ^{99m}TcMAA, technetium-99m-labeled macroaggregated albumin.

Reprinted from Rodriguez-Roisin R, Krowka MJ, Herve P, Fallon MB. Pulmonary hepatic-vascular disorders (PHD). Eur Respir J 2004;24(5):873.

abnormalities. A characteristic feature of PAH, which is commonly seen in POPH, is the plexiform lesion. It is a dilated pulmonary artery whose normal structure has been replaced by an intraluminal plexus of endothelial calls and slit-like vascular channels [2]. In an autopsy study of 12 patients with POPH, four patterns of pulmonary artery disease were described: medial hypertrophy, thrombosis, plexiform lesions, and the coexistence of plexiform and thrombotic lesions [21]. Examples of typical lesions are seen in Figs. 1–4 [23].

Pathophysiology and pathogenesis

At the present time, the pathogenesis of POPH is not fully understood. Two things known at the present time are that the development of POPH appears to be independent of the cause of the portal hypertension [24], and the severity of the underlying portal hypertension or liver disease does not appear to correlate with the severity of the PAH [19].

It appears that three vascular abnormalities combine to cause the vascular obstruction that leads to the increase in PVR seen in POPH: an imbalance of vasomediators leading to vasoconstriction, endothelial damage leading to remodeling, with associated proliferation of endothelium and smooth muscle, and in situ microthrombosis. A proposed mechanism for POPH starts with the increased blood flow of portal hypertension and liver disease causing vascular wall shear stress, which activates a cascade of events that may eventually lead to the characteristic histopathologic changes of POPH [8]. However, among patients with increased blood flow not secondary to portal hypertension (such as a result of an atrial septal defect of the ostium secundum type), the incidence of PAH is variable, suggesting other factors play a role in POPH. What these factors are still represents a quandary.

It is likely that a complex interaction of vascular proliferative and angiogenetic mediators with endothelial and smooth muscle responses plays a role if the development of POPH [9]. Increased levels of

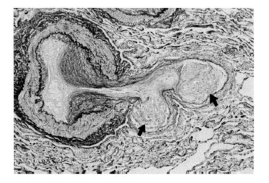

Fig. 1. Plexogenic type. Lung explant from a 37-year-old woman with stage IV primary biliary cirrhosis who underwent combined heart-lung-liver transplantation. Parent pulmonary artery (*left*) shows medial hypertrophy, as well as intimal fibroelastosis at the origin of the arterial branch. The branch (*right*) is involved by two microaneurysms (*arrows*) that contain plexiform lesions (Verhoeff–van Gieson). (*Reprinted from* Krowka MJ, Edwards WD. A spectrum of pulmonary vascular pathology in portopulmonary hypertension. Liver Transpl 2000;6(2):241; with permission.)

endothelin-1 (ET-1), a potent vasoconstrictor produced by both the pulmonary endothelium and the liver, has been shown to play a role in the pathogenesis of idiopathic PAH, as well as other types of secondary PAH [25,26]. Increased levels of ET-1 have been reported in patients with liver disease and ascites [27,28]. This raises the possibility of the role of ET-1 in POPH.

The presence of portosystemic shunts may allow the shunting of vasoactive compounds

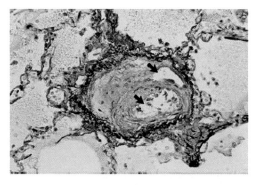

Fig. 3. Thrombotic type. Post–liver transplantation autopsy specimen of the lung (day 7) from a 46-year-old man with hepatitis C liver disease and cirrhosis. The muscular pulmonary arteriole is obstructed by a recanalized thrombus, showing two small residual lumens (*arrows*) (Verhoeff–van Gieson). (*Reprinted from* Krowka MJ, Edwards WD. A spectrum of pulmonary vascular pathology in portopulmonary hypertension. Liver Transpl 2000;6(2):241; with permission.)

from the splanchnic circulation to the pulmonary circulation. This would thereby allow these substances to escape liver metabolism, which may play a role in the development of POPH [6,14,29]. Examples of vasoconstrictors that are found in elevated concentrations include prostaglandin $F_2\alpha$ and thromboxane B_2 and angiotensin 1, all of which are potent vasoconstrictors and may be involved in POPH [30]. In contrast, prostacyclin

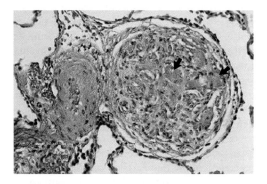

Fig. 2. Plexogenic type. Autopsy specimen from a 55-year-old woman with cryptogenic cirrhosis. This highly obstructive plexiform lesion is acutely occluded by platelet-fibrin thrombi (*pink homogeneous material, arrows*) (hematoxylin-eosin). (*Reprinted from* Krowka MJ, Edwards WD. A spectrum of pulmonary vascular pathology in portopulmonary hypertension. Liver Transpl 2000;6(2):241; with permission.)

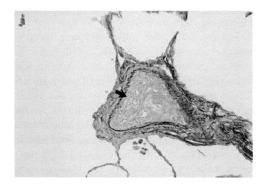

Fig. 4. Fibrotic type. Post–liver transplantation autopsy specimen of the lung (day 9) from a 54-year-old man with alcoholic cirrhosis and alpha₁-antitrypsin deficiency (*ZZ phenotype*). The muscular pulmonary arteriole is completely occluded by an old dense fibrous plug (*arrow*), presumably of thrombotic origin (Verhoeff–van Geison). (*Reprinted from* Krowka MJ, Edwards WD. A spectrum of pulmonary vascular pathology in portopulmonary hypertension. Liver Transpl 2000;6(2):241; with permission.)

synthase, the enzyme responsible for the production of prostacyclin, a potent vasodilator, is decreased in the lungs of patients with POPH [31]. In addition, the decrease in liver phagocytosis secondary to the development of the portosystemic shunts allows circulating bacteria and bacterial endotoxins from the gastrointestinal tract to enter the pulmonary circulation. This leads to increased pulmonary phagocytosis, which releases numerous cytokines into the extracellular milieu [2]. It has been suggested that this induction of pulmonary intravascular macrophages, often seen in cirrhotic patients, may contribute to the development of POPH [32].

While some genetic polymorphisms have been associated with various types of PAH, at the current time no genetic relationships specific to POPH have been identified [2,33]. However, a multicenter National Institutes of Health–funded study is under way to address the issue of genetic associations in the setting of POPH and HPS [4]. Identification of genetic polymorphisms in POPH would likely play an important role in future treatment considerations of selected patients.

Clinical features

In the early stages of POPH, patients may be asymptomatic or only have symptoms of their underlying portal hypertension. This then requires that the health care providers treating these patients must have a high clinical suspicion for pulmonary hypertension, especially in patients undergoing evaluation for LT.

The most common initial symptom in those patients who are symptomatic is dyspnea on exertion. However, dyspnea in a patient with underlying liver disease can stem from a myriad of etiologies [6]. These include, but are not limited to, cardiomyopathy, hepatic hydrothorax, restriction from tense ascites, parenchymal lung disease, deconditioning, and muscle wasting. Other symptoms, especially as the severity of the POPH progresses, include peripheral edema, fatigue, dyspnea at rest, hemoptysis, and orthopnea. Later, even more worrisome symptoms include chest discomfort and syncope [8]. However, some patients may remain asymptomatic, and identification of disease may be serendipitous [34].

On physical examination, appreciable findings generally depend on the severity of POPH. In mild disease, findings may be notable only for signs of underlying liver disease, such as jaundice, spider telangiectasias, lower extremity edema, and ascites. However, as the severity of the POPH progresses, findings of right-sided cardiac dysfunction, as well as volume overload, become more apparent. These include jugular venous distension, accentuated P2 component with widened splitting of the second heart sound, right ventricular heave, a murmur of tricuspid regurgitation, a murmur of pulmonic insufficiency (Graham Steell murmur), and a pulsatile liver.

Arterial blood gases may reveal mild-to-moderate hypoxemia, an increased alveolar-arterial oxygen gradient, and a decreased carbon dioxide level. A PCO_2 value less than 30 mmHg has been suggested as an indicator of PAH in patients with portal hypertension [35]. The decrease in arterial oxygenation was found to be significantly worse on patients with POPH when compared with a cohort of liver transplant patients with normal right ventricular systolic pressures [36]. This hypoxemia was not found to be a result of clinically significant intracardiac or intrapulmonary shunting.

Electrocardiography typically suggests right atrial enlargement, right ventricular hypertrophy, or right axis deviation [10]. Later EKG findings can include a right bundle-branch block, as well as T-wave inversions in leads V1 to V4 [8,37]. Pulmonary function testing (PFT) may reveal a decreased diffusing capacity. PFT is equally important in excluding significant airflow obstruction. A mild restrictive pattern may be present [38]. Chest radiography may be normal, or may reveal prominent pulmonary vasculature, as well as signs of right-sided cardiac hypertrophy [6]. Increased vascularity is frequently seen in the upper lobes [39]. Ventilation/perfusion scanning may reveal a "mosaic" pattern, but specific segmental perfusion abnormalities should prompt evaluation for pulmonary emboli [2].

A recent publication documents the differing appearance of POPH as compared with idiopathic PAH on pulmonary angiogram [40]. As can be seen in Figs. 5 and 6, tapering of the peripheral arteries and sparse arborization ("pruned tree" appearance) were more commonly seen in the patients with idiopathic PAH as compared with the POPH patients [40]. In POPH, the pulmonary arteries were dilated near the segmental arteries, which were narrowed in idiopathic PAH.

Evaluation

Identification of POPH in patients with underlying portal hypertension or liver disease is

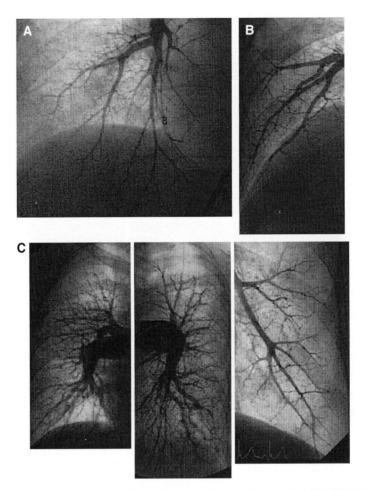

Fig. 5. (*A, B, C*) Pulmonary angiograms in patients with portopulmonary hypertension (PPHTN). The degree of sparse arborization and tapering on wedged pulmonary angiography was more moderate in PPHTN than in idiopathic pulmonary artery hypertension (IPAH) (see Fig. 6). The central pulmonary arteries are dilated near the subsegmental arteries, which are narrow in IPAH. (*Reprinted from* Sakuma M, Souma S, Kitamukai O, et al. Portopulmonary hypertension: hemodynamics, pulmonary aniography, and configuration of the heart. Circ J 2005;69(11):1389; with permission.)

critical not only to guide medical therapy, but also to assess appropriate candidacy for LT. All patients undergoing evaluation for LT should be screened for POPH because mortality in patients with moderate to severe POPH is increased during the perioperative period [2,41]. Therefore, the advisability and timing of transplantation may be influenced by POPH, and it is unacceptable to make the diagnosis in the operating room during transplantation [12].

Evaluation of patients with liver disease or portal hypertension with complaints suggestive of PAH (such as dyspnea on exertion) should begin with a thorough history and physical examination. The screening procedure of choice is a two-dimensional transthoracic echocardiogram (TTE). The echocardiogram can be done in conjunction with a number of other tests as previously mentioned, such as EKG, chest radiography, and PFT. Findings on TTE that are suggestive of POPH (in the setting of portal hypertension) include increased tricuspid peak regurgitant jet velocity, pulmonic valve insufficiency, paradoxical septal motion, right ventricular hypertrophy and dilatation, and an increased right ventricular systolic pressure (RVSP) estimate. The RVSP is calculated from the peak tricuspid regurgitant velocity using the modified Bernoulli equation and an estimate of the right atrial pressure [9].

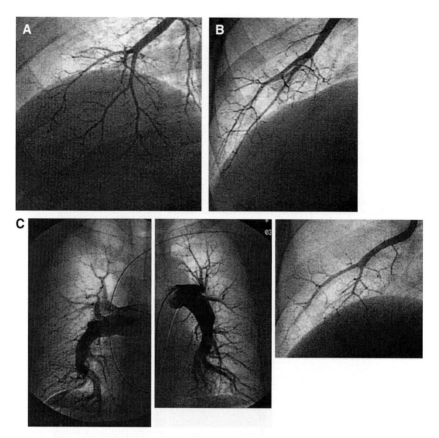

Fig. 6. (*A*, *B*, *C*) Pulmonary angiograms in patients with IPAH. Sparse arborization and tapering are marked compared with patients with PPHTN (see Fig. 5). Central pulmonary arteries are dilated. (*Reprinted from* Sakuma M, Souma S, Kitamukai O, et al. Portopulmonary hypertension: hemodynamics, pulmonary aniography, and configuration of the heart. Circ J 2005;69(11):1389; with permission.)

TTE was found to have a sensitivity of 97% and a specificity of 77% in the diagnosis of moderate to severe PAH in patients undergoing LT evaluation [42]. In another series of patients undergoing LT evaluation, when using an RVSP cutoff of 40 mmHg, sensitivity, specificity, positive predictive value, and negative predictive value of TTE were 80%, 96%, 60%, and 98%, respectively [43].

To accurately measure RVSP, a tricuspid regurgitant jet must be present. However, this is not found in 10% to 20% of patients with elevated right ventricular pressures [44]. Because of this, one study proposes using the pulmonary acceleration time (PAT) as an alternative method of screening for pulmonary hypertension [45]. The PAT is measured from the Doppler pulmonary artery flow velocity tracing as the time from the onset of ejection to the time of peak velocity.

Normal PAT values are usually higher than 120 ms, with a decrease in the setting of PAH. The authors found that a PAT less than 100 ms had a sensitivity of 100% and a specificity of 96% for detecting POPH.

Regardless of the echocardiographic technique used to screen for PAH in patients with liver disease or portal hypertension, TTE cannot distinguish between true POPH (increased PVR) and PAH caused by a hyperdynamic state (normal/ low PVR). Therefore, the gold standard for diagnosis of POPH is right heart catheterization (RHC) [8,42,46]; however, no consensus exists as to exactly what echocardiographic finding is indicative of the need to proceed to RHC [4,42,47].

Recent data from the Mayo Clinic substantiate advising any patient undergoing LT evaluation with an RVSP greater than 50 mmHg to have RHC [4,11]. Even using this cutoff of RVSP greater than 50 mmHg, one third of patients had normal PVR at time of RHC. Importantly, no patients with significant POPH remained unidentified by this cutoff. If TTE cannot be performed for any reason, RHC should be completed.

RHC allows accurate measurement of the mPAP, PAOP, CO, and documentation of an elevated PVR. As stated previously, PVR is calculated by the formula: $PVR = [(mPAP - PAOP) \div CO] \times 80$. If clinically indicated, left-heart catheterization can be performed concurrently to exclude coronary artery or left ventricular disease. This information would also be important if considering LT.

During RHC, acute vasodilator testing is usually performed, using either intravenous epoprostenol or inhaled nitric oxide (NO). This is done to aide in the determination of vasodilator responsiveness and to assess change in PAOP. A decrease in mPAP and the PVR of more than 20%, with no increase in the CO, can be considered a significant vasodilatory response [48,49]. The goal of this testing is to aid in determining staging severity and therapeutic expectations, and not to assess for the ability to use calcium channel blocker therapy, which is the traditional indication for this procedure in PAH. This change is because calcium channel blockers are contraindicated in portal hypertension, and therefore POPH, as will be discussed further. An increase in PAOP with vasodilator challenge may have prognostic significance. Of note, a positive vasodilator response cannot predict survival, either with or without LT.

In patients with POPH, the acute vasodilatory effect of epoprostenol appears to be greater than that of NO. It has been hypothesized that this may be because of persistent endogenous excess NO production [50–52]. Accordingly, changes in hemodynamics should take into account the agent used to provoke the response.

Medical management

At the present time, there are no major long-term studies or guidelines on the use of pharmacotherapy in POPH [4,6]. No randomized, controlled clinical trial (RCT) has been conducted for the purpose of POPH management. Likely secondary to the rarity of POPH, treatment of this disease has been empirical. Therefore, the usual approach in treating PAH from any cause has been to initiate therapy when the patient is both symptomatic and has an elevated mPAP (>35 mmHg) as well as an increased PVR [33].

Patients who are diagnosed with mild POPH frequently have no signs or symptoms of PAH. In these patients, specific treatment of POPH is not generally required [24]. Regular follow-up, along with repeat TTE, is strongly recommended to follow for progression of the disease. In addition, even mild POPH can pose a danger in certain situations, such as surgery.

General therapy for all patients with POPH usually includes diuretics, which function by reducing the increased intravascular volume commonly present with liver disease. In addition, diuresis can reduce CO by decreasing right ventricular preload. Furosemide and/or spironolactone are the traditional diuretics of choice [2].

Mild-moderate arterial hypoxemia is a common finding in POPH, as previously discussed. Theoretically, hypoxemia may worsen PAH through pulmonary vasoconstriction, and therefore supplemental oxygen should be considered for all patients with hypoxemia to maintain oxygen saturation higher than 90% at all times [2].

Transjugular intrahepatic portosytemic shunting (TIPS) has no role in the treatment of POPH, and may acutely increase preload, thereby increasing CO and mPAP. Transient increases (doubling) of PVR have been documented [2]. Such acute change in hemodynamics may place additional stress on an already dysfunctional right ventricle in the setting of moderate to severe POPH.

Anticoagulation, which is often prescribed for other populations with PAH for its ability to slow disease progression, is traditionally not recommended in patients with POPH [2,53,54]. This is because of the inherent risk of hemorrhagic complications in patients with underlying liver disease and portal hypertension, especially with prior history of gastrointestinal bleeding. In addition, the patients' underlying liver disease often leads to abnormalities in their clotting factors, and therefore these patients are often auto-anticoagulated.

Digoxin has been shown to enhance CO in the acute setting in patients with idiopathic PAH [55]. It may have a role in POPH, but this has not yet been studied. However, caution must be paid to possible hypokalemia in patients who are receiving diuretics.

Calcium channel blockers, which are often first-line vasodilators in patients who have a positive response to acute vasodilator challenge during RHC are contraindicated in POPH, for they may further increase the hepatic venous pressure gradient [56,57]. It is postulated that such medications may exacerbate mesenteric vasodilatation that, in turn, results in higher flow into the portal circulation. This higher flow increases the portal vascular pressure, thus worsening the pressure difference between the portal and hepatic veins. Gastroesophageal varices, known to develop when this gradient rises to greater than 12 mmHg, may become more problematic.

Beta-blockers can have a variety of effects in patients with POPH. A few case reports demonstrate improvement in PAH in patients with portal hypertension [58,59]. However, a more recent report documents a significant worsening in exercise capacity and pulmonary hemodynamics in POPH patients receiving beta-blocking medication [60]. At the present time, beta-blockers would not be regularly recommended in all POPH patients, but addressed on a case-by-case basis.

There is only one case report describing the successful use of nitrates in POPH, therefore it is impractical to draw any conclusions at the present time [61].

Intravenous (IV) epoprostenol is currently the best-studied drug in POPH. In the largest series to date, IV epoprostenol was shown to improve the mPAP and the PVR in both the acute and long-term settings [62]. Smaller series have shown similar results [63,64]; however, whether this improvement in hemodynamics is translated to an improvement in survival at the current time is unclear. Preliminary data indicate that IV epoprostenol plus LT in highly selected patients does improve survival [4].

IV epoprostenol is not an easy treatment to administer, for its continuous intravenous delivery system requires permanent central venous access, and its use is prone to complications. Another concern with this drug are reports of progressive splenomegaly with worsening thrombocytopenia [65]. However, recent data from the Mayo Clinic does not demonstrate a statistically significant decrease in platelet count in a large cohort of patients with POPH treated with IV epoprostenol [66].

Other prostanoids have become available for the treatment of PAH, as well as for POPH. These agents hold promise in that they are delivered through a variety of ways, including orally, subcutaneously, or by inhalation, and therefore do not offer the complications of a continued central venous infusion. However, at the current time, the data on these agents include case reports and small case series only. To date, no prospective, RCTs have been undertaken for POPH.

The dual endothelin receptor antagonist, bosentan (Tracleer), is an oral agent approved by the Food and Drug Administration (FDA) in 2002 for treatment of PAH. The concern with this agent is that it may cause a transient increase in liver function enzymes, of significant concern in the POPH population. However, a number of case reports have described its successful use in POPH. The largest series of 11 patients with POPH treated with bosentan resulted in a significant reduction in PVR with no adverse effects on liver function enzymes [67].

Another oral agent used in the treatment of POPH is the phosphodiesterase-5 inhibitor, sildenafil (Revatio), which was approved by the FDA in 2005 for the treatment of PAH. Sildenafil blocks the degradation of cyclic guanosine monophosphate, the second messenger of NO, thereby prolonging NO-mediated vasodilatation. In other forms of PAH, sildenafil increases CO, and decreases both mPAP and PVR, without major adverse effects [68,69]. A recent series of 14 patients with POPH treated with sildenafil (in addition their current therapy) demonstrated an increase in 6-minute walk distance, as well as an improvement in pulmonary hemodynamics at 3 months, in 12 of 14 patients, with no major adverse effects [70]. Combination therapy with prostacyclin medication appeared to have a better long-term improvement (12 months) than sildenafil alone. This series lends evidence to the use of sildenafil in patients with POPH despite the already increased endogenous NO production seen in liver disease.

Although evidence-based guidelines based on RCTs are lacking, based on the successful experiences with idiopathic PAH, treatment of POPH patients with IV epoprostenol, oral bosentan (in highly selected cases), and oral sildenafil, or a combination of these agents, appears reasonable.

Liver transplantation

Traditional thinking has held that POPH is a contraindication for LT. This is opposite of HPS, which is an indication for LT. However, in a highly selected subset of patients with POPH, LT may be beneficial.

The presence of POPH increases the risk for perioperative, as well as long-term, morbidity and mortality associated with LT [71]. As mPAP and PVR increase, so does the mortality associated with LT [72]. Many, if not all, LT centers consider mPAP higher than 50 mmHg to be an absolute contraindication to transplantation [2]. Potential candidates must be evaluated at centers experienced in the management of POPH.

Clinical assessment protocols before LT must include an algorithmic approach to the identification of POPH. One proposed algorithm for patients undergoing LT evaluation uses a screening TTE, followed by RHC, if the RVSP is more than 50 mmHg, and then categorizes patients into the aforementioned POPH severity classes (Table 3) [2].

For LT candidates documented to have moderate to severe POPH (mPAP >35 mmHg) who will have vasodilator treatment initiated, the goal of treatment should be to reduce the mPAP to less than 35 mmHg, and the PVR to less than 400 dynes/s/cm^{-5} before proceeding to LT [2]. The reason for this is that previous data have demonstrated no increased mortality risk when the mPAP is less than 35 mmHg [12,38]. A recent report from the Baylor College of Medicine demonstrated that in eight patients with POPH as their only contraindication to LT, pretreatment with intravenous epoprostenol caused a significant improvement in their cardiopulmonary hemodynamics, allowing 75% to be listed for LT [73].

The resolution of symptoms after LT may be slow, and may take months to years to completely resolve [6,74]. There have been reports of persistence of progression of PAH after LT [75–77]. Recurrence of PAH following failure of the transplanted liver has also been reported [78].

During the surgery of LT, patients with POPH are at high risk for complications. The most critical times during the surgery include anesthesia induction, pre- and post–graft reperfusion, and during the immediate postoperative period [79]. Patients may need the support of intraoperative vasodilators. However, most of these data come from the time period before aggressive screening and treatment of POPH before arriving in the operating room.

A multicenter database was organized at 10 LT centers to identify and track patients with POPH being evaluated for LT between 1996 and 2001 [80]. The database showed that the in-hospital LT mortality was 36% in POPH patients, reemphasizing the need for accurate preoperative assessments. Death in these patients generally resulted from right-sided heart failure [72].

A very small subset of patients may benefit from multiorgan transplantation, whether liver-lung or liver-heart-lung. However, only a minimum of case reports exist in the literature and no recommendation concerning multiorgan transplantation can be made at the current time [81,82].

One important question to be addressed is how POPH should affect the Model for End-Stage Liver Disease (MELD) score. The provision of additional MELD points to expedite LT (MELD "exception") for POPH is controversial. As previously mentioned, with no apparent increased mortality risk when the mPAP is less than 35 mmHg, there appears to be a window of transplant opportunity in POPH, suggesting that the MELD "exception" has merit [4]. Further study regarding this transplant priority issue in the setting of POPH is needed.

Prognosis

Survival from time of diagnosis is difficult to predict. As compared with idiopathic PAH, patients with POPH appear to have a substantially shorter survival rate [14]. This was demonstrated in a survival analysis by Kawut and colleagues [83] in 2005, which showed a higher risk for death in patients with POPH as compared with patients with idiopathic PAH, after adjustment for age and

Table 3
Sample algorithm for pulmonary hemodynamic assessment via right heart catheterization before LT[a]

mPAP <35 mmHg	Proceed to LT
mPAP ≥ 35 to ≤ 50 mmHg	If PVR <240, proceed to LT (volume excess/hyperdynamic circulation)
mPAP ≥ 35 to ≤ 50 mmHg	If PVR >240, higher risk LT Initiate vasodilator therapy before LT
mPAP >50 mmHg	LT contraindicated Initiate or continue vasodilator therapy

Abbreviations: LT, liver transplantation; mPAP, mean pulmonary artery pressure (mmHg); PVR, pulmonary vascular resistance (dynes/s/cm^{-5}); RVSP, right ventricular systolic pressure.

[a] Patients proceed to right heart catheterization if screening transthoracic Doppler echocardiography demonstrates RVSP >50 mmHg and/or right ventricular dysfunction.

ethnicity (Fig. 7). Preliminary data from the Mayo Clinic demonstrate survival after 1, 2, and 5 years in patients with POPH is 71%, 58%, and 44%, respectively, regardless of LT status [84]. Causes of death reflect the underlying diseases, and include right-sided cardiac failure, sudden cardiac death, gastrointestinal bleeding, and small bowel perforation [19,62,85].

In the pre-LT era, cardiac index appeared to be the most significant prognostic variable [8]. Right ventricular impairment is often an indication of advanced PAH, and patients with this dysfunction may have elevated brain natriuretic peptide (BNP) levels. A persistently elevated BNP in a patient with PAH is a poor prognostic factor, and is associated with increased mortality [86]. This is more pronounced if the patient is already receiving treatment for PAH [87].

Follow-up

Patients with POPH should be followed with clinical assessments, as well as echocardiography, on a regular basis to screen for progression of disease. The 6-minute walk test, a useful prognostic tool in patients with idiopathic PAH, may not be as useful in patients with POPH, owing to complications of their underlying liver disease, including ascites and lower extremity edema [6]. However, serial RHC may be necessary for accurate assessment of pulmonary hemodynamics in patients with POPH.

Unique cases

POPH and HPS are two distinct diseases, with completely different mechanisms of action. However, case reports can be found that describe the spontaneous resolution of HPS, followed by the development of PAH over many months [88–91]. This transition has mainly occurred in the setting of cirrhosis with cessation of alcohol use. Case reports also exist that demonstrate the development of POPH after LT in patients with preexisting HPS [92]. Only one published case has suggested the transition from POPH to HPS [93].

Pediatric considerations

POPH is not a disease unique to adults, but affects the pediatric population as well. A recent report in *The Journal of Pediatrics* summarizes the clinical course of seven patients with POPH [94]. Causes of underlying portal hypertension included biliary atresia, cavernous transformation of the portal vein, primary sclerosing cholangitis, and cryptogenic cirrhosis. The median interval between diagnosis of portal hypertension and POPH was 12.1 years. The symptoms that prompted evaluation for POPH were subtle and included a new heart murmur, dyspnea, and syncope. Pediatric patients being evaluated for LT must be screened for POPH, just as adults with portal hypertension are, including echocardiogram. In this series, 4 of 7 patients died, suggesting that just as we strive to identify adult patients with

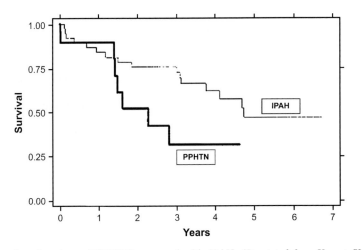

Fig. 7. Adjusted survivor functions of PPHTN compared with IPAH. (*Reprinted from* Kawut SM, Taichman DB, Ahya VN, et al. Hemodynamics and survival of patients with portopulmonary hypertension. Liver Transpl 2005;11(9): 1109; with permission.)

POPH, we must do the same with the pediatric population [95].

Summary

POPH is characterized by the obstruction of pulmonary arterial blood flow as a consequence of portal hypertension. This obstruction is more than simple vasoconstriction of the pulmonary vasculature, as pathologic changes such as plexogenic arteriopathy can be demonstrated. As this vasculopathy progresses, pulmonary vascular resistance increases to the point of right-sided heart failure, and eventually death [4].

The absence of a good animal model coupled with the rarity of POPH has not allowed further advances in the pathogenesis, diagnosis, and treatment of this disease. Just now, researchers are attempting to establish this animal model, typified by a recent article by Loureiro-Silva and colleagues [96], which illustrates the effect of sildenafil on NO in cirrhotic rat livers.

Clinically, multicenter trials need to be undertaken for the treatment of POPH. One possibility to gain more knowledge would be to not exclude patients with POPH from pharmaceutical trials of PAH. In addition, more elucidation on the safety and efficacy of LT in POPH patients is needed.

Documenting a relationship between genetic polymorphisms and POPH has potential therapeutic implications as well. If such abnormalities can be detected in patients before the development of POPH, innovative measures may be undertaken to prevent full-blown disease [4]. Ultimately, prevention would be the best treatment for this difficult, rare disease.

References

[1] Naeye RL. "Primary" pulmonary hypertension with coexisting portal hypertension. A retrospective study of six cases. Circulation 1960;22:376–84.
[2] Rodriguez-Roisin R, Krowka MJ, Herve P, et al. Pulmonary-hepatic vascular disorders (PHD). Eur Respir J 2004;24(5):861–80.
[3] Mantz FA Jr, Craige E. Portal axis thrombosis with spontaneous portacaval shunt and resultant cor pulmonale. AMA Arch Pathol 1951;52(1):91–7.
[4] Krowka MJ. Evolving dilemmas and management of portopulmonary hypertension. Semin Liver Dis 2006;26:265–72.
[5] Simonneau G, Galie N, Rubin LJ, et al. Clinical classification of pulmonary hypertension. J Am Coll Cardiol 2004;43(12 Suppl S):5S–12S.
[6] Budhiraja R, Hassoun PM. Portopulmonary hypertension: a tale of two circulations. Chest 2003;123(2):562–76.
[7] Cohen MD, Rubin LJ, Taylor WE, et al. Primary pulmonary hypertension: an unusual case associated with extrahepatic portal hypertension. Hepatology 1983;3(4):588–92.
[8] Herve P, Lebrec D, Brenot F, et al. Pulmonary vascular disorders in portal hypertension. Eur Respir J 1998;11(5):1153–66.
[9] Swanson KL, Krokwa MJ. Portopulmonary hypertension. In: Mandel J, Taichman D, editors. Pulmonary vascular disease. Philadelphia: Elsevier, Inc.; 2006. p. 132–41.
[10] Kuo PC, Plotkin JS, Johnson LB, et al. Distinctive clinical features of portopulmonary hypertension. Chest 1997;112(4):980–6.
[11] Krowka MJ, Swanson KL, Frantz RP, et al. Portopulmonary hypertension: results from a 10-year screening algorithm. Hepatology 2006;44(6):1502–10.
[12] Krowka MJ, Plevak DJ, Findlay JY, et al. Pulmonary hemodynamics and perioperative cardiopulmonary-related mortality in patients with portopulmonary hypertension undergoing liver transplantation. Liver Transpl 2000;6(4):443–50.
[13] Castro M, Krowka MJ. Hepatopulmonary syndrome. A pulmonary vascular complication of liver disease. Clin Chest Med 1996;17(1):35–48.
[14] Mandell MS, Groves BM. Pulmonary hypertension in chronic liver disease. Clin Chest Med 1996;17(1):17–33.
[15] McDonnell PJ, Toye PA, Hutchins GM. Primary pulmonary hypertension and cirrhosis: are they related? Am Rev Respir Dis 1983;127(4):437–41.
[16] Taura P, Garcia-Valdecasas JC, Beltran J, et al. Moderate primary pulmonary hypertension in patients undergoing liver transplantation. Anesth Analg 1996;83(4):675–80.
[17] Ramsay MA, Simpson BR, Nguyen AT, et al. Severe pulmonary hypertension in liver transplant candidates. Liver Transpl Surg 1997;3(5):494–500.
[18] Abenhaim L. The International Primary Pulmonary Hypertension Study (IPPHS). Chest 1994;105(2 Suppl):37S–41S.
[19] Hadengue A, Benhayoun MK, Lebrec D, et al. Pulmonary hypertension complicating portal hypertension: prevalence and relation to splanchnic hemodynamics. Gastroenterology 1991;100(2):520–8.
[20] Rich S, Dantzker DR, Ayres SM, et al. Primary pulmonary hypertension. A national prospective study. Ann Intern Med 1987;107(2):216–23.
[21] Edwards BS, Weir EK, Edwards WD, et al. Coexistent pulmonary and portal hypertension: morphologic and clinical features. J Am Coll Cardiol 1987;10(6):1233–8.
[22] Wagenvoort CA, Mulder PG. Thrombotic lesions in primary plexogenic arteriopathy. Similar pathogenesis or complication? Chest 1993;103(3):844–9.

[23] Krowka MJ, Edwards WD. A spectrum of pulmonary vascular pathology in portopulmonary hypertension. Liver Transpl 2000;6(2):241–2.

[24] Hoeper MM, Krowka MJ, Strassburg CP. Portopulmonary hypertension and hepatopulmonary syndrome. Lancet 2004;363(9419):1461–8.

[25] Bernardi M, Gulberg V, Colantoni A, et al. Plasma endothelin-1 and -3 in cirrhosis: relationship with systemic hemodynamics, renal function and neurohumoral systems. J Hepatol 1996;24(2):161–8.

[26] Gerbes AL, Moller S, Gulberg V, et al. Endothelin-1 and -3 plasma concentrations in patients with cirrhosis: role of splanchnic and renal passage and liver function. Hepatology 1995;21(3):735–9.

[27] Moore K, Wendon J, Frazer M, et al. Plasma endothelin immunoreactivity in liver disease and the hepatorenal syndrome. N Engl J Med 1992; 327(25):1774–8.

[28] Benjaminov FS, Prentice M, Sniderman KW, et al. Portopulmonary hypertension in decompensated cirrhosis with refractory ascites. Gut 2003;52(9): 1355–62.

[29] Flemale A, Sabot JP, Popijn M, et al. Pulmonary hypertension associated with portal thrombosis. Eur J Respir Dis 1985;66(3):224–8.

[30] Tokiwa K, Iwai N, Nakamura K, et al. Pulmonary hypertension as a fatal complication of extrahepatic portal hypertension. Eur J Pediatr Surg 1993;3(6): 373–5.

[31] Tuder RM, Cool CD, Geraci MW, et al. Prostacyclin synthase expression is decreased in lungs from patients with severe pulmonary hypertension. Am J Respir Crit Care Med 1999;159(6):1925–32.

[32] Keyes JW Jr, Wilson GA, Quinonest JD. An evaluation of lung uptake of colloid during liver imaging. J Nucl Med 1973;14(9):687–91.

[33] Hoeper MM, Rubin LJ. Update in pulmonary hypertension 2005. Am J Respir Crit Care Med 2006; 173(5):499–505.

[34] Murata K, Shimizu A, Takase K, et al. Asymptomatic primary pulmonary hypertension associated with liver cirrhosis. J Gastroenterol 1997;32(1):102–4.

[35] Kuo PC, Plotkin JS, Gaine S, et al. Portopulmonary hypertension and the liver transplant candidate. Transplantation 1999;67(8):1087–93.

[36] Swanson KL, Krowka MJ. Arterial oxygenation associated with portopulmonary hypertension. Chest 2002;121(6):1869–75.

[37] Krowka MJ. Hepatopulmonary syndrome versus portopulmonary hypertension: distinctions and dilemmas. Hepatology 1997;25(5):1282–4.

[38] Castro M, Krowka MJ, Schroeder DR, et al. Frequency and clinical implications of increased pulmonary artery pressures in liver transplant patients. Mayo Clin Proc 1996;71(6):543–51.

[39] Chan T, Palevsky HI, Miller WT. Pulmonary hypertension complicating portal hypertension: findings on chest radiographs. AJR Am J Roentgenol 1988; 151(5):909–14.

[40] Sakuma M, Souma S, Kitamukai O, et al. Portopulmonary hypertension: hemodynamics, pulmonary angiography, and configuration of the heart. Circ J 2005;69(11):1386–93.

[41] Murray KF, Carithers RL Jr. AASLD practice guidelines: evaluation of the patient for liver transplantation. Hepatology 2005;41(6):1407–32.

[42] Kim WR, Krowka MJ, Plevak DJ, et al. Accuracy of doppler echocardiography in the assessment of pulmonary hypertension in liver transplant candidates. Liver Transpl 2000;6(4):453–8.

[43] Colle IO, Moreau R, Godinho E, et al. Diagnosis of portopulmonary hypertension in candidates for liver transplantation: a prospective study. Hepatology 2003;37(2):401–9.

[44] Yock PG, Popp RL. Noninvasive estimation of right ventricular systolic pressure by Doppler ultrasound in patients with tricuspid regurgitation. Circulation 1984;70(4):657–62.

[45] Torregrosa M, Genesca J, Gonzalez A, et al. Role of Doppler echocardiography in the assessment of portopulmonary hypertension in liver transplantation candidates. Transplantation 2001;71(4):572–4.

[46] Krowka MJ. Portopulmonary hypertension: diagnostic advances and caveats. Liver Transpl 2003; 9(12):1336–7.

[47] Cotton CL, Gandhi S, Vaitkus PT, et al. Role of echocardiography in detecting portopulmonary hypertension in liver transplant candidates. Liver Transpl 2002;8(11):1051–4.

[48] Krowka MJ. Pulmonary hypertension: diagnostics and therapeutics. Mayo Clin Proc 2000;75(6): 625–30.

[49] Gaine S. Pulmonary hypertension. JAMA 2000; 284(24):3160–8.

[50] Findlay JY, Harrison BA, Plevak DJ, et al. Inhaled nitric oxide reduces pulmonary artery pressures in portopulmonary hypertension. Liver Transpl Surg 1999;5(5):381–7.

[51] Whittle BJ, Moncada S. Nitric oxide: the elusive mediator of the hyperdynamic circulation of cirrhosis? Hepatology 1992;16(4):1089–92.

[52] Morales-Blanhir J, Santos S, de Jover L, et al. Clinical value of vasodilator test with inhaled nitric oxide for predicting long-term response to oral vasodilators in pulmonary hypertension. Respir Med 2004; 98(3):225–34.

[53] Fuster V, Steele PM, Edwards WD, et al. Primary pulmonary hypertension: natural history and the importance of thrombosis. Circulation 1984;70(4): 580–7.

[54] Rich S, Kaufmann E, Levy PS. The effect of high doses of calcium-channel blockers on survival in primary pulmonary hypertension. N Engl J Med 1992; 327(2):76–81.

[55] Rich S, Seidlitz M, Dodin E, et al. The short-term effects of digoxin in patients with right ventricular dysfunction from pulmonary hypertension. Chest 1998; 114(3):787–92.

[56] Ota K, Shijo H, Kokawa H, et al. Effects of nifedipine on hepatic venous pressure gradient and portal vein blood flow in patients with cirrhosis. J Gastroenterol Hepatol 1995;10(2):198–204.

[57] Navasa M, Bosch J, Reichen J, et al. Effects of verapamil on hepatic and systemic hemodynamics and liver function in patients with cirrhosis and portal hypertension. Hepatology 1988;8(4):850–4.

[58] Boot H, Visser FC, Thijs JC, et al. Pulmonary hypertension complicating portal hypertension. A case report with suggestions for a different therapeutic approach. Eur Heart J 1987;8(6):656–60.

[59] Buchhorn R, Hulpke-Wette M, Wessel A, et al. Beta-blocker therapy in an infant with pulmonary hypertension. Eur J Pediatr 1999;158(12):1007–8.

[60] Provencher S, Herve P, Jais X, et al. Deleterious effects of beta-blockers on exercise capacity and hemodynamics in patients with portopulmonary hypertension. Gastroenterology 2006; 130(1):120–6.

[61] Ribas J, Angrill J, Barbera JA, et al. Isosorbide-5-mononitrate in the treatment of pulmonary hypertension associated with portal hypertension. Eur Respir J 1999;13(1):210–2.

[62] Krowka MJ, Frantz RP, McGoon MD, et al. Improvement in pulmonary hemodynamics during intravenous epoprostenol (prostacyclin): a study of 15 patients with moderate to severe portopulmonary hypertension. Hepatology 1999;30(3):641–8.

[63] McLaughlin VV, Genthner DE, Panella MM, et al. Compassionate use of continuous prostacyclin in the management of secondary pulmonary hypertension: a case series. Ann Intern Med 1999;130(9): 740–3.

[64] Kuo PC, Johnson LB, Plotkin JS, et al. Continuous intravenous infusion of epoprostenol for the treatment of portopulmonary hypertension. Transplantation 1997;63(4):604–6.

[65] Findlay JY, Plevak DJ, Krowka MJ, et al. Progressive splenomegaly after epoprostenol therapy in portopulmonary hypertension. Liver Transpl Surg 1999;5(5):362–5.

[66] Golbin JM, Krowka MJ. Effect of prostacyclins on thrombocytopenia in portopulmonary hypertension. Presented at the 2006 Pulmonary Hypertension Association International Conference. Minneapolis, MN, June 23–25, 2006.

[67] Hoeper MM, Halank M, Marx C, et al. Bosentan therapy for portopulmonary hypertension. Eur Respir J 2005;25(3):502–8.

[68] Michelakis E, Tymchak W, Lien D, et al. Oral sildenafil is an effective and specific pulmonary vasodilator in patients with pulmonary arterial hypertension: comparison with inhaled nitric oxide. Circulation 2002;105(20):2398–403.

[69] Ghofrani HA, Wiedemann R, Rose F, et al. Sildenafil for treatment of lung fibrosis and pulmonary hypertension: a randomised controlled trial. Lancet 2002;360(9337):895–900.

[70] Reichenberger F, Voswinckel R, Steveling E, et al. Sildenafil treatment for portopulmonary hypertension. Eur Respir J 2006;28(3):563–7.

[71] De Wolf AM, Scott VL, Gasior T, et al. Pulmonary hypertension and liver transplantation. Anesthesiology 1993;78(1):213–4.

[72] Krowka MJ, Mandell MS, Ramsay MA, et al. Hepatopulmonary syndrome and portopulmonary hypertension: a report of the multicenter liver transplant database. Liver Transpl 2004;10(2): 174–82.

[73] Sussman N, Kaza V, Barshes N, et al. Successful liver transplantation following medical management of portopulmonary hypertension: a single-center series. Am J Transplant 2006;6(9):2177–82.

[74] Levy MT, Torzillo P, Bookallil M, et al. Case report: delayed resolution of severe pulmonary hypertension after isolated liver transplantation in a patient with cirrhosis. J Gastroenterol Hepatol 1996;11(8): 734–7.

[75] Rafanan AL, Maurer J, Mehta AC, et al. Progressive portopulmonary hypertension after liver transplantation treated with epoprostenol. Chest 2000; 118(5):1497–500.

[76] Mandell MS, Groves BM, Duke J. Progressive plexogenic pulmonary hypertension following liver transplantation. Transplantation 1995;59(10): 1488–90.

[77] Prager MC, Cauldwell CA, Ascher NL, et al. Pulmonary hypertension associated with liver disease is not reversible after liver transplantation. Anesthesiology 1992;77(2):375–8.

[78] Kett DH, Acosta RC, Campos MA, et al. Recurrent portopulmonary hypertension after liver transplantation: management with epoprostenol and resolution after retransplantation. Liver Transpl 2001; 7(7):645–8.

[79] Csete M. Intraoperative management of liver transplant patients with pulmonary hypertension. Liver Transpl Surg 1997;3(4):454–5.

[80] Mandall MS, Krowka MJ. Formation of a national database on pulmonary hypertension and hepatopulmonary syndrome in chronic liver disease. Anesthesiology 1997;87(2):450–1.

[81] Dennis CM, McNeil KD, Dunning J, et al. Heart-lung-liver transplantation. J Heart Lung Transplant 1996;15(5):536–8.

[82] Pirenne J, Verleden G, Nevens F, et al. Combined liver and (heart-)lung transplantation in liver transplant candidates with refractory portopulmonary hypertension. Transplantation 2002;73(1):140–2.

[83] Kawut SM, Taichman DB, Ahya VN, et al. Hemodynamics and survival of patients with portopulmonary hypertension. Liver Transpl 2005;11(9): 1107–11.

[84] Swanson KL, Wiesner RH, Rosen CB, et al. Pulmonary vascular complications of liver disease: survival analysis of 140 patients evaluated at Mayo Clinic. Hepatology 2003;38(4 Suppl 1):219A.

[85] Robalino BD, Moodie DS. Association between primary pulmonary hypertension and portal hypertension: analysis of its pathophysiology and clinical, laboratory and hemodynamic manifestations. J Am Coll Cardiol 1991;17(2):492–8.

[86] Nagaya N, Nishikimi T, Uematsu M, et al. Plasma brain natriuretic peptide as a prognostic indicator in patients with primary pulmonary hypertension. Circulation 2000;102(8):865–70.

[87] Leuchte HH, Holzapfel M, Baumgartner RA, et al. Characterization of brain natriuretic peptide in long-term follow-up of pulmonary arterial hypertension. Chest 2005;128(4):2368–74.

[88] Mal H, Burgiere O, Durand F, et al. Pulmonary hypertension following hepatopulmonary syndrome in a patient with cirrhosis. J Hepatol 1999;31(2):360–4.

[89] Shah T, Isaac J, Adams D, et al. Development of hepatopulmonary syndrome and portopulmonary hypertension in a paediatric liver transplant patient. Pediatr Transplant 2005;9(1):127–31.

[90] Jones FD, Kuo PC, Johnson LB, et al. The coexistence of portopulmonary hypertension and hepatopulmonary syndrome. Anesthesiology 1999;90(2):626–9.

[91] Umeda A, Tagawa M, Kohsaka T, et al. Hepatopulmonary syndrome can show spontaneous resolution: possible mechanism of portopulmonary hypertension overlap? Respirology 2006;11(1):120–3.

[92] Martinez-Palli G, Barbera JA, Taura P, et al. Severe portopulmonary hypertension after liver transplantation in a patient with preexisting hepatopulmonary syndrome. J Hepatol 1999;31(6):1075–9.

[93] Tasaka S, Kanazawa M, Nakamura H, et al. An autopsied case of primary pulmonary hypertension complicated by hepatopulmonary syndrome [in Japanese] Nihon Kyobu Shikkan Gakkai Zasshi 1995; 33(1):90–4.

[94] Condino AA, Ivy DD, O'Connor JA, et al. Portopulmonary hypertension in pediatric patients. J Pediatr 2005;147(1):20–6.

[95] Krowka MJ. Many faces of portopulmonary hypertension. J Pediatr 2005;147(1):3–4.

[96] Loureiro-Silva MR, Iwakiri Y, Abraldes JG, et al. Increased phosphodiesterase-5 expression is involved in the decreased vasodilator response to nitric oxide in cirrhotic rat livers. J Hepatol 2006;44(5): 886–93.

Clin Chest Med 28 (2007) 219–232

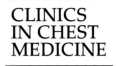

Pulmonary Hypertension Associated with Chronic Respiratory Disease

Reda E. Girgis, MB, BCh*, Stephen C. Mathai, MD, MHS

Division of Pulmonary and Critical Care Medicine, Johns Hopkins University, 1830 East Monument Street, 5th Floor, Baltimore, MD 21205, USA

Pulmonary hypertension (PH) is a well-recognized complication of chronic respiratory disease (Box 1). The Third World Symposium on Pulmonary Arterial Hypertension grouped these conditions under the heading "Pulmonary Hypertension Associated with Lung Diseases and/or Hypoxemia" [1]. A more accurate term is *chronic respiratory disease*, because extrapulmonary conditions that cause hypoventilation are included in this category. Moreover, although alveolar hypoxia probably plays an important role, it has become increasingly clear that these disorders do not simply represent chronic hypoxic PH. These conditions represent significant proportion of PH. In the authors' referral clinic, one fifth of all patients who have PH had an underlying respiratory disease. In a national survey of hospital discharge diagnoses, respiratory diseases were listed as the principal diagnosis in 28% of cases where PH was reported from 2000 through 2002 [2]. Recent investigations have described the prevalence and clinical correlates of PH in these conditions and highlight its impact on functional capacity and survival [3–6]. The recent availability of new pharmacologic agents for pulmonary arterial hypertension [7] has generated renewed interest in this problem, although the potential efficacy of medical therapy remains to be determined. This article provides an overview of the most common respiratory diseases associated with PH and recommendations for the diagnostic evaluation and treatment.

Chronic obstructive pulmonary disease

The exact prevalence of PH in chronic obstructive pulmonary disease (COPD) is unclear, but it is more common among patients who have severe airflow limitation. In a recent large French series of patients referred for lung volume reduction surgery or transplantation with a mean force expiratory volume in 1 second (FEV_1) of 24% predicted, half had a mean pulmonary artery pressure (MPAP) greater than 25 mm Hg [8]. On average, PH is mild in severity (25–35 mm Hg MPAP) with preserved right ventricular function. However, a small subset of patients who have severe PH associated with modest obstruction seems to exist. Chaouat and colleagues [3] observed an MPAP of 40 mm Hg or more in 27 of 998 patients who had COPD. Eleven patients (1.1%) had no other identifiable cause for the PH. The median FEV_1 in this group was 50% predicted, but diffusing capacity for carbon monoxide (DL_{CO}) was extremely low and emphysema was prominent on high-resolution CT. A strikingly similar finding was reported by Thabut and coworkers [8], who used a cluster analysis to identify 16 of 215 patients who had advanced COPD with severe PH (MPAP of 40 ± 10 mm Hg) that contrasted with moderate obstruction (FEV_1 of 49% ± 12% predicted). In both studies, patients who had severe PH had profound hypoxemia without hypercapnia.

Despite the usually moderate nature of PH in COPD, it clearly has an adverse impact on survival. Numerous studies have shown increased mortality; however, whether PH is an independent predictor or a reflection of underlying disease severity remains unclear. The group in Strasbourg, France

---

* Corresponding author.

E-mail address: rgirgis@jhmi.edu (R.E. Girgis).

doi:10.1016/j.ccm.2006.11.006

Box 1. Respiratory diseases causing pulmonary hypertension

Obstructive lung disease
Chronic obstructive pulmonary disease (COPD)
Cystic fibrosis/bronchiectasis
Obliterative bronchiolitis

Interstitial lung disease
Connective tissue disease–related
Idiopathic interstitial pneumonias
    Idiopathic pulmonary fibrosis
    Nonspecific interstitial pneumonia
    Others
Sarcoidosis
Langerhans cell histiocytosis
Lymphangioleiomyomatosis
Others

Alveolar hypoventilation
Obesity–hypoventilation syndrome
Thoracic cage disorders
    Kyphoscoliosis
Neuromuscular disease

Sleep-disordered breathing
Obstructive sleep apnea (OSA)
Central sleep apnea
Overlap syndrome (COPD in combination with OSA)

Chronic exposure to high altitude
Developmental abnormalities/neonatal lung disease

reported a 5-year survival rate of 36% among patients whose MPAP exceeded 25 mm Hg, compared with 62% among those who did not have PH. Pulmonary function and blood gas variables were not predictive of survival [9]. In their analysis of severe PH cases with MPAP of 40 mm Hg or more, Chaouat and colleagues [3] found that the 5-year survival rate was less than 20%.

Vascular remodeling

The lack of reversibility in response to oxygen or nitric oxide inhalation indicates that acute hypoxic vasoconstriction is not the primary determinant and that structural changes, such as vascular remodeling, account for PH. Although numerous studies have shown a relationship between PH and partial pressure of oxygen, arterial (Pao_2), the correlation is weak. Chronic hypoxia

induces neomuscularization of previously nonmuscularized pulmonary arterioles and medial hypertrophy of small muscular pulmonary arteries. These changes are observed in chronic mountain dwellers. A prominent feature of the vascular remodeling of COPD-related PH is intimal thickening caused by longitudinally oriented smooth muscle cells with abundant extracellular deposition of collagen and elastin (intimal fibroelastosis). These changes have also been described in patients who have mild, normoxemic COPD who do not have PH and in asymptomatic smokers [10]. Small vessel thrombi or emboli may also occur. Medial hypertrophy is often observed in established PH [11], but may also be seen when PH is absent.

Mechanisms for vascular remodeling

Many pathogenetic pathways proposed in pulmonary arterial hypertension have been similarly implicated in PH associated with lung disease. Pulmonary arterial rings of patients who have COPD have impaired endothelial-dependent vasodilatation [12], and expression of endothelial nitric oxide synthase is reduced in advanced disease and asymptomatic smokers [13]. Exhaled nitric oxide has been shown to be reduced in patients who have COPD and PH [14]. A link may also exist between certain polymorphisms in the nitric oxide synthase gene and PH in COPD [15]. Other endothelial-derived mediators may be involved. Excretion of prostacyclin metabolites are decreased in patients who have COPD with PH, but not in those who do not [16]. Studies of circulating endothelin-1 have yielded conflicting results, whereas pulmonary vascular expression is increased in established PH [17] but not in early disease [13]. Smokers and patients who have moderate COPD have been shown to have enhanced expression of vascular endothelial growth factor in vascular smooth muscle, and this correlates with arterial wall thickness [18]. Recent studies suggest an important role for serotonin (5-HT) and its transporter (5-HTT) in the vascular smooth muscle hyperplasia of PH. The 5-HTT LL genotype, which is linked with greater 5-HTT expression, was associated with significantly higher pulmonary artery pressure in patients who have COPD compared with the other polymorphisms [19]. A correlation has been shown between small airway inflammation and vascular remodeling [20]. Increased CD8 lymphocytes were detected in the adventitia of small muscular arteries of patients who had mild COPD and in smokers, and correlated with intimal thickening and endothelial dysfunction. These findings suggest that smoking may have direct effects on the pulmonary vasculature.

The presence of alveolar hypoventilation from any cause, with consequent hypercapnia, acts synergistically with hypoxia to induce pulmonary vasoconstriction and vascular remodeling. The accompanying increase in hydrogen ion concentration seems to be the key factor [11]. Hypercapnia promotes renal salt and water retention through multiple mechanisms, which can cause edema in the absence of cardiac dysfunction [21].

Mechanical factors

Pulmonary artery wedge pressure is often mildly elevated, but correlates with MPAP [8,22]. This finding may reflect underlying left ventricular diastolic dysfunction. Loss of capillaries from emphysematous destruction of alveolar walls was previously believed to be an important mechanism of PH in emphysema. However, PH is not related to total alveolar surface area or radiographic lung density [11]. Advanced airflow limitation may increase intra-alveolar pressures, leading to compression of intra-alveolar vessels. A frequently overlooked factor is the effect of increased alveolar pressure and hyperinflation resulting from advanced airflow limitation. In contrast to the systemic circulation in which the capillaries offer minimal resistance, the pulmonary capillary bed accounts for more than half the total pulmonary vascular resistance [23]. These alveolar vessels can therefore be compressed by high alveolar pressure. Hyperinflation would stretch these vessels, leading to further narrowing. This effect becomes evident during hyperventilation, when pulmonary artery pressure and pulmonary vascular resistance can increase dramatically [24]. Analysis of passive pressure/flow curves in patients who have COPD, where flow is increased with either unilateral pulmonary artery balloon occlusion or dobutamine infusion, shows an increased extrapolated pressure intercept, suggesting vascular closure [25,26]. Under these circumstances, the driving pressure across the pulmonary circulation is not pulmonary artery pressure minus left atrial pressure, but rather pulmonary artery pressure minus this "critical closing pressure." The latter may be elevated as a result of alveolar pressure exceeding left atrial pressure (ie, in West zone 2 conditions) or increased

vascular recoil from remodeling [25]. Ignoring an elevated closing pressure could lead to the erroneous conclusion that pulmonary vascular resistance is increased, when in fact the slope of the pressure/flow curve may be normal.

Interstitial lung diseases

Connective tissue diseases

Interstitial lung disease is the most common pulmonary manifestation of scleroderma (systemic sclerosis). The impact of concomitant PH on the course of interstitial lung disease in systemic sclerosis is becoming increasingly appreciated. A typical pattern is that of mild dyspnea in the setting of stable or slowly declining pulmonary function tests over many years. An abrupt worsening of symptoms, hypoxemia, and DL_{CO} heralds the onset of PH. A recent review of 619 patients by the Johns Hopkins Scleroderma Center showed that the prevalence of PH increased with worsening restrictive ventilatory defect. Among patients who had mild restriction (total lung capacity, 65%–79% predicted), 22% had an estimated right ventricular systolic pressure (RVSP) on echocardiography of more than 45 mm Hg, whereas 30% and 47% of those who had moderate and severe restriction (total lung capacity < 50%), respectively, showed echocardiographic evidence of PH. Long-term survival of patients who had combined PH and restriction was similar to that of those who had isolated PH, and significantly worse than that of those who had an isolated restrictive defect [27].

Idiopathic pulmonary fibrosis

PH is becoming increasingly recognized as an important complication of idiopathic pulmonary fibrosis (IPF). Among 79 consecutive patients evaluated for lung transplantation, 32% had an MPAP more than 25 mm Hg [4]. These patients manifested a greater degree of hypoxemia and reduced exercise capacity compared with those who did not have PH, yet lung volumes were similar. Moreover, a sizable proportion of unselected patients who had IPF have moderate to severe PH. Leuchte and colleagues [28] reported that 6 of 28 consecutive patients who had IPF had an MPAP of more than 35 mm Hg. In these patients, rapid clinical deterioration associated with right heart failure can occur, which is often unrelated to progression of the underlying parenchymal process.

Pulmonary vascular involvement has important physiologic consequences in interstitial lung
disease and other lung diseases. In the presence of
a normal ventilation/perfusion (V/Q) relationship,
a fall in mixed venous partial pressure of oxygen
(Po$_2$), resulting from decreased cardiac output,
has little impact on arterial oxygenation. With increasing V/Q mismatch and intrapulmonary
shunting, mixed venous Po$_2$ becomes an important determinant of Pao$_2$. Diffusion limitation is
also a key factor, particularly with exercise [29],
and is similarly magnified by a reduction in mixed
venous oxygen. Agusti and coworkers [29] showed
that the increase in MPAP, decline in Pao$_2$, and
V/Q inequality during exercise are related to
structural vascular changes that prevent the redis-
tribution of blood away from poorly ventilated
units. PH is clearly a poor prognostic factor in
IPF. In the series by Lettieri and coworkers [4],
the 1-year mortality rate was 29% compared
with 6% in patients who had no PH. Similarly, investigators at the Mayo Clinic observed a median
survival of 0.7 years in patients who had IPF and
an RVSP on echocardiography of more than
50 mm Hg, compared with a survival of more
than 4 years for those who had an RVSP of less
than 50 mm Hg [30].

Pathologically, the vasculopathy of IPF consists of medial and intimal changes similar to those
observed in COPD. In addition, the intimal lesions
can progress to acellular fibrosis with luminal
obliteration (Fig. 1) [31]. Destruction of lung tissue
with loss of vasculature and fibrosis of vessels in
affected regions is considered an important

mechanism. Fibrotic areas have markedly reduced
vascular density, and endothelial cell markers are
absent from fibroblastic foci [32]. A weak correlation with Pao$_2$ suggests a role for hypoxia [33].
However, the pattern of vascular remodeling, the
lack of reversibility with oxygen, and the occurrence of PH in patients who have only mild hypoxemia all point away from hypoxia as the primary
cause. Moreover, because PH can magnify hypoxemia, interpretation of correlations between Pao$_2$
and pulmonary artery pressure is problematic.
Alterations in certain vasoactive mediators have
been proposed. Endothelin is prominently expressed in IPF lungs with more intense vascular
endothelial expression in those who have PH
[34]. Arterial endothelin-1 levels are elevated in
interstitial lung disease, are higher among those
who have PH, and correlate with MPAP [35].

Sarcoidosis, Langerhans cell histiocytosis, and lymphangioleiomyomatosis

Although sarcoidosis, Langerhans cell histiocytosis, and lymphangioleiomyomatosis are considered interstitial lung diseases, they have been
grouped separately [1] because of the direct vascular involvement by the specific pathognomonic
features of each disorder and the frequent occurrence of severe PH. Active vascular granulomatous inflammation or healed lesions are very
common in sarcoidosis, involving both arteries
and veins [36]. However, the prevalence of PH in
a recent echocardiographic survey in a Japanese
population was less than 6% [37]. The extent of
vascular involvement is related to the degree of
parenchymal disease, corresponding to the clinical
association of PH with reduced lung volumes and
advanced radiographic stage [37–39]. However,
a subset of patients who have severe PH without
significant fibrosis clearly seems to exist. In
reviewing their experience with 22 patients, Nunes
and colleagues [38] found that 15 had radiographic stage IV disease. The remaining 7 had
a mean total lung capacity of 84% predicted and
an average MPAP of 52 mm Hg. Diffusing capacity and Pao$_2$ were significantly reduced in both
groups compared to patients who had sarcoidosis
and no PH who were matched for radiographic
stage [38]. As with other lung diseases, PH is an
ominous complication in sarcoidosis, associated
with reduced functional capacity, increased oxygen requirement, and higher mortality [6]. Among
patients who have sarcoidosis who were listed for
lung transplantation in the United States from

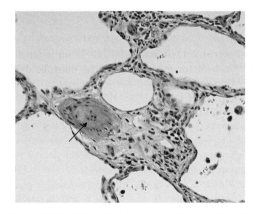

Fig. 1. PH in idiopathic pulmonary fibrosis. Vascular
intimal fibrosis with luminal obliteration (*arrow*) in a region involved by interstitial fibrosis and chronic inflammation. Courtesy of Rubin Tuder, MD, Baltimore, MD.

1995 to 2002, 74% had an MPAP more than 25 mm Hg and 36% had an MPAP of 40 mm Hg or more [6]. Patients who died while awaiting lung transplantation had an average MPAP of 41 mm Hg compared with 32 mm Hg among survivors, whereas forced vital capacity and FEV_1 showed no difference [40]. In a smaller cohort, no survivors had a right atrial pressure of 15 mm Hg or more, whereas 45% of patients dying while on the waiting list had an elevated right atrial pressure; on multivariate analysis, this was the only significant risk factor for mortality [41].

A prominent proliferative, inflammatory vasculopathy with occasional Langerhans cells involving both arteries and veins is well described in Langerhans cell histiocytosis. Fartoukh and colleagues [42] reported on 21 consecutive patients referred for lung transplantation, all with severe PH (average MPAP of 59 mm Hg). Although advanced parenchymal disease was present, no relationship was found between pulmonary function and MPAP. Moreover, vascular remodeling was observed in regions unaffected by parenchymal lesions, and progressed on serial lung biopsies independent of the interstitial and bronchiolar processes.

Despite the pathognomonic proliferation of smooth muscle cells around bronchovascular structures in lymphangioleiomyomatosis, severe pulmonary hypertension seems uncommon. The presence of an altered cardiovascular response to exercise in some patients, however, points to pulmonary vascular involvement [43].

Sleep-disordered breathing

Episodic and potentially dramatic increases in pulmonary artery pressure accompany apneic episodes in obstructive sleep apnea (OSA), particularly during rapid eye movement sleep [44]. This finding has been largely attributed to hypoxia, although other factors related to large swings in intrathoracic pressure may also be important, such as increased venous return and left ventricular afterload [45]. In contrast to certain animal models, however, intermittent hypoxia does not generally produce PH in humans [46]. The relationship between OSA and PH was reviewed recently [47]. The prevalence of PH (defined as MPAP ≥ 20 mm Hg) has been estimated to be around 20%. However, most cases of PH associated with OSA are mild, with MPAP generally less than 25 to 30 mm Hg. Even severe OSA is unlikely to be the sole cause of clinically important PH.

Increasing body mass index and more severe nocturnal desaturation are linked to PH in OSA, whereas the relationship with the apnea–hypopnea index is minor [48,49]. Patients who have OSA and PH have consistently been shown to have altered daytime lung function compared with those who do not have PH. These include lower forced vital capacity, FEV_1, and Pao_2, and higher arterial partial pressure of carbon dioxide ($Paco_2$) [49]. Most studies have not excluded patients with associated COPD (overlap syndrome) and the obesity–hypoventilation syndrome (OHS), two commonly associated conditions that can independently cause PH and augment the propensity for OSA to contribute to PH.

The Strasbourg group recently reviewed their experience with these subsets of patients [50]. Among 181 patients who had pure severe OSA (mean apnea–hypopnea index, 73/h) and no comorbid conditions, MPAP was 15 ± 5 mm Hg and only 9% had an MPAP of 20 mm Hg or more. In contrast, 27 patients with OHS, defined as a body mass index more than 30 and $Paco_2$ more than 45 mm Hg, had an MPAP of 23 ± 10 mm Hg, and 59% had an MPAP of 20 mm Hg or more. Overlap patients had intermediate values. Abnormal daytime lung function and gas exchange are likely to be associated with vascular remodeling. Reduced vessel caliber would magnify the effects of an obstructive apnea on pulmonary hemodynamics. Diurnal PH in OSA is associated with an enhanced pressor response to hypoxia [44] and an altered pressure–flow relationship [51] consistent with vascular remodeling.

Another common comorbidity in OSA that probably contributes to PH is left heart disease [52]. OSA is an established risk factor for systemic hypertension [53], which is frequently associated with left ventricular diastolic dysfunction, and recently, OSA was identified as an independent risk factor for left ventricular diastolic dysfunction defined by echocardiography [54]. Moreover, Arias and colleagues [55] reported that 9 of 10 patients who had OSA and PH and no other cardiac risk factors had left ventricular diastolic dysfunction compared with 4 of 13 patients who had no PH. Pulmonary artery wedge pressure is frequently elevated in PH associated with OSA, and in one study, directly correlated with pulmonary artery pressure [56]. Therefore, although mild PH is common in OSA, comorbidities, such as abnormal daytime pulmonary function and left heart disease, likely contribute to its pathogenesis.

Diagnostic evaluation of pulmonary hypertension in respiratory disease

Clinicians traditionally have not aggressively pursued the diagnosis of PH in chronic respiratory diseases, largely because of the lack of specific therapy. However, the increasing array of drugs for pulmonary arterial hypertension may potentially be useful in treating these conditions. A diagnostic evaluation for PH is also clinically important to (1) identify other treatable causes for PH (eg, left heart disease, chronic thromboembolic disease), (2) help delineate the basis for symptoms, (3) provide prognostic information that may guide decisions, such as lung transplantation, and (4) guide the aggressiveness of certain interventions, such as oxygen supplementation and nocturnal positive pressure ventilation.

Routine clinical assessments

Although symptoms clearly overlap, dyspnea and fatigue that seem disproportionate to the degree of respiratory impairment may suggest superimposed PH. Physical signs may often be obscured by hyperinflation or obesity. Enlargement of the central pulmonary arteries on chest radiograph increases the likelihood that PH is present, but is not accurate enough to make a confident diagnosis. Electrocardiographic signs of cor pulmonale are also predictive but have low sensitivity [57].

A main pulmonary artery diameter of 29 mm or larger on CT was a good predictor for PH in parenchymal lung disease, with sensitivity and specificity of 84% and 75%, respectively [58]. The combination of main pulmonary artery enlargement and a segmental artery/bronchus ratio of more than one increased the specificity to 100%. The presence of ground-glass attenuation and septal lines in a polygonal network were found to be more frequent in sarcoidosis with PH versus no PH [38]. The authors attributed these radiographic findings to pulmonary venous obstruction.

Correlations between the degree of obstructive or restrictive ventilatory defect and PH are modest. The DL_{CO}, which is mainly determined by the pulmonary capillary blood volume, is often severely reduced when PH complicates lung disease. Among patients who had emphysema and were being considered for lung volume reduction, DL_{CO} was the only pulmonary function variable that correlated with pulmonary vascular resistance [22]. The DL_{CO} corrected for alveolar volume seems to be a more sensitive indicator of pulmonary vascular involvement in IPF [29]. Severe hypoxemia may also suggest PH.

Echocardiography

The diagnostic accuracy of echocardiography is considerably lower in patients who have PH associated with respiratory disease compared with those who have pulmonary arterial hypertension [59]. Estimating RVSP is not possible in a high percentage of patients because of anatomic factors, particularly hyperinflation. When RVSP can be estimated, it is often inaccurate, frequently more than 10 to 20 mm Hg different from the measured value at right heart catheterization. In contrast, adequate visualization of the right ventricle is possible in most patients. The absence of right ventricular abnormalities had a negative predictive value of 90% [59]. Surprisingly, the specificity was low at 57%, yielding a positive predictive value of only 39%. The basis for this observation is unclear. Right ventricular strain may result from exercise-induced PH. Alternatively, the more negative intrathoracic pressure of interstitial lung disease and large pressure swings of COPD increase right ventricular afterload without altering intravascular pressure referenced to atmospheric. Other indices may be useful, such as the right ventricular outflow tract acceleration time and isovolumic relaxation time [60].

Cardiac MRI is a superior imaging technique to echocardiography, particularly for the right ventricle. MRI technology is rapidly evolving and may be an ideal noninvasive assessment for PH and right ventricular function, but it has not been studied in lung diseases.

Brain natriuretic peptide

The plasma brain natriuretic peptide (BNP) level may be helpful in detecting PH in chronic lung disease. In a heterogeneous group of patients who had chronic lung disease, plasma BNP was 297 ± 54 pg/mL among 47 patients who had moderate to severe PH (MPAP > 35 mm Hg) compared with 26 ± 4 pg/mL in the remaining 129 patients [5]. Using a cut-off value of 33 pg/mL, the sensitivity and specificity for moderate to severe PH was 87% and 81%, respectively. The ability of an elevated BNP to predict mortality was similar to an MPAP of 35 mm Hg.

Right heart catheterization

Given the limited usefulness of noninvasive techniques, right heart catheterization is required to confidently diagnose PH, particularly when results of noninvasive testing are equivocal. Moreover, right heart catheterization is essential to determine the severity of PH. Although this procedure is extremely safe when performed by an experienced clinician, it should only be performed when the results will influence subsequent management because of the discomfort, expense, and risks involved (Fig. 2). An acute vasodilator challenge is only of academic interest in patients who have respiratory disease. This testing is useful in pulmonary arterial hypertension to identify candidates for a therapeutic trial of calcium channel blockers. These agents were studied in patients who had lung disease–related PH and were uniformly found to have no meaningful benefit or to have adverse consequences.

Exercise testing

When resting pulmonary hemodynamics are normal, moderate exercise during right heart catheterization or echocardiography may uncover exercise-induced PH. However, normal values for exercise pulmonary artery pressure are not well defined and changes in left heart filling pressures are difficult to gauge. Moreover, the clinical significance of isolated exercise-induced PH is not clear. Oxygen desaturation with exercise frequently accompanies PH associated with lung disease and has been correlated with survival [61]. Formal cardiopulmonary exercise testing may be useful in distinguishing a ventilatory versus cardiovascular origin of exercise intolerance [62].

Sleep studies

A low threshold should exist for obtaining a polysomnogram. Although the importance of isolated nocturnal desaturation in the pathogenesis of PH is controversial, performing overnight oximetry in patients who have established PH and mild daytime hypoxemia (PaO_2 of 60–70 mm Hg) seems prudent. Exercise-induced desaturation cannot be used to predict nocturnal desaturation [63].

Lung biopsy

In the setting of known PH, radiographic and pulmonary function manifestations of an underlying lung disease can be mild, as illustrated in Fig. 3. Transbronchial lung biopsy entails

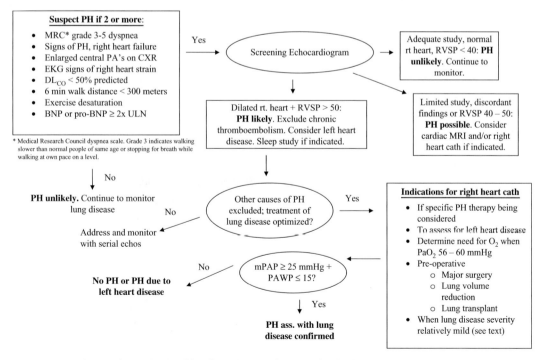

Fig. 2. Diagnostic algorithm for pulmonary hypertension in chronic respiratory disease.

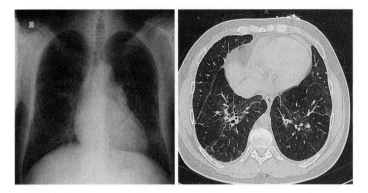

Fig. 3. Chest radiograph and thin section CT showing mild fibrotic changes at the lung bases with minimal bronchiectasis and enlarged central pulmonary arteries. The patient was a 43-year-old male who had known PH (mean pulmonary artery pressure, 44 mm Hg; cardiac index, 1.74 L/min/m^2; right atrial pressure, 14; pulmonary artery wedge pressure, 10). Total lung capacity 83% of predicted, FEV_1/forced vital capacity ratio 0.78, DL_{CO} 46% predicted, resting room air PaO_2 78 mm Hg. Pulmonary hypertension and right ventricular dysfunction progressed over 3 years despite therapy with epoprostenol, whereas no changes occurred in lung volumes or chest radiograph. Explanted lungs at lung transplantation showed fibrotic nonspecific interstitial pneumonia. Pulmonary arteries showed intimal thickening and medial hypertrophy, but no plexiform or concentric intimal lesions characteristic of pulmonary arterial hypertension.

increased risk for bleeding with PH and may not yield a diagnosis. Although the complication rate of surgical lung biopsy is low, the presence of PH, and particularly right heart dysfunction, increases the risk [64]. When clinical features are atypical for pulmonary arterial hypertension, a lung biopsy may provide useful information, such as detection of granulomatous or interstitial lung disease.

Treatment of pulmonary hypertension associated with chronic respiratory disease

Conventional modalities

Oxygen therapy and positive pressure ventilation

Correction of hypoxemia with long-term oxygen therapy clearly improves survival in COPD, but only modest, if any, improvements in pulmonary hemodynamics occur. Long-term oxygen therapy prevents progression of PH in COPD [65,66]. Although no data support the use of long-term oxygen therapy in other hypoxemic lung diseases [67], most clinicians prescribe it, particularly with complicating PH for which a PaO_2 of less than 60 mm Hg is required for Medicare coverage, compared with less than 56 mm Hg in the absence of PH. The efficacy of supplemental oxygen for nocturnal or exercise-induced desaturation with resting daytime PaO_2 of 60 mm Hg or more is unclear. Among patients who had COPD and mild PH (average MPAP of 25 mm Hg) at baseline,

Fletcher and coworkers [68] found reduced survival with isolated nocturnal desaturation. In a randomized trial, patients treated with nocturnal oxygen experienced a reduction in MPAP of 4 mm Hg over 3 years compared with an increase of 4 mm in a sham-treated control group [69], but no difference in survival [68]. A subsequent study by the group in Strasbourg, France found no difference in change in pulmonary artery pressure over time, survival, or subsequent need for long-term oxygen therapy among patients who had COPD with average baseline MPAP of 18 to 20 mm Hg [70]. Oxygen use consistently has been shown to improve exercise capacity with isolated exercise-induced desaturation and to reduce the concomitant rise in pulmonary artery pressure [71]. Thus, in the setting of PH, oxygen may be beneficial for treating nocturnal or exercise-induced hypoxemia when resting daytime saturation exceeds 89%.

Successful amelioration of OSA with continuous positive airway pressure [72,73] or weight loss [74] often leads to improvement in the mild degree of PH that is typically observed in severe OSA. In alveolar hypoventilation caused by restrictive thoracic cage disorders, restoration of daytime gas exchange variables toward normal with nocturnal noninvasive positive-pressure ventilation significantly lowered MPAP from 33 to 25 mm Hg after 1 year [75]. In contrast, patients who had COPD and a comparable degree of arterial blood gas derangements did not show hemodynamic improvement, suggesting that vascular remodeling is a more important factor [75]. Serial data on pulmonary hemodynamics in response to noninvasive positive-pressure ventilation are lacking in other hypoventilation syndromes, but this modality has been shown to improve clinical outcomes in obesity–hypoventilation [76] and neuromuscular disease [77]. Thus, optimization of nocturnal ventilation with consequent improvement in daytime gas exchange seems to be a worthwhile goal in the management of pulmonary hypertension associated with extra-pulmonary causes of hypoventilation.

Therapy directed toward underlying lung disease

Efforts to reverse or halt progression of the underlying disorder may impact the PH. Several anecdotal cases of response to corticosteroid therapy have been reported with sarcoidosis-related PH, particularly those without advanced fibrosis [38], again supporting the presence of direct vascular involvement by granulomatous inflammation. Bronchodilators may be helpful in treating COPD by reducing hyperinflation and large swings in intrathoracic pressure [62]. Theophylline may enhance ventricular performance and reduce pulmonary vascular resistance [20], but caution is required in the setting of heart failure because its clearance is impaired.

Other conventional management

Diuretics are useful in managing right heart failure. Digoxin use remains controversial in the absence of concomitant left heart failure or atrial fibrillation. Supraventricular tachyarrhythmias are poorly tolerated in the setting of a hypertrophied, noncompliant right ventricle, which is more dependent on effective atrial contraction for adequate filling. Restoring sinus rhythm often leads to the resolution of right heart failure. Care should be taken to avoid negative inotropes, such as β-blockers and calcium channel antagonists, in the presence of right ventricular dysfunction. Vaccination against influenza and pneumococcus and early, aggressive treatment of respiratory tract infections are important because pneumonia is poorly tolerated.

Specific therapy for pulmonary hypertension

When PH persists after therapy for the underlying lung disease has been optimized, an important, although unanswered, clinical question is whether therapy directly targeting the pulmonary vasculature has a role. Two primary concerns arise when considering this approach. First, pulmonary vasodilators may attenuate hypoxic vasoconstriction in poorly ventilated units, thereby worsening V/Q matching and hypoxemia [78]. Second, nonselective vasodilators may induce a decline in systemic vascular resistance but have no or minimal effect on pulmonary vascular resistance. Cardiac output would therefore be unable to increase, leading to systemic hypotension and potentially exacerbating or precipitating right ventricular ischemia and worsening right heart failure [79]. Simple vasorelaxants such as calcium channel blockers can reduce pulmonary artery pressure and pulmonary vascular resistance in COPD-related PH, but this effect is short-lived [80], has no clinical benefit, and occurs at the expense of worsening gas exchange [81]. Adverse consequences have also been described in interstitial lung disease–related PH, including systemic hypotension [78].

The explosion of effective newer therapies for pulmonary arterial hypertension [7] in the past decade has generated considerable interest in the potential usefulness of these agents in PH associated with chronic respiratory disease [82,83]. Unfortunately, no controlled, randomized clinical trials of chronic use have been conducted in this population. Published experience has consisted of anecdotal case reports or acute dosing.

Intravenous prostanoids share the same potential as calcium channel blockers to induce systemic hypotension and V/Q mismatching. In patients who had COPD, acute respiratory failure, and MPAP more than 30 mm Hg, intravenous epoprostenol induced transient nonselective vasodilatation and worsened oxygenation [84]. The group from Giessen, Germany observed equal reductions in systemic and pulmonary vascular resistance along with an increase in intrapulmonary shunt during acute challenge with epoprostenol in advanced pulmonary fibrosis [78,85]. However, successful long-term outcomes have been described in patients who have scleroderma with moderate interstitial lung disease [86] and sarcoidosis [87].

Delivery of pharmacologic agents through inhalation is an attractive modality because vasodilatation to poorly ventilated lung units and systemic hemodynamic effects are minimized. Olschewski and colleagues [78] showed a significant reduction in the ratio between pulmonary and systemic vascular resistance and no effect on pulmonary shunt flow with aerosolized prostacyclin. However, the potential for hypotension and worsening oxygenation remains, particularly with higher doses [88], likely representing "spill over" into the systemic circulation. Anecdotal cases of sustained benefit with inhaled iloprost have been reported in cystic fibrosis [89] and connective tissue disease–related interstitial lung disease [78].

Despite the widespread use of the endothelin receptor antagonist bosentan for treating pulmonary arterial hypertension, reports on its use in PH associated with respiratory disease have been sparse. Successful outcomes have been presented for COPD [83] and sarcoidosis [90]. In both cases, the severity of PH seemed to be disproportionate to the degree of pulmonary function abnormalities. Given the putative role of endothelin in fibrosis [91], bosentan has recently been studied in randomized, placebo-controlled clinical trials in IPF and scleroderma-related interstitial lung disease in the absence of overt PH. Neither study met the primary end point of an improvement in 6-minute walk distance after 12 months [92]. However, no worsening in oxygenation occurred with bosentan, suggesting that any adverse impact on V/Q matching is minimal. Moreover, in the IPF trial, a trend occurred toward a reduction in a combined secondary end point of time to death or clinical deterioration (36% in placebo versus 23% for bosentan group; $P < .08$) and a significant difference in this end point among the subset of patients who had biopsy-proven IPF (38% versus 12%; $P = .005$).

An increasing number of reports have recently assessed agents targeting the nitric oxide–cyclic guanosine monophosphate (cGMP) pathway in PH associated with respiratory disease. Acute administration of inhaled nitric oxide is capable of inducing selective pulmonary vasodilation in PH of diverse origins, including parenchymal lung disease [93]. Inhaled nitric oxide is rapidly scavenged and inactivated by hemoglobin, accounting for the absence of systemic effects. In patients who have COPD, in whom hypoxemia is primarily caused by V/Q imbalance, inhaled nitric oxide can worsen arterial PaO_2 as a result of increased perfusion to poorly ventilated units [94]. This effect can be prevented by concomitant use of supplemental oxygen. In a 3-month randomized, controlled, open-label study, Vonbank and colleagues [95] compared "pulsed" inhaled nitric oxide in combination with oxygen versus oxygen alone in 40 patients who had COPD and were hypoxemic with an MPAP of more than 25 mm Hg. Mean pulmonary artery pressure and pulmonary vascular resistance decreased significantly from 28 to 21 mm Hg

and 277 to 173 dyne/s/cm^5, respectively, in the inhaled nitric oxide group compared with no change in the control group. Arterial oxygenation was unchanged, but mean $PaCO_2$ decreased from 56 to 50 mm Hg, suggesting improved perfusion to better ventilated units. Although 39% of patients treated with inhaled nitric oxide reported subjective improvement compared with 13% of controls, no significant difference could be detected in maximal oxygen consumption. Although some success has been reported with long-term treatment with inhaled nitric oxide in IPF [96] and a small series of sarcoidosis-related PH [97], it is unlikely to become a useful modality because of the limited benefits observed and the cumbersome nature of the delivery device.

The phosphodiesterase type V inhibitor sildenafil increases cGMP, the second messenger of nitric oxide. The effects of a single 50-mg dose were comparable to those of inhaled nitric oxide on hemodynamics and showed a trend toward improved PaO_2 in patients who had pulmonary fibrosis and an MPAP more than 35 mm Hg [85]. Two recent small series suggest that hemodynamics and exercise capacity in patients who have COPD and IPF-related PH can improve after 8 to 12 weeks of therapy [98,99]. Gas exchange parameters were not reported.

Lung transplantation

Because of the extremely poor prognosis of advanced PH complicating chronic lung disease and the lack of proven therapies, appropriate candidates should be referred promptly for lung transplantation. The recently implemented Lung Allocation Scoring system of the United Network for Organ Sharing places a heavy emphasis on the presence of PH and high oxygen requirements [100]. These patients, particularly those who have IPF, will likely receive a relatively high score and, consequently, an organ offer soon after listing.

When is the pulmonary hypertension disproportionate to the degree of lung disease?

The pulmonary vascular response can vary widely among individuals exposed to similar insults. From a clinical practice perspective, the question is whether the PH is completely the result of the respiratory condition and therefore treatment should be focused on the latter, or, to some extent, does an independent pulmonary vascular process exist that can be targeted by specific PH therapies. Some general guidelines can be constructed based on the reported severity of PH occurring in the setting of various conditions. PH can be classified as mild (MPAP of 25–34 mm Hg), moderate (MPAP of 35–44 mm Hg) or severe (MPAP $\geq$ 45 mm Hg, or any degree of PH accompanied by evidence of right ventricular failure).

Significant PH is rare in pure OSA, although moderate PH is common in the setting of chronic alveolar hypoventilation. PH complicating COPD and other obstructive lung diseases is not expected unless the FEV_1 is less than 50% of predicted and is typically mild to moderate. In interstitial lung disease, moderate to severe PH typically occurs in the setting of advanced parenchymal disease, wherein the total lung capacity or forced vital capacity is less than 50% of predicted or with extensive radiographic changes. Advanced PH in the presence of underlying lung disease of less severity raises the possibility of a primary vasculopathy that is at least partly independent from the underlying parenchymal process. Conceptually, the likelihood that PH-specific drug therapy would be efficacious is highest in these cases. In these situations, the authors would consider a carefully monitored trial of pulmonary arterial hypertension drug therapy. Randomized clinical trials are required to assess the usefulness of these agents.

Summary

PH is a common, although often overlooked, complication of chronic respiratory diseases. Although often mild and overshadowed by the underlying condition, PH and right ventricular dysfunction can dominate the clinical picture, particularly in certain interstitial lung diseases. A diagnosis of PH has important prognostic implications and helps delineate the basis for symptoms. Further research is needed to improve the diagnostic accuracy of noninvasive testing and to understand the pathogenesis of PH associated with respiratory disease. Newer therapies for PAH have not been studied in this setting and their role remains to be defined. Lung transplantation should be considered early for patients who have advanced PH complicating chronic lung disease.

References

[1] Simonneau G, Galie N, Rubin LJ, et al. Clinical classification of pulmonary hypertension. J Am Coll Cardiol 2004;43(12 Suppl S):5S–12S.

[2] Hyduk A, Croft JB, Ayala C, et al. Pulmonary hypertension surveillance—United States, 1980–2002. MMWR Surveill Summ 2005;54(5):1–28.

[3] Chaouat A, Bugnet AS, Kadaoui N, et al. Severe pulmonary hypertension and chronic obstructive pulmonary disease. Am J Respir Crit Care Med 2005;172(2):189–94.

[4] Lettieri CJ, Nathan SD, Barnett SD, et al. Prevalence and outcomes of pulmonary arterial hypertension in advanced idiopathic pulmonary fibrosis. Chest 2006;129(3):746–52.

[5] Leuchte HH, Baumgartner RA, Nounou ME, et al. Brain natriuretic peptide is a prognostic parameter in chronic lung disease. Am J Respir Crit Care Med 2006;173(7):744–50.

[6] Shorr AF, Helman DL, Davies DB, et al. Pulmonary hypertension in advanced sarcoidosis: epidemiology and clinical characteristics. Eur Respir J 2005;25(5):783–8.

[7] Rubin LJ. Pulmonary arterial hypertension. Proc Am Thorac Soc 2006;3(1):111–5.

[8] Thabut G, Dauriat G, Stern JB, et al. Pulmonary hemodynamics in advanced COPD candidates for lung volume reduction surgery or lung transplantation. Chest 2005;127(5):1531–6.

[9] Oswald-Mammosser M, Weitzenblum E, Quoix E, et al. Prognostic factors in COPD patients receiving long-term oxygen therapy. Importance of pulmonary artery pressure. Chest 1995;107(5):1193–8.

[10] Santos S, Peinado VI, Ramirez J, et al. Characterization of pulmonary vascular remodeling in smokers and patients with mild COPD. Eur Respir J 2002;19(4):632–8.

[11] MacNee W. Pathophysiology of cor pulmonale in chronic obstructive pulmonary disease. Part one. Am J Respir Crit Care Med 1994;150(3):833–52.

[12] Dinh-Xuan AT, Higenbottam TW, Clelland CA, et al. Impairment of endothelium-dependent pulmonary-artery relaxation in chronic obstructive lung disease. N Engl J Med 1991;324(22): 1539–47.

[13] Barbera JA, Peinado VI, Santos S, et al. Reduced expression of endothelial nitric oxide synthase in pulmonary arteries of smokers. Am J Respir Crit Care Med 2001;164(4):709–13.

[14] Clini E, Cremona G, Campana M, et al. Production of endogenous nitric oxide in chronic obstructive pulmonary disease and patients with cor pulmonale. Correlates with echo-Doppler assessment. Am J Respir Crit Care Med 2000;162(2 Pt 1): 446–50.

[15] Yildiz P, Oflaz H, Cine N, et al. Gene polymorphisms of endothelial nitric oxide synthase enzyme associated with pulmonary hypertension in patients with COPD. Respir Med 2003;97(12):1282–8.

[16] Christman BW, McPherson CD, Newman JH, et al. An imbalance between the excretion of thromboxane and prostacyclin metabolites in pulmonary hypertension. N Engl J Med 1992;327(2):70–5.

[17] Giaid A, Yanagisawa M, Langleben D, et al. Expression of endothelin-1 in the lungs of patients with pulmonary hypertension. N Engl J Med 1993;328(24):1732–9.

[18] Santos S, Peinado VI, Ramirez J, et al. Enhanced expression of vascular endothelial growth factor in pulmonary arteries of smokers and patients with moderate chronic obstructive pulmonary disease. Am J Respir Crit Care Med 2003;167(9): 1250–6.

[19] Eddahibi S, Chaouat A, Morrell N, et al. Polymorphism of the serotonin transporter gene and pulmonary hypertension in chronic obstructive pulmonary disease. Circulation 2003;108(15): 1839–44.

[20] Barbera JA, Peinado VI, Santos S. Pulmonary hypertension in chronic obstructive pulmonary disease. Eur Respir J 2003;21(5):892–905.

[21] MacNee W. Pathophysiology of cor pulmonale in chronic obstructive pulmonary disease. Part two. Am J Respir Crit Care Med 1994;150(4): 1158–68.

[22] Scharf SM, Iqbal M, Keller C, et al. Hemodynamic characterization of patients with severe emphysema. Am J Respir Crit Care Med 2002;166(3): 314–22.

[23] Shepard JM, Gropper MA, Nicolaysen G, et al. Lung microvascular pressure profile measured by micropuncture in anesthetized dogs. J Appl Physiol 1988;64(2):874–9.

[24] Harris P, Segel N, Green I, et al. The influence of the airways resistance and alveolar pressure on the pulmonary vascular resistance in chronic bronchitis. Cardiovasc Res 1968;2(1):84–92.

[25] McGregor M, Sniderman A. On pulmonary vascular resistance: the need for more precise definition. Am J Cardiol 1985;55(1):217–21.

[26] Naeije R, Barbera JA. Pulmonary hypertension associated with COPD. Crit Care 2001;5(6):286–9.

[27] Chang B, Wigley FM, White B, et al. Scleroderma patients with combined pulmonary hypertension and interstitial lung disease. J Rheumatol 2003; 30(11):2398–405.

[28] Leuchte HH, Neurohr C, Baumgartner R, et al. Brain natriuretic peptide and exercise capacity in lung fibrosis and pulmonary hypertension. Am J Respir Crit Care Med 2004;170(4):360–5.

[29] Agusti AG, Roca J, Gea J, et al. Mechanisms of gas-exchange impairment in idiopathic pulmonary fibrosis. Am Rev Respir Dis 1991;143(2):219–25.

[30] Nadrous HF, Pellikka PA, Krowka MJ, et al. Pulmonary hypertension in patients with idiopathic pulmonary fibrosis. Chest 2005;128(4):2393–9.

[31] Heath D, Smith P. Disorders of the vascular system. In: Thurlbeck WM, editor. Pathology of the lung. Stuttgart (Germany): Thieme Medical Publishers; 1988. p. 687–750.

[32] Ebina M, Shimizukawa M, Shibata N, et al. Heterogeneous increase in CD34-positive alveolar capillaries in idiopathic pulmonary fibrosis. Am J Respir Crit Care Med 2004;169(11):1203–8.

[33] Weitzenblum E, Ehrhart M, Rasaholinjanahary J, et al. Pulmonary hemodynamics in idiopathic pulmonary fibrosis and other interstitial pulmonary diseases. Respiration 1983;44(2):118–27.

[34] Giaid A, Michel RP, Stewart DJ, et al. Expression of endothelin-1 in lungs of patients with cryptogenic fibrosing alveolitis. Lancet 1993;341(8860): 1550–4.

[35] Trakada G, Nikolaou E, Pouli A, et al. Endothelin-1 levels in interstitial lung disease patients during sleep. Sleep Breath 2003;7(3):111–8.

[36] Takemura T, Matsui Y, Saiki S, et al. Pulmonary vascular involvement in sarcoidosis: a report of 40 autopsy cases. Hum Pathol 1992;23(11): 1216–23.

[37] Handa T, Nagai S, Miki S, et al. Incidence of pulmonary hypertension and its clinical relevance in patients with sarcoidosis. Chest 2006;129(5): 1246–52.

[38] Nunes H, Humbert M, Capron F, et al. Pulmonary hypertension associated with sarcoidosis: mechanisms, haemodynamics and prognosis. Thorax 2006;61(1):68–74.

[39] Sulica R, Teirstein AS, Kakarla S, et al. Distinctive clinical, radiographic, and functional characteristics of patients with sarcoidosis-related pulmonary hypertension. Chest 2005;128(3):1483–9.

[40] Shorr AF, Davies DB, Nathan SD. Predicting mortality in patients with sarcoidosis awaiting lung transplantation. Chest 2003;124(3):922–8.

[41] Arcasoy SM, Christie JD, Pochettino A, et al. Characteristics and outcomes of patients with sarcoidosis listed for lung transplantation. Chest 2001;120(3):873–80.

[42] Fartoukh M, Humbert M, Capron F, et al. Severe pulmonary hypertension in histiocytosis X. Am J Respir Crit Care Med 2000;161(1):216–23.

[43] Taveira-DaSilva AM, Stylianou MP, Hedin CJ, et al. Maximal oxygen uptake and severity of disease in lymphangioleiomyomatosis. Am J Respir Crit Care Med 2003;168(12):1427–31.

[44] Niijima M, Kimura H, Edo H, et al. Manifestation of pulmonary hypertension during REM sleep in obstructive sleep apnea syndrome. Am J Respir Crit Care Med 1999;159(6):1766–72.

[45] Schafer H, Hasper E, Ewig S, et al. Pulmonary haemodynamics in obstructive sleep apnoea: time course and associated factors. Eur Respir J 1998; 12(3):679–84.

[46] Zielinski J. Effects of intermittent hypoxia on pulmonary haemodynamics: animal models versus studies in humans. Eur Respir J 2005;25(1):173–80.

[47] Atwood CW, Jr., McCrory D, Garcia JG, et al. Pulmonary artery hypertension and sleep-disordered breathing: ACCP evidence-based clinical practice guidelines. Chest 2004;126(1 Suppl): 72S–7S.

[48] Bady E, Achkar A, Pascal S, et al. Pulmonary arterial hypertension in patients with sleep apnoea syndrome. Thorax 2000;55(11):934–9.

[49] Chaouat A, Weitzenblum E, Krieger J, et al. Pulmonary hemodynamics in the obstructive sleep apnea syndrome. Results in 220 consecutive patients. Chest 1996;109(2):380–6.

[50] Kessler R, Chaouat A, Schinkewitch P, et al. The obesity-hypoventilation syndrome revisited: a prospective study of 34 consecutive cases. Chest 2001; 120(2):369–76.

[51] Sajkov D, Wang T, Saunders NA, et al. Daytime pulmonary hemodynamics in patients with obstructive sleep apnea without lung disease. Am J Respir Crit Care Med 1999;159(5 Pt 1):1518–26.

[52] Shamsuzzaman AS, Gersh BJ, Somers VK. Obstructive sleep apnea: implications for cardiac and vascular disease. JAMA 2003;290(14):1906–14.

[53] Peppard PE, Young T, Palta M, et al. Prospective study of the association between sleep-disordered breathing and hypertension. N Engl J Med 2000; 342(19):1378–84.

[54] Arias MA, Garcia-Rio F, Alonso-Fernandez A, et al. Obstructive sleep apnea syndrome affects left ventricular diastolic function: effects of nasal continuous positive airway pressure in men. Circulation 2005;112(3):375–83.

[55] Arias MA, Garcia-Rio F, Alonso-Fernandez A, et al. Pulmonary hypertension in obstructive sleep apnoea: effects of continuous positive airway pressure: a randomized, controlled cross-over study. Eur Heart J 2006;27(9):1106–13.

[56] Sanner BM, Doberauer C, Konermann M, et al. Pulmonary hypertension in patients with obstructive sleep apnea syndrome. Arch Intern Med 1997;157(21):2483–7.

[57] Oswald-Mammosser M, Oswald T, Nyankiye E, et al. Non-invasive diagnosis of pulmonary hypertension in chronic obstructive pulmonary disease. Comparison of ECG, radiological measurements, echocardiography and myocardial scintigraphy. Eur J Respir Dis 1987;71(5):419–29.

[58] Tan RT, Kuzo R, Goodman LR, et al. Utility of CT scan evaluation for predicting pulmonary hypertension in patients with parenchymal lung disease. Medical College of Wisconsin Lung Transplant Group. Chest 1998;113(5):1250–6.

[59] Arcasoy SM, Christie JD, Ferrari VA, et al. Echocardiographic assessment of pulmonary hypertension in patients with advanced lung disease. Am J Respir Crit Care Med 2003;167(5):735–40.

[60] Tramarin R, Torbicki A, Marchandise B, et al. Doppler echocardiographic evaluation of pulmonary artery pressure in chronic obstructive pulmonary disease. A European multicentre study. Working Group on Noninvasive Evaluation of Pulmonary Artery Pressure. European Office of the World Health Organization, Copenhagen. Eur Heart J 1991;12(2):103–11.

[61] Flaherty KR, Andrei AC, Murray S, et al. Idiopathic pulmonary fibrosis: prognostic value of changes in physiology and six minute hallwalk. Am J Respir Crit Care Med 2006;174(7):803–9.

[62] Naeije R. Pulmonary hypertension and right heart failure in COPD. Monaldi Arch Chest Dis 2003; 59(3):250–3.

[63] Fletcher EC, Luckett RA, Miller T, et al. Exercise hemodynamics and gas exchange in patients with chronic obstruction pulmonary disease, sleep desaturation, and a daytime PaO2 above 60 mm Hg. Am Rev Respir Dis 1989;140(5):1237–45.

[64] Riley DJ. Risk of surgical lung biopsy in idiopathic interstitial pneumonias. Chest 2005;127(5): 1485–6.

[65] Weitzenblum E, Sautegeau A, Ehrhart M, et al. Long-term course of pulmonary arterial pressure in chronic obstructive pulmonary disease. Am Rev Respir Dis 1984;130(6):993–8.

[66] Zielinski J, Tobiasz M, Hawrylkiewicz I, et al. Effects of long-term oxygen therapy on pulmonary hemodynamics in COPD patients: a 6-year prospective study. Chest 1998;113(1):65–70.

[67] Crockett AJ, Cranston JM, Antic N. Domiciliary oxygen for interstitial lung disease. Cochrane Database Syst Rev 2001;(3): CD002883.

[68] Fletcher EC, Donner CF, Midgren B, et al. Survival in COPD patients with a daytime PaO2 greater than 60 mm Hg with and without nocturnal oxyhemoglobin desaturation. Chest 1992;101(3): 649–55.

[69] Fletcher EC, Luckett RA, Goodnight-White S, et al. A double-blind trial of nocturnal supplemental oxygen for sleep desaturation in patients with chronic obstructive pulmonary disease and a daytime PaO2 above 60 mm Hg. Am Rev Respir Dis 1992;145(5):1070–6.

[70] Chaouat A, Weitzenblum E, Kessler R, et al. Outcome of COPD patients with mild daytime hypoxaemia with or without sleep-related oxygen desaturation. Eur Respir J 2001;17(5):848–55.

[71] Fujimoto K, Matsuzawa Y, Yamaguchi S, et al. Benefits of oxygen on exercise performance and pulmonary hemodynamics in patients with COPD with mild hypoxemia. Chest 2002;122(2):457–63.

[72] Alchanatis M, Tourkohoriti G, Kakouros S, et al. Daytime pulmonary hypertension in patients with obstructive sleep apnea: the effect of continuous positive airway pressure on pulmonary hemodynamics. Respiration 2001;68(6):566–72.

[73] Sajkov D, Wang T, Saunders NA, et al. Continuous positive airway pressure treatment improves pulmonary hemodynamics in patients with obstructive sleep apnea. Am J Respir Crit Care Med 2002;165(2):152–8.

[74] Valencia-Flores M, Orea A, Herrera M, et al. Effect of bariatric surgery on obstructive sleep apnea and hypopnea syndrome, electrocardiogram, and

pulmonary arterial pressure. Obes Surg 2004;14(6): 755–62.

[75] Schonhofer B, Barchfeld T, Wenzel M, et al. Long term effects of non-invasive mechanical ventilation on pulmonary haemodynamics in patients with chronic respiratory failure. Thorax 2001;56(7): 524–8.

[76] Olson AL, Zwillich C. The obesity hypoventilation syndrome. Am J Med 2005;118(9):948–56.

[77] Aboussouan LS, Khan SU, Meeker DP, et al. Effect of noninvasive positive-pressure ventilation on survival in amyotrophic lateral sclerosis. Ann Intern Med 1997;127(6):450–3.

[78] Olschewski H, Ghofrani HA, Walmrath D, et al. Inhaled prostacyclin and iloprost in severe pulmonary hypertension secondary to lung fibrosis. Am J Respir Crit Care Med 1999;160(2):600–7.

[79] Gomez A, Bialostozky D, Zajarias A, et al. Right ventricular ischemia in patients with primary pulmonary hypertension. J Am Coll Cardiol 2001; 38(4):1137–42.

[80] Agostoni P, Doria E, Galli C, et al. Nifedipine reduces pulmonary pressure and vascular tone during short- but not long-term treatment of pulmonary hypertension in patients with chronic obstructive pulmonary disease. Am Rev Respir Dis 1989; 139(1):120–5.

[81] Melot C, Hallemans R, Naeije R, et al. Deleterious effect of nifedipine on pulmonary gas exchange in chronic obstructive pulmonary disease. Am Rev Respir Dis 1984;130(4):612–6.

[82] Higenbottam T. Pulmonary hypertension and chronic obstructive pulmonary disease: a case for treatment. Proc Am Thorac Soc 2005;2(1):12–9.

[83] Maloney JP. Advances in the treatment of secondary pulmonary hypertension. Curr Opin Pulm Med 2003;9(2):139–43.

[84] Archer SL, Mike D, Crow J, et al. A placebo-controlled trial of prostacyclin in acute respiratory failure in COPD. Chest 1996;109(3):750–5.

[85] Ghofrani HA, Wiedemann R, Rose F, et al. Sildenafil for treatment of lung fibrosis and pulmonary hypertension: a randomised controlled trial. Lancet 2002;360(9337):895–900.

[86] Strange C, Bolster M, Mazur J, et al. Hemodynamic effects of epoprostenol in patients with systemic sclerosis and pulmonary hypertension. Chest 2000;118(4):1077–82.

[87] McLaughlin VV, Genthner DE, Panella MM, et al. Compassionate use of continuous prostacyclin in the management of secondary pulmonary hypertension: a case series. Ann Intern Med 1999; 130(9):740–3.

[88] Walmrath D, Schneider T, Pilch J, et al. Effects of aerosolized prostacyclin in severe pneumonia.

Impact of fibrosis. Am J Respir Crit Care Med 1995;151(3 Pt 1):724–30.

[89] Tissieres P, Nicod L, Barazzone-Argiroffo C, et al. Aerosolized iloprost as a bridge to lung transplantation in a patient with cystic fibrosis and pulmonary hypertension. Ann Thorac Surg 2004;78(3): e48–50.

[90] Foley RJ, Metersky ML. Successful treatment of sarcoidosis-associated pulmonary hypertension with bosentan. Respiration 2005 [Epub ahead of print].

[91] Clozel M, Salloukh H. Role of endothelin in fibrosis and anti-fibrotic potential of bosentan. Ann Med 2005;37(1):2–12.

[92] ATS presentation highlights strong rationale for a morbidity/mortality study with bosentan in Idiopathic Pulmonary Fibrosis (IPF). Allschwil, Switzerland: Actelion, May 23, 2006 [press release].

[93] Krasuski RA, Warner JJ, Wang A, et al. Inhaled nitric oxide selectively dilates pulmonary vasculature in adult patients with pulmonary hypertension, irrespective of etiology. J Am Coll Cardiol 2000;36(7):2204–11.

[94] Barbera JA, Roger N, Roca J, et al. Worsening of pulmonary gas exchange with nitric oxide inhalation in chronic obstructive pulmonary disease. Lancet 1996;347(8999):436–40.

[95] Vonbank K, Ziesche R, Higenbottam TW, et al. Controlled prospective randomised trial on the effects on pulmonary haemodynamics of the ambulatory long term use of nitric oxide and oxygen in patients with severe COPD. Thorax 2003;58(4): 289–93.

[96] Yung GL, Kriett JM, Jamieson SW, et al. Outpatient inhaled nitric oxide in a patient with idiopathic pulmonary fibrosis: a bridge to lung transplantation. J Heart Lung Transplant 2001; 20(11):1224–7.

[97] Preston IR, Klinger JR, Landzberg MJ, et al. Vasoresponsiveness of sarcoidosis-associated pulmonary hypertension. Chest 2001;120(3):866–72.

[98] Alp S, Skrygan M, Schmidt WE, et al. Sildenafil improves hemodynamic parameters in COPD-an investigation of six patients. Pulm Pharmacol Ther 2006;19(6):386–90.

[99] Madden BP, Allenby M, Loke TK, et al. A potential role for sildenafil in the management of pulmonary hypertension in patients with parenchymal lung disease. Vascul Pharmacol 2006;44(5):372–6.

[100] Egan TM, Murray S, Bustami RT, et al. Development of the new lung allocation system in the United States. Am J Transplant 2006;6(5 Pt 2): 1212–27.

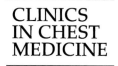

CLINICS
IN CHEST
MEDICINE

Clin Chest Med 28 (2007) 233–241

Pulmonary Hypertension Associated with Left-Sided Heart Disease

Ronald J. Oudiz, MD[a,b,*]

[a]David Geffen School of Medicine at UCLA, CA, USA
[b]Department of Medicine, Division of Cardiology, Liu Center for Pulmonary Hypertension,
Los Angeles Biomedical Research Institute at Harbor-UCLA Medical Center,
1124 West Carson Street, #405, Torrance, CA 90502-2006, USA

Pulmonary hypertension (PH) may be a relatively common hemodynamic finding in patients who have left-sided heart disease (LHD); its presence is usually associated with increased morbidity and mortality [1–15]. Not uncommonly, patients who have systolic and diastolic left ventricular (LV) cardiomyopathic processes develop PH with varying degrees of hemodynamic and clinical severity. It is unknown precisely how many patients in the United States have PH due to LHD; however, in subgroups of patients, such as those who have symptomatic aortic stenosis, PH has been found to be present in up to 65% [4,5]. PH is a predictor of mortality in disorders such as postmyocardial infarction [2], idiopathic dilated cardiomyopathy (DCM) [6,14], and postcardiac transplantation [1,16,17], even when the PH is reversible [3,18].

Classification of pulmonary hypertension

In an attempt to unify the classification of various forms of PH among scientists and clinicians, a consensus meeting of PH experts was convened in 2003, known as the 3rd World Symposium on Pulmonary Arterial Hypertension [19]. At this meeting, experts revised the original consensus-based PH classification system [20], incorporating all forms of PH, including pulmonary arterial hypertension (PAH) and PH due to LHD (Box 1)

[21]. Within the category of pulmonary venous hypertension, two subcategories of PH are recognized: PH due to left-sided (left atrial and/or LV) heart disease, and PH due to left-sided (mitral and/or aortic) valvular heart disease. Overlapping clinical scenarios can be present, however, including coexisting PAH and pulmonary venous hypertension, and this is often a source of confusion and controversy because there is limited information in the medical literature and texts addressing these scenarios.

Left-sided heart diseases leading to pulmonary venous hypertension

Box 2 lists the various forms of LHD that have the potential for causing PH. In these patients, PH results from increased LV or left atrial filling pressure and is highly correlated with Doppler echocardiographic evidence of diastolic dysfunction [22]. In patients who have systolic LV dysfunction, the presence of PH is not only related to the associated diastolic dysfunction but is also influenced by the degree of associated mitral regurgitation present [23]. In patients who have diastolic dysfunction, the curve for LV diastolic pressure in relation to volume (ie, diastolic compliance curve, Fig. 1) is shifted upward and to the left [6], with a resultant increase in diastolic LV filling pressure (and thus elevated left atrial and pulmonary venous pressure).

The various underlying pathologic mechanisms in LHD that result in an elevated hydrostatic pressure in the pulmonary veins commonly lead to passive elevation of pulmonary arterial pressure

---

* Department of Cardiology, Liu Center for Pulmonary Hypertension, Los Angeles Biomedical Research Institute at Harbor-UCLA Medical Center, 1124 West Carson Street, #405, Torrance, CA 90502-2006.

E-mail address: oudiz@humc.edu

Box 1. Revised clinical classification of pulmonary hypertension

1. Pulmonary arterial hypertension (PAH)
   1.1. Idiopathic PAH
   1.2. Familial PAH
   1.3. Associated with PAH
       1.3.1. Collagen vascular disease
       1.3.2. Congenital systemic-to-pulmonary shunts
       1.3.3. Portal hypertension
       1.3.4. HIV infection
       1.3.5. Drugs and toxins
       1.3.6. Other (thyroid disorders, glycogen storage disease, Gaucher's disease, hereditary
              hemorrhagic telangiectasia, hemoglobinopathies, myeloproliferative disorders,
              splenectomy)
   1.4. Associated with significant venous or capillary involvement
       1.4.1. Pulmonary veno-occlusive disease
       1.4.2. Pulmonary capillary hemangiomatosis
   1.5. Persistent pulmonary hypertension of the newborn

2. Pulmonary hypertension with left heart disease
   2.1. Left-sided atrial or ventricular heart disease
   2.2. Left-sided valvular heart disease

3. Pulmonary hypertension associated with lung diseases or hypoxemia
   3.1. Chronic obstructive pulmonary disease
   3.2. Interstitial lung disease
   3.3. Sleep-disordered breathing
   3.4. Alveolar hypoventilation disorders
   3.5. Chronic exposure to high altitude
   3.6. Developmental abnormalities

4. Pulmonary hypertension due to chronic thrombotic or embolic disease
   4.1. Thromboembolic obstruction of proximal pulmonary arteries
   4.2. Thromboembolic obstruction of distal pulmonary arteries
   4.3. Nonthrombotic pulmonary embolism (tumor, parasites, foreign material)

5. Miscellaneous (sarcoidosis, histiocytosis X, lymphangiomatosis, compression of
   pulmonary vessels [adenopathy, tumor, fibrosing mediastinitis])

From Simmoneau G, Galie N, Rubin LJ, et al. Clinical classification of pulmonary hypertension. J Am
Coll Cardiol 2004;43:6S. Copyright © 2004, reprinted with permission from American College of Cardiology Foundation.

(PAP). "Reactive" pulmonary vasoconstriction can occur and subsequent pulmonary vascular "remodeling" may ensue, leading to irreversible pulmonary vascular disease [18]. This remodeling has been postulated to be a result of changes in the elastic fibers of the pulmonary arterial wall, intimal fibrosis, and medial hypertrophy—changes similar to those seen in idiopathic PAH [24].

The importance of the right ventricle in patients who have LHD should be recognized, particularly in those patients who have LV systolic dysfunction due to idiopathic DCM. La Vecchia and colleagues [25] studied 92 patients who had DCM and 61 patients who had ischemic cardiomyopathy. Although the mean PAP was similar in the two groups, right ventricular (RV) dysfunction was noted in 65% of the DCM group and in only 16% in the ischemic cardiomyopathy group, compatible with a more diffuse cardiomyopathic process in the DCM group. The investigators however, stated, "one unresolved issue is whether RV dysfunction has a different meaning

Box 2. Left-sided heart diseases leading to pulmonary venous hypertension

1. Left ventricular systolic dysfunction
    1.1. Ischemic
    1.2. Nonischemic
        1.2.1. Familial/idiopathic dilated cardiomyopathy
        1.2.2. Valvular/volume overload
            1.2.2.1. Mitral regurgitation
            1.2.2.2. Aortic regurgitation
            1.2.2.3. Aortic stenosis
            1.2.2.4. Mitral stenosis

2. Left ventricular diastolic dysfunction
    2.1. Restrictive and constrictive cardiomyopathies
    2.2. Hypertensive and hypertrophic cardiomyopathy
    2.3. Diastolic dysfunction of the elderly/idiopathic?

3. Reduced left atrial compliance [78]

and, possibly, a different impact on prognosis according to etiology of heart failure." Thus, when PH is present in patients who have DCM, it may be impossible to define the relative contributions of the PH per se to the overall cardiac performance.

Finally, a number of extrinsic influences (including hormonal and other growth factors) and the sympathetic nervous system may superimpose their effects to modulate the final "trophic influence" on the cardiovascular system.

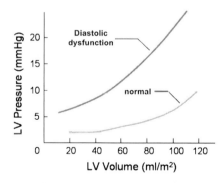

Fig. 1. LV diastolic compliance curves in normal patients and patients who have diastolic dysfunction. In patients who have normal LV diastolic function, as LV diastolic volume increases, LV diastolic pressure rises slowly. When diastolic function is impaired, a more rapid rise in LV diastolic pressure occurs as diastolic volume increases.

Pulmonary hypertension "out of proportion" to left-sided heart disease

The transpulmonary gradient (TPG), defined as the mean PAP minus the pulmonary capillary wedge pressure, is usually low (<12 mm Hg) [1,26] in cases of LHD with PH, signifying that the elevation in PAP is passive. From a purely academic standpoint, even when the TPG is high, "isolated pulmonary arteriopathy cannot be diagnosed" [27]. It is well-known, however, that in some individuals who have LHD, the PAP is elevated out of proportion to that expected by the elevated left atrial pressure. In these cases, the TPG is elevated, often above 25 to 30 mm Hg. In such cases, it is thought that an intrinsic abnormality in the pulmonary arterial circulation exists due to underlying disease of the pulmonary circulation or to or an abnormal pulmonary arterial vasoconstrictor response [26].

The issue is further clouded when RV function is taken into account (see earlier discussion) and when the interactions between RV dilation and LV diastolic function are considered. In many patients who have PH, LV filling is impaired [28,29]; however, the mechanism of this impairment is unclear and controversial. Some researchers have proposed a mechanical basis for LV impairment, postulating that the dilated right ventricle physically impairs left ventricle filling. Gan and coworkers [30] recently found that stroke volume correlated with LV end-diastolic volume and LV septal curvature but not with RV end-diastolic volume or mean PAP. Other investigators, however, have found no effect of mechanical compression by the right ventricle when PH is present [31].

Prognosis of pulmonary hypertension in patients who have left-sided heart disease

A study of nearly 200 patients who had left-sided heart failure showed PH to be an independent predictor of mortality [32]. This study also showed that when pulmonary artery pressure is followed over time, an increase in mean PAP of 30% or greater was incrementally predictive of poor prognosis beyond that of a single hemodynamic measurement.

In patients who have LV systolic dysfunction, pulmonary venous pressure is elevated to varying degrees, with higher left atrial and resultant higher pulmonary venous pressure seen in patients who have overt clinical heart failure and pulmonary edema [33–35]. The presence of elevated PAP is common in these patients and improves with treatment of the heart failure. Drugs such as diuretics [36], angiotensin-converting enzyme inhibitors [37], angiotensin receptor antagonists [38], nitrates [39,40], hydralazine [41], nesiritide [42], and inotropic agents [43] have been demonstrated to reduce PAP.

After myocardial infarction, the presence of PH is highly predictive of mortality. Møller and colleagues [2] studied 536 patients who underwent echocardiography after myocardial infarction. These investigators found that mortality increased linearly with RV systolic pressure, independent of LV ejection fraction (LVEF), LV diastolic function, and mitral regurgitation severity.

In patients undergoing cardiac transplantation, pretransplant PH predicts mortality. Butler and colleagues [3] reported pretransplant hemodynamics in 182 patients undergoing cardiac transplantation. Using a cutoff of 16 mm Hg, the TPG was found to be elevated in 25% of patients who died during the follow-up period compared with only 6% of survivors (odds ratio for risk of dying: 4.93). Similarly, the odds ratio for risk of dying was 5.93 for patients who had a systolic PAP greater than 50 mm Hg compared with patients whose PAP was less than 30 mm Hg.

Patients who have hemodynamically significant mitral stenosis have chronically elevated left atrial pressure and often develop chest pain, dyspnea, and hemoptysis [44]. In these patients, the degree of PH correlates with the severity of their disease [15]. In many instances, after relief of the mitral stenosis by valvuloplasty [45] or by valve replacement [11], the PAP may remain elevated despite the return of left atrial pressure to normal. In these patients, it has been hypothesized that intrinsic pulmonary vascular disease developed due to the long-standing shear forces across the pulmonary vascular bed associated with the chronic passive elevation in PAP, possibly related to a circulating "vasoconstrictive factor" [46].

Diagnostic approach

For screening purposes, echocardiography is commonly performed when PH is suspected, and in such cases, it is recommended as a first-line test by PH experts [27]. Echocardiography offers the ability to noninvasively estimate PAP and can help identify LHD. In addition to evaluation of LV systolic and valvular function, echocardiography can identify patients who have isolated LV diastolic dysfunction, an increasingly prevalent

clinical condition, especially in the aging population [47]. Some investigators favor this noninvasive approach to catheterization when evaluating PH in cardiac transplant candidates [48].

Cardiac catheterization is required for definitive diagnosis in all cases of PH. Although echocardiography plays a role in the diagnosis of PH [27], considerable variation in PAP estimates exists [49]. Further, echocardiography cannot accurately determine left atrial (and therefore pulmonary venous) pressure.

To calculate the TPG in patients who have PH, right-sided heart catheterization must be performed. In cases in which PH is found and LHD is suspected by history, physical findings, or echocardiography, left-sided heart catheterization should probably also be performed; however, a consensus on how to proceed has not been established. Some experts, for example, will perform acute vasoreactivity testing of the pulmonary vascular bed in a manner similar to what is done for PAH [50] in hopes of predicting long-term outcome and response to therapy. With the advent of newer drugs to treat pulmonary arterial hypertension, this testing may be particularly important because these drugs have been shown to improve outcome when used in patients who have PAH (ie, PH without LHD [51–56]). Only limited data exist, however, on the evaluation of the use of some of these drugs in cases of PH with LHD. In some trials that have used potent pulmonary arterial vasodilators in patients who have PH due to LHD, outcomes have been variable (see later discussion) and, thus, their role in such cases remains unknown.

Cardiopulmonary exercise testing has been increasingly used for diagnosing and managing patients who have systolic [1,57] and diastolic [58,59] LV dysfunction and PH [60,61]. This noninvasive modality serves to characterize the nature of the exercise limitation in these patients and provides prognostic information [57] and a basis for follow-up after treatment. Further, it can help determine when a pulmonary vascular limit to exercise is present [61].

In some instances, in patients who have LHD, the presence of PH and related RV dysfunction can help determine whether the PH is simply related to increased pulmonary venous pressure or it is "out of proportion" to the patient's LHD. Ghio and colleagues [62] performed right heart catheterization in 379 consecutive patients who had heart failure and were referred to their institution. All patents had moderate to severe chronic heart failure, an LVEF less than 35%, and primary

DCM or ischemic cardiomyopathy. These investigators found that RV ejection fraction predicted mortality independent of the presence or absence of PH, suggesting that it is the effect on the right ventricle rather than the increase in PAP itself that determines the mortality risk or need for cardiac transplantation. Another study of patients who had moderate heart failure and LVEF less than 45% demonstrated similar findings [63].

Treatment

In most patients who have LHD and associated PH, the initial therapy should focus on the underlying LHD rather than the PH (which by itself may reduce or normalize PA pressure [36–39, 41,43]). There are no drugs approved by the Food and Drug Administration that have a specific indication for the treatment of PH associated with LHD. In addition, only a small number of studies of novel treatments have focused on treating PH in these patients.

Currently, for patients who have idiopathic PAH and associated PAH, conditions in which LHD is absent (see Box 1), treatment is focused

on three therapeutic targets using the following classes of drugs: (1) prostacyclin analogs, (2) endothelin receptor antagonists, and (3) drugs targeting the nitric oxide pathway (nitric oxide and phosphodiesterase [PDE]-5 inhibitors). These drugs have been shown to improve various clinical parameters in patients who have PAH over the short- and long-term, including exercise capacity and hemodynamics. These studies, however, excluded patients who had LHD. Few studies have examined these drugs in PH associated with LHD (Table 1).

There are limited studies evaluating prostacyclin analogs in patients who have LHD. These studies were designed based on the concept that cyclic AMP–mediated effects on vascular smooth muscle would produce vasodilation. An acute study by Brown and colleagues used the inhaled prostacyclin analog iloprost to evaluate preoperative reversibility of pulmonary vascular resistance in cardiac transplantation patients [64], with results similar to inhaled nitric oxide [65].

Short-term studies evaluating prostacyclin analogs in LHD have demonstrated increases in LVEF [66] and salutary hemodynamic changes

Table 1
Pulmonary hypertension drugs studied in left-sided heart disease

Drug	Type	Primary end point	Outcome	Comments	Reference
Epoprostenol	Prostacyclin analog	LVEF	Acute increase in LVEF	Long-term use not evaluated	[66]
Epoprostenol	Prostacyclin analog	Not stated	Acute improvement in hemodynamics	Long-term use not evaluated	[67]
Epoprostenol	Prostacyclin analog	Time until death	Mortality worse	Trial terminated early	[71]
Epoprostenol, iloprost	Prostacyclin analog	Myocardial ischemia	Myocardial ischemia induced	—	[69]
Iloprost	Prostacyclin analog	Vasoreactivity	Safe to use	Given by inhalation	[64]
Nitric oxide	Vasodilator	Vasoreactivity	Safe to use	—	[65]
Darusentan	Endothelin receptor antagonist	LV end-systolic volume (MRI) at 24 wk	No change	—	[72]
Tezosentan	Endothelin receptor antagonist	Oxygen saturation at 1 h	No change	Worse outcome with higher dose	[73]
Bosentan	Endothelin receptor antagonist	Change in clinical status after 26 wk	No change	Pilot trial; study terminated early	[74]
Sildenafil	PDE-5 inhibitor	Exercise heart rate	Exercise heart rate blunted	—	[75]
Sildenafil	PDE-5 inhibitor	Not stated	Several variables acutely improved	Long-term use not evaluated	[76]

[67], with reductions in right and left atrial filling pressures and systemic and pulmonary vascular resistance [68]. Thus, a case could be made to use epoprostenol to treat patients who have combined LHD and PH; however, there have been theoretic concerns of these drugs having adverse effects in the coronary circulation [69] and concerns regarding elevations in pulmonary capillary pressure [70] and acute pulmonary edema. Longer-term studies of epoprostenol in LHD, such as the Flolan International Randomized Survival Trial (FIRST) trial [71] studying patients with refractory heart failure, showed increased mortality compared with conventional therapy. The FIRST Data and Safety Monitoring Committee terminated this trial early because subjects receiving epoprostenol experienced a trend toward decreased survival.

In the Endothelin A Receptor Antagonist Trial in Heart Failure trial [72], 642 patients who had LVEF less than 35% and chronic, stable heart failure symptoms (New York Heart Association [NYHA] class II–IV) despite the use of standard congestive heart failure drugs were randomized to the endothelin receptor antagonist darusentan or to placebo. After 24 weeks of treatment, there was no change in the primary end point, LV end-systolic volume, or any secondary end points (concentrations of norepinephrine, epinephrine, and serum aldosterone). The primary end point was chosen as a marker for LV remodeling; invasive pressures were not evaluated.

Another endothelin antagonist study (the Randomized Intravenous Tezosentan, or RITZ-5, study) evaluated the ability of acutely administered intravenous tezosentan versus placebo to improve oxygen saturation at 1 hour in patients who had pulmonary edema. No change in oxygen saturation was seen; outcome was worse with higher doses of tezosentan [73].

More recently, a pilot study evaluating the effects of the endothelin receptor antagonist bosentan in patients who had NYHA IIIB-IV symptoms [74] was terminated early due to the occurrence of liver function abnormalities and a failure of the drug to effect a change in clinical status at interim analysis.

The use of the PDE-5 inhibitor sildenafil has recently gained attention in its use for PAH [51] and LHD [75,76]. Bocchi and colleagues [75] demonstrated that sildenafil decreased resting heart rate and blunted the exercise-induced increase in heart rate compared with placebo in patients who had LHD. Guazzi and colleagues [76] studied the acute effects of sildenafil in 16

subjects who had LHD. They found a significant decrease in PAP and a significant increase in aerobic capacity as measured by peak VO_2. Nevertheless, there are concerns that long-term PDE-5 inhibition might produce unwanted adverse events perhaps similar to those seen with milrinone, a PDE-3 inhibitor [77].

Summary

The presence of PH in patients who have LHD predicts a poor outcome; however, no study to date has demonstrated long-term benefit from drugs specifically designed to improve pulmonary hemodynamics. There are currently no consensus recommendations on the management of PH when coexisting LHD is present. The underlying cause of LHD should be treated first. When PH appears to be out of proportion to the degree of LHD, cautious use of drugs approved for PAH may ameliorate some of the signs and symptoms of PH; however, theoretic and practical concerns limit any formal recommendations at this time. Further studies of novel agents to treat PH in patients with LHD are warranted.

References

[1] Costanzo MR, Augustine S, Bourge R, et al. Selection and treatment of candidates for heart transplantation: a statement for health professionals from the Committee on Heart Failure and Cardiac Transplantation of the Council on Clinical Cardiology, American Heart Association. Circulation 1995;92: 3593–612.

[2] Møller JE, Hillis GS, Oh JK, et al. Prognostic importance of secondary pulmonary hypertension after acute myocardial infarction. Am J Cardiol 2005;96:199–203.

[3] Butler J, Stankewicz MA, Wu J, et al. Pre-transplant reversible pulmonary hypertension predicts higher risk for mortality after cardiac transplantation. J Heart Lung Transplant 2005;24:170–7.

[4] Johnson LW, Hapanowicz MB, Buonanno C, et al. Pulmonary hypertension in isolated aortic stenosis. Hemodynamic correlations and follow-up. J Thorac Cardiovasc Surg 1988;95:603–7.

[5] Faggiano P, Antonini-Canterin F, Ribichini F, et al. Pulmonary artery hypertension in adult patients with symptomatic valvular aortic stenosis. Am J Cardiol 2000;85:204–8.

[6] Grzybowski J, Bilinska ZT, Ruzyllo W, et al. Determinants of prognosis in nonischemic dilated cardiomyopathy. J Card Fail 1996;2:77–85.

[7] Emanuel R. Valvotomy in mitral stenosis with extreme pulmonary vascular resistance. Br Heart J 1963;25:119–25.

[8] Najafi H, Dye W, Javid H, et al. Mitral valve replacement: review of seven years experience. Am J Cardiol 1969;24:386–92.

[9] Zener JC, Hancock EW, Shumway NE, et al. Regression of extreme pulmonary hypertension after mitral valve surgery. Am J Cardiol 1972;30:820–6.

[10] Ward C, Hancock BW. Extreme pulmonary hypertension caused by mitral valve disease: natural history and results of surgery. Br Heart J 1975;37: 74–8.

[11] Chaffin JS, Daggett WM. Mitral valve replacement: a nine-year follow-up of risks and survival. Ann Thorac Surg 1978;27:312–9.

[12] Cevese PG, Gallucci V, Valfre C, et al. Pulmonary hypertension in mitral valve surgery. J Cardiovasc Surg 1980;21:7–10.

[13] Scott WC, Miller DC, Haverich A, et al. Operative risk of mitral valve replacement: discriminant analysis of 1329 procedures. Circulation 1985;72: II-108–19.

[14] Abramson SV, Burke JF, Kelly JJ, et al. Pulmonary hypertension predicts mortality and morbidity in patients with dilated cardiomyopathy. Ann Intern Med 1992;116:888–95.

[15] Walston A, Peter RH, Morris JJ, et al. Clinical implications of pulmonary hypertension in mitral stenosis. Am J Cardiol 1973;32:650–5.

[16] Erickson KW, Constanzo-Nordin MR, O'Sullivan EJ, et al. Influence of preoperative transpulmonary gradient on late mortality after orthotopic heart transplantation. J Heart Lung Transplant 1990;9: 526–37.

[17] Hosenpud JD, Bennett LE, Keck BM, et al. The Registry of the International Society of Heart and Lung Transplantation: seventeenth official report—2000. J Heart Lung Transplant 2000;19:909–31.

[18] Delgado JF, Conde E, Sanchez V, et al. Pulmonary vascular remodeling in pulmonary hypertension due to chronic heart failure. Eur J Heart Fail 2005; 7:1011–6.

[19] Proceedings of the 3rd World Symposium on Pulmonary Arterial Hypertension. Venice, Italy, June 23–25, 2003. J Am Coll Cardiol 2004;43:1S–90S.

[20] Fishman AP. Clinical classification of pulmonary hypertension. Clin Chest Med 2001;22:385–91.

[21] Simonneau G, Galie N, Rubin LJ, et al. Clinical classification of pulmonary hypertension. J Am Coll Cardiol 2004;43:5S–12S.

[22] Lipkin DP, Poole-Wilson PA. Symptoms limiting exercise in chronic heart failure. Br Med J 1986; 292:1030–1.

[23] Enriquez-Sarano M, Rossi A, Seward JB, et al. Determinants of pulmonary hypertension in left ventricular dysfunction. J Am Coll Cardiol 1997; 29:153–9.

[24] Gaine S. Pulmonary hypertension. JAMA 2000;284: 3160–8.

[25] La Vecchia L, Zanolla L, Varotto L, et al. Reduced right ventricular ejection fraction as a marker for idiopathic dilated cardiomyopathy compared with ischemic left ventricular dysfunction. Am Heart J 2001;142:181–9.

[26] Dalen JE, Dexter L, Ockene IS, et al. Precapillary pulmonary hypertension: its relationship to pulmonary venous hypertension. Trans Am Clin Climatol Assoc 1974;86:207–18.

[27] McGoon M, Gutterman D, Steen V, et al. Screening, early detection, and diagnosis of pulmonary arterial hypertension: ACCP evidence-based clinical practice guidelines. Chest 2004;126:14S–34S.

[28] Louie EK, Rich S, Brundage BH. Doppler echocardiographic assessment of impaired left ventricular filling in patients with right ventricular pressure overload due to primary pulmonary hypertension. J Am Coll Cardiol 1986;8:1298–306.

[29] Moustapha A, Kaushik V, Diaz S, et al. Echocardiographic evaluation of left-ventricular diastolic function in patients with chronic pulmonary hypertension. Cardiology 2001;95:96–100.

[30] Gan CT, Lankhaar JW, Marcus JT, et al. Impaired left ventricular filling due to right-to-left ventricular interaction in patients with pulmonary arterial hypertension. Am J Physiol Heart Circ Physiol 2006;290:H1528–33.

[31] Nootens M, Wolfkiel CJ, Chomka EV, et al. Understanding right and left ventricular systolic function and interactions at rest and with exercise in primary pulmonary hypertension. Am J Cardiol 1995;75: 374–7.

[32] Grigioni F, Potena L, Galie N, et al. Prognostic implications of serial assessments of pulmonary hypertension in severe chronic heart failure. J Heart Lung Transplant 2006;25:1241–6.

[33] Staub NC. Pulmonary edema. Physiol Rev 1974;54: 678–811.

[34] Drake RE, Doursout MF. Pulmonary edema and elevated left atrial pressure: four hours and beyond. News Physiol Sci 2002;17:223–6.

[35] Otto CM, Davis KB, Reid CL, et al. Relation between pulmonary artery pressure and mitral stenosis severity in patients undergoing balloon mitral commissurotomy. Am J Cardiol 1993;71:874–8.

[36] Silke B. Haemodynamic impact of diuretic therapy in chronic heart failure. Cardiology 1994;84(Suppl 2): 115–23.

[37] Ader R, Chatterjee K, Ports T, et al. Immediate and sustained hemodynamic and clinical improvement in chronic heart failure by an oral angiotensin converting enzyme inhibitor. Circulation 1980;61: 931–7.

[38] Regitz-Zagrosek V, Neuss M, Fleck E. Effects of angiotensin receptor antagonists in heart failure: clinical and experimental aspects. Eur Heart J 1995; 16(Suppl N):86–91.

[39] Franciosa JA, Cohn JN. Effect of isosorbide dinitrate on response to submaximal and maximal exercise in patients with congestive heart failure. Am J Cardiol 1979;43:1009–14.

[40] Schneeweiss A. Comparative evaluation of isosorbide-5-mononitrate and nitroglycerin in chronic congestive heart failure. Am J Cardiol 1988;61: 19E–21E.

[41] Chatterjee K. Hydralazine in heart failure. Herz 1983;8:187–98.

[42] Colucci WS, Elkayam U, Horton DP, et al. Intravenous nesiritide, a natriuretic peptide, in the treatment of decompensated congestive heart failure. Nesiritide Study Group. N Engl J Med 2000;343: 246–53.

[43] Mauro VF, Mauro LS. Use of intermittent dobutamine infusion in congestive heart failure. Drug Intell Clin Pharm 1986;20:919–24.

[44] Rothenberg AJ, Clark JG, Muenster JJ, et al. The natural history of mitral stenosis. Dis Chest 1969; 55(1):3–6.

[45] Levine MJ, Weinstein JS, Diver DJ, et al. Progressive improvement in pulmonary vascular resistance after percutaneous mitral valvuloplasty. Circulation 1989;79:1061–7.

[46] Wood P. Pulmonary hypertension with special reference to the vasoconstrictive factor. Br Heart J 1958;4:557–70.

[47] Aurigemma GP, Gaasch WH. Clinical practice: diastolic heart failure. N Engl J Med 2004;351: 1097–105.

[48] Stein JH, Neumann A, Preston LM, et al. Echo for hemodynamic assessment of patients with advanced heart failure and potential heart transplant recipients. J Am Coll Cardiol 1997;30:1765–72.

[49] Rich S, D'Alonzo GE, Dantzker DR, et al. Magnitude and implications of spontaneous hemodynamic variability in primary pulmonary hypertension. Am J Cardiol 1985;55:159–63.

[50] Sitbon O, Humbert M, Jais X, et al. Long-term response to calcium channel blockers in idiopathic pulmonary arterial hypertension. Circulation 2005; 111:3105–11.

[51] Galie N, Ghofrani HA, Torbicki A, et al. Sildenafil Use in Pulmonary Arterial Hypertension (SUPER) Study Group. Sildenafil citrate therapy for pulmonary arterial hypertension. N Engl J Med 2005; 353:2148–57.

[52] Barst RJ, Rubin LJ, McGoon MD, et al. Survival in primary pulmonary hypertension with long-term continuous intravenous prostacyclin. Ann Intern Med 1994;121:409–15.

[53] Rubin LJ, Badesch DB, Barst RJ, et al. Bosentan therapy for pulmonary arterial hypertension. N Engl J Med 2002;346:896–903.

[54] Simonneau G, Barst RJ, Galie N, et al. Continuous subcutaneous infusion of treprostinil, a prostacyclin analogue, in patients with pulmonary arterial hypertension: a double-blind, randomized, placebo-controlled trial. Am J Respir Crit Care Med 2002;165:800–4.

[55] Shapiro SM, Oudiz RJ, Cao T, et al. Primary pulmonary hypertension: improved long-term effects and survival with continuous intravenous epoprostenol infusion. J Am Coll Cardiol 1997;30: 343–9.

[56] McLaughlin VV, Oudiz RJ, Frost A, et al. Randomized study of adding inhaled iloprost to existing bosentan in pulmonary arterial hypertension. Am J Respir Crit Care Med 2006;174:1257–63.

[57] Mancini DM, Eisen H, Kussmaul W, et al. Value of peak oxygen consumption for optimal timing of cardiac transplantation in ambulatory patients with heart failure. Circulation 1991;83:778–86.

[58] Packer M. Abnormalities of diastolic function as a potential cause of exercise intolerance in chronic heart failure. Circulation 1990;81(Suppl 2):III 78–86.

[59] Kitzman DW, Higginbotham MB, Cobb FR, et al. Exercise intolerance in patients with heart failure and preserved left ventricular systolic function: failure of the Frank-Starling mechanism. J Am Coll Cardiol 1991;17:1065–72.

[60] Sun XG, Hansen JE, Oudiz RJ, et al. Exercise pathophysiology in patients with primary pulmonary hypertension. Circulation 2001;104:429–35.

[61] Markowitz DH, Systrom DM. Diagnosis of pulmonary vascular limit to exercise by cardiopulmonary exercise testing. J Heart Lung Transplant 2004;23: 88–95.

[62] Ghio S, Gavazzi A, Campana C, et al. Independent and additive prognostic value of right ventricular systolic function and pulmonary artery pressure in patients with chronic heart failure. J Am Coll Cardiol 2001;37:183–8.

[63] De Groote P, Millaire A, Foucher-Hossein C, et al. Right ventricular ejection fraction is an independent predictor of survival in patients with moderate heart failure. J Am Coll Cardiol 1998;32:948–54.

[64] Braun S, Schrotter H, Schmeisser A, et al. Evaluation of pulmonary vascular response to inhaled iloprost in heart transplant candidates with pulmonary venous hypertension. Int J Cardiol 2007;115:67–72.

[65] Fojon S, Fernandez-Gonzalez C, Sanchez-Andrade J, et al. Inhaled nitric oxide through a noninvasive ventilation device to assess reversibility of pulmonary hypertension in selecting recipients for heart transplant. Transplant Proc 2005;37:4028–30.

[66] Virgolini I, Auinger C, Weissel M, et al. Increase in left ventricular ejection fraction (LVEF) induced by PGE1 and PGI2. Prog Clin Biol Res 1989;301:463–7.

[67] Yui Y, Nakajima H, Kawai C, et al. Prostacyclin therapy in patients with congestive heart failure. Am J Cardiol 1982;50:320–4.

[68] Dzau VJ, Swartz SL, Creager MA. The role of prostaglandins in the pathophysiology of and therapy for congestive heart failure. Heart Fail 1986;2:6–13.

[69] Bugiardini R, Galvani M, Ferrini D, et al. Myocardial ischemia during intravenous prostacyclin administration: hemodynamic findings and precautionary measures. Am Heart J 1987;113:234–40.

[70] Haywood GA, Sneddon JF, Bashir Y, et al. Adenosine infusion for the reversal of pulmonary

vasoconstriction in biventricular failure. A good test but a poor therapy. Circulation 1992;86:896–902.

[71] Califf RM, Adams KF, McKenna WJ, et al. A randomized controlled trial of epoprostenol therapy for severe congestive heart failure: the Flolan International Randomized Survival Trial (FIRST). Am Heart J 1997;134:44–54.

[72] Anand I, McMurray J, Cohn JN, et al. Long-term effects of darusentan on left-ventricular remodelling and clinical outcomes in the Endothelin A Receptor Antagonist Trial in Heart Failure (EARTH): randomised, double-blind, placebo-controlled trial. Lancet 2004;364:347–54.

[73] Kaluski E, Kobrin I, Zimlichman R, et al. RITZ-5: randomized intravenous TeZosentan (an endothelin-A/B antagonist) for the treatment of pulmonary edema: a prospective, multicenter, double-blind, placebo-controlled study. J Am Coll Cardiol 2003; 41:204–10.

[74] Packer M, McMurray J, Massie BM, et al. Clinical effects of endothelin receptor antagonism with bosentan in patients with severe chronic heart failure: results of a pilot study. J Card Fail 2005; 11:12–20.

[75] Bocchi EA, Guimarâes G, Mocelin A, et al. Sildenafil effects on exercise, neurohormonal activation, and erectile dysfunction in congestive heart failure. A double blind, placebo-controlled, randomized study followed by a prospective treatment for erectile dysfunction. Circulation 2002;106:1097–103.

[76] Guazzi M, Tumminello G, Di Marco F, et al. The effects of phosphodiesterase-5 inhibition with sildenafil on pulmonary hemodynamics and diffusion capacity, exercise ventilatory efficiency, and oxygen uptake kinetics in chronic heart failure. J Am Coll Cardiol 2004;44:2339–48.

[77] Packer M, Carver JR, Rodeheffer RJ, et al, the PROMISE Study Research Group. Effect of oral milrinone on mortality in severe chronic heart failure. N Engl J Med 1991;325:1468–75.

[78] Pilote L, Huttner I, Marpole D, et al. Stiff left atrial syndrome. Can J Cardiol 1988;4:255–7.

ELSEVIER
SAUNDERS

Clin Chest Med 28 (2007) 243–253

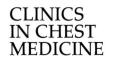

CLINICS
IN CHEST
MEDICINE

Congenital Heart Disease Associated Pulmonary Arterial Hypertension

Michael J. Landzberg, MD

Boston Adult Congenital Heart (BACH) and Pulmonary Hypertension Group, Children's Hospital,
Brigham and Women's Hospital, Beth Israel Deaconess Medical Center, Harvard University,
300 Longwood Avenue, Boston, MA 02115-5724, USA

Congenital heart disease (CHD) is currently the world's leading birth defect, with incidence estimated at 8 per 1000 live births, which corresponds to approximately 1 million or more North American adults and a similar number of children with CHD. Although survival for individuals with CHD continues to improve because of advances in anatomic understanding and care, the functional capacity of patients who have CHD often remains limited when compared with age-matched controls. Pulmonary arterial hypertension (PAH) associated with CHD (CHD-PAH) is one of the most common causes of severe morbidity and premature mortality in patients who have CHD, with an estimated prevalence of CHD-PAH in patients never receiving indicated surgeries of 30% versus 15% in patients who have CHD who received such surgeries [1–3].

Conceptions about CHD-PAH are in evolution, with CHD-PAH previously classified within the "primary (currently, "idiopathic") pulmonary hypertension" grouping. With more recent understanding of potentially differing pathogenetic mechanisms, therapeutic goals, treatment plans, and outcomes compared with idiopathic PAH, however, recategorization has occurred as a unique entity within the more global PAH (Group 1) category [4]. Subcategories have been designated based on complexity and size of shunt defects, association with additional extracardiac anomalies, and status of anatomic repairs. Most recently, an expanded subcategorization has been proposed, which allows for further classification based on anatomy (defects above and below the tricuspid valve and clarification of specific types of complex disease), the presence of myocardial restriction as evidenced by equalization of pressure between chambers, and direction of shunt (left-to-right, right-to-left, balanced) (Box 1) [5].

CHD-PAH occurs in several different scenarios:

1. "Dynamic" PAH related to high shunt flow and responding to control of the shunt ("preoperative" PAH)
2. Late, postoperative, PAH
3. Shunt reversal or "Eisenmenger physiology"
4. Immediate postoperative or "reactive" PAH
5. States previously considered to have normal (or mild elevation of) pulmonary vascular resistance, with unusual congenital defects, in which hemodynamics and well-being are contingent on maintenance of lowest possible pulmonary vascular resistance

These forms of CHD-PAH are discussed separately in this article.

Dynamic pulmonary arterial hypertension

The original descriptions of PAH associated with systemic-to-pulmonary arterial shunts demonstrated that type and size of the underlying anatomic defect and the magnitude of shunt flow are risk factors for the development of PAH [6].

E-mail address: michael.landzberg@cardio.
chboston.org

doi:10.1016/j.ccm.2006.12.004

chestmed.theclinics.com

Box 1. Proposed revised classification of congenital systemic-to-pulmonary shunts associated with pulmonary arterial hypertension

1. Type
    1.1 Simple pre-tricuspid shunts
        1.1.1 Atrial septal defect
            1.1.1.1 Ostium secundum
            1.1.1.2 Sinus venosus

        1.1.2 Total or partial unobstructed anomalous pulmonary venous return

    1.2 Simple post-tricuspid shunts
        1.2.1 Ventricular septal defect
        1.2.2 Patent ductus arteriosus

    1.3 Combined shunts (describe combination and define predominant defect)

    1.4 Complex CHD
        1.4.1 Atrioventricular septal defects
            1.4.1.1 Partial (ostium primum atrial septal defect)
            1.4.1.2 Complete

        1.4.2 Truncus arteriosus
        1.4.3 Single ventricle physiology with unobstructed pulmonary blood flow
        1.4.4 Transposition of the great arteries with Ventricular septal defect (without pulmonary stenosis) and/or patent ductus arteriosus
        1.4.5 Other

2. Dimensions (specify for each defect if more than one congenital heart defect)
    2.1 Hemodynamic
        2.1.1 Restrictive (pressure gradient across the defect)
        2.1.2 Nonrestrictive

    2.2 Anatomic
        2.2.1 Small to moderate (atrial septal defect ≤2.0 cm and ventricular septal defect ≤1.0 cm)
        2.2.2 Large (atrial septal defect >2.0 cm and ventricular septal defect >1.0 cm)

3. Direction of shunt
    3.1 Predominantly systemic-to-pulmonary
    3.2 Predominantly pulmonary-to-systemic
    3.3 Bidirectional

4. Associated extracardiac abnormalities

5. Repair status
    5.1 Unoperated
    5.2 Palliated (specify type of operation(s), age at surgery)
    5.3 Repaired (specify type of operation(s), age at surgery)

From Galie N. Classification of patients with congenital systemic-to-pulmonary shunts associated with pulmonary arterial hypertension: current status and future directions. In: Beghetti M, editor. Pulmonary arterial hypertension related to congenital heart disease. Munich (Germany): Elsevier GmbH; 2006. p. 15; with permission.

Pulmonary vascular histology resembled that described in idiopathic PAH, with medial thickening and plexiform lesions in severe cases [7]. Animal studies of surgically induced shunts to increase pulmonary blood flow or pulmonary arterial pressure suggest that both contribute to increased shear stress and structural changes [8,9]. Increased expression of numerous mediators and receptors also has been observed in the pulmonary arteries of shunted animals, including endothelin-1 and ET_B receptors with or without increased expression of ET_A receptors [10], angiotensin-II and the angiotensin A and B receptors [11], vascular endothelial growth factor (VEGF) with or without its Flk-1/KDR receptors [12] and transforming growth factor (TGFβ-1) with the ALK1 receptor (Box 2) [13]. Expression of signaling molecules, such as calcium-dependent K+ channels [14], phosphodiesterase 5 [15], inducible nitric oxide synthase, angiopoietin-1, MCP-1, intercellular adhesion molecule (ICAM), and tenascin, is also increased and that of BMPR1A, BMPR2, and N-cGMP is decreased in animal models of pulmonary overcirculation [11,16,17]. These experimental studies and recent evidence in humans [18] suggest that endothelin plays a key pathogenetic role in the development and sustenance of CHD-PAH [19–22].

Clinically, specific anatomic lesions carry differing risks for development of PAH (Box 3), with highest potential occurring in unrepaired truncus arteriosus as compared with ventricular and atrial septal defects at moderate and relatively low risk, respectively. Whether the variation in these risks is related to shunt flow or an underlying genetic predisposition, such as an abnormality in BMPR-II [23] is unknown. The nature of the anatomic abnormality also determines the age at presentation, with high pressure, high volume shunting (atrioventricular septal defect, truncus arteriosus, transposition of the great vessels, large patent ductus arteriosus and ventricular septal defects) having risk of earliest presentation, particularly in the presence of trisomy 21.

Surgical experience has suggested that the changes that occur with shunt-mediated PAH are reversible, as long as the surgery is performed before pulmonary vascular changes are "fixed." This determination of when lesions are "fixed" remains consensus opinion rather than rigorously tested standard. Most centers with expertise in the management of patients who have CHD-PAH tend to rely on catheterization-based calculations of pulmonary blood flow (Qp) with isolation of all sources of Qp, individualized measurements of resistance in isolated lung segments, and direct measurement of pulmonary venous pressure to assess PAH reversibility and the likelihood of surgical success. (Patients who have congenital

---

Box 2. Vasoactive mediators and signaling molecules implicated in the pathogenesis of pulmonary arterial hypertension associated with congenital heart disease

Vasoactive mediators
   Endothelin-1 and endothelin
      receptors A and B
   Angiotensin II and angiotensin
      receptors
   Vascular endothelial growth factor
      and the flk1/tdr receptor

Signaling pathways
   Calcium-dependent K+ channels
   Increased phosphodiesterase 5
      activity
   Decreased nitric oxide synthase
      activity
   Angiopoietin 1
   Tenascin
   Diminished function of
   BMPR1A
   BMPR2

Abbreviation: BMPR, bone morphogenic protein receptor.

Box 3. Risk factors for development of pulmonary arterial hypertension in patients who have congenital heart disease

Type of defect
   High risk: truncus arteriosus,
      atrioventricular canal defect
   Moderate risk: ventricular septal
      defect
   Low risk: atrial septal defect

Size of defect
Flow rate of shunt

cardiopulmonary disease may have intrinsic or developed multiple systemic venous or systemic arterial sources of pulmonary blood flow, potentially with different oxygen saturation and content, or pulmonary arterial or venous narrowings—or isolated resistance-based restriction to pulmonary blood flow—in individual segments. Physically isolating each affected contributor to pulmonary blood flow, measuring beyond physical obstructions, potentially controlling or temporarily occluding sources of blood flow so as to allow a single source in calculating its resistance, and combining resistances in this circulation constructed in parallel [$1/R_{total} = 1/R_1 + 1/R_2 + 1/R_3...$] may be necessary for most accurate assessment of Qp and pulmonary vascular resistance [PVR]. At rare times, the measure of absolute Qp falls beyond the capabilities of cardiopulmonary catheterization, and measure of relative Qp via magnetic resonance must be combined with temporally close measure of pressures at catheterization, so as to estimate PVR). Many centers use a preoperative PVR <15 Wood units and pulmonary/systemic resistance ratio ≤2/3 as thresholds associated with better surgical outcomes [24], but individual institutions vary on these thresholds, often modifying them according to the specific anatomic lesion and responses to acute vasodilator testing.

An important concept with regard to predicting the outcome of surgery, especially in borderline cases, is that PVR is flow dependent. High shunt flows can recruit pulmonary vasculature (thereby reducing PVR). With the elimination of shunt, these additionally recruited vascular beds may "de-recruit," no longer accommodating the increased blood flow, and PVR (and hence PA pressure) may fall less than would be predicted based on the reduction of blood flow alone. It should not be assumed that PVR will necessarily fall in proportion to the reduction in shunt and pulmonary blood flow.

Patients with advanced disease deemed to be at high surgical risk still may be considered for staged procedures. Strategies that use combinations of aggressive pharmacotherapy (ie, infused prostacyclins, oral endothelin antagonists, or phosphodiesterase inhibitors) and catheter or surgically based reduction of pulmonary blood flow [25] or graded septostomy (or both) can be used in an attempt to halt the inflammation-like pathologic changes caused by the damaging effects of sustained high pressure and shear stress contributing to progression of the pulmonary vascular disease or to increase systemic output, albeit typically at the price of increased systemic arterial cyanosis. Patients are reassessed periodically, and if functional or hemodynamic status improves, surgery can be reconsidered. This decision to ultimately repair shunting depends on whether pulmonary vascular disease or shunting is thought to be more detrimental at the time of assessment for the individual. Although some patients have been reported to achieve hemodynamic stabilization and improved functional status and survival with these strategies, they have yet to be established in controlled trials.

Late postoperative pulmonary hypertension

Late postoperative pulmonary hypertension, perhaps the least well understood of all CHD-PAH syndromes, is distinguished from "reactive" PAH in that it refers to development or persistence of pulmonary hypertension after the immediate postoperative period despite what seems to be adequate surgical repair. Typically, this condition is attributed to timing of anatomic shunt correction that is too late, miscalculation of the likelihood of surgical correction, or longstanding effects of stable but elevated right ventricular afterload that leads to recalcitrant remodeling. Care must be taken to exclude additional pulmonary hypertension (PHT) triggers (including pulmonary venous hypertension, pericardial constriction, ventilatory lung diseases, chronic macro or in situ thromboembolic diseases, portal hypertension, and pharmacologic toxin exposures), particularly triggers believed to occur with increased frequency in this population (caused by specific physiologies intrinsic to particular cardiac defects, with resultant long-term abnormalities of loading conditions, valvular function, or hepatic congestion). In these situations, aggressive medical therapy of these factors with diuretics, agents that promote cardiac remodeling (angiotensin-converting enzyme inhibitors or calcium channel blockers), removal of pericardial constraint, targeted therapy of portal hypertension, and anticoagulation can conceivably promote reversal of pulmonary vascular changes over subsequent months to years. In their absence, therapeutic options for late postoperative CHD-PAH remain similar to those for idiopathic PAH, with focus on chronic use of pulmonary vasoactive agents such prostacyclins, endothelin receptor antagonists, or phosphodiesterase V inhibitors, with assessment of potential for lung (or heart-lung) transplantation (albeit with greater risk than the idiopathic PAH population).

Eisenmenger physiology

First termed "Eisenmenger physiology" by Wood [6] in 1958, this classification of CHD-PAH refers to the development of bidirectional or a predominant right-to-left shunt accompanied by oxygen-unresponsive hypoxemia and PAH in patients born with large systemic-to-pulmonary shunts. Although first reported in "simple lesions," such as atrial and ventricular septal defects and patent ductus arteriosus, Eisenmenger physiology is also seen in more "complex lesions," such as atrioventricular septal defects, conoventricular defects, including truncus arteriosus and tetralogy of Fallot and its variants, and single-ventricle lesions. Although it tends to be recognized in the middle of the second decade of life, Eisenmenger physiology may be recognized first during the changes in hemodynamic loading that occur with pregnancy. Whether additional triggers of PAH other than intravascular shunt are required for development of Eisenmenger physiology remains debated.

Dyspnea on exertion is the most common presenting symptom of patients who have Eisenmenger physiology, followed by palpitations, edema and fluid retention, hemoptysis, and syncope [6]. Patients who have Eisenmenger physiology encounter increasing morbidity through the successive decades of life, with declining survival. Eisenmenger physiology is also associated with more unique complications compared with patients who have idiopathic or other forms of associated PAH:

- Hypoxemia-related secondary erythrocytosis (frequently associated with iron deficiency caused by increased red-cell turnover) leads to increased blood viscosity and intravascular "sludging." Additional damage to the cerebrovascular circulation, kidneys (glomerular, tubular, and interstitial function may be altered), and pulmonary circulation (in the form of in situ thromboses or frank pulmonary emboli) can occur.

- Intravascular fluid retention and elevated systemic venous pressure may alter hepatic function.

- Concomitant congenital skeletal abnormalities and restrictive thoracic disease may contribute to hypoxemia.

- Hyperuricemia may cause gout.
- The occurrence of clinical bleeding disorders is debated.
- True cardiac ischemic chest pain, usually caused by right ventricular ischemia as a result of excessive right ventricular wall tension, coronary arterial compression by a dilated pulmonary artery, or atherosclerosis, may occur with exertion or at rest.

For patients who have Eisenmenger physiology, progressive right ventricular failure and premature death are the rule. The immediate causes of death include sudden death (likely caused by tachy- or bradyarrhythmias), recalcitrant right ventricular failure, hemoptysis (typically caused by bronchial arterial rupture or pulmonary infarction), and complications during pregnancy. Because of the direct communication of the systemic venous and arterial circulations, strokes caused by systemic "paradoxical" embolization and brain abscesses also contribute to morbidity and mortality [26–28]. Poor functional class, decreasing subpulmonary or subsystemic ventricular function, elevated uric acid, worsening systemic hypoxemia, and declining multiorgan system function are all predictors of mortality for patients who have Eisenmenger physiology [29]. (Recall that in CHDs, the morphologic right ventricle is not necessarily contracting underneath the pulmonary circulation, and similarly, the morphologic left ventricle does not necessarily connect to the systemic circulation. The ventricle that serves as a conduit to the lungs is best described as the "subpulmonary ventricle," whereas the ventricle that supplies the systemic arterial circulation is denoted the "subsystemic ventricle.")

Similar to all forms of CHD-PAH, diagnosis of Eisenmenger physiology requires precise anatomic imaging, shunt definition, and elimination of additional confounding triggers for PHT. Precise anatomic definition has been aided by marked advances in diagnostic multidimensional echocardiographic, CT, and MRI techniques. Because of moderately frequent limitations in echocardiographic "windows" (ability to obtain appropriate or optimal viewing planes) and concerns over radiation exposure, coupled with technique-specific ability to best assess ventricular dimensions, valvular regurgitation, tissue characteristics, and site-specific flow quantification, cardiac MRI plays an increasingly important role in congenital cardiac diagnosis. Primary indications for cardiac MRI include failure of other techniques to provide complete and consistent data, support of diagnostic catheterization or surgery, and use of the technique-specific abilities listed previously (ie, flow, volume, and tissue characteristics). Because of the vast array of available imaging potentials and sequences and the complexity and—at times—unpredictability of patient physiology and anatomy, preprocedural planning and trained clinician presence, interaction, and procedural supervision are required for production and interpretation of meaningful data [30]. In addition to imaging, cardiac catheterization in centers that specialize in the intricacies of CHD-PHT and the acute support of such patients is mandatory to safely and accurately establish the severity of PAH, exclude additional confounders, quantify shunting, and test therapeutic potentials.

In the past, the lack of safe and effective therapies for Eisenmenger physiology led many clinicians to advocate a nonaggressive approach to treatment. The emphasis was on educated consumerism with avoidance of destabilizing situations, such as large fluid shifts, alterations in catecholamines, extreme fatigue, high altitude, cigarette and other smoke exposures, changes in renal or hepatic function, and pregnancy. Reversible contributing factors, such as anemia related to iron deficiency, electrolyte disorders, arrhythmias, and infection, were (and still are) treated aggressively (Box 4).

All procedures in patients who have Eisenmenger physiology require careful team planning because patients are at increased risk for morbidity and mortality even with the simplest of interventions. The type and mode of anesthetic administration should be optimized for individual patients by individuals skilled in treating patients who have Eisenmenger physiology. Air filters are generally used on all venous catheters to minimize the risk of cerebral air embolism, although controversy exists regarding the benefit of this approach compared with meticulous guarding of all intravenous administration systems.

Erythrocytosis tends to remain stable in cyanotic patients, and alterations in serum hemoglobin more often reflect other problems, such as infections, nutritional alterations, or changes in fluid volume. Prophylactic phlebotomy or erythropheresis plays no role in patient management. Studies that determine the role of iron store repletion and optimization of serum hemoglobin and blood viscosity (with or without phlebotomy) in lowering the occurrence of other organ system damage or thrombosis have not been conducted [31,32].

Box 4. Potentially preventable or reversible factors that contribute to deterioration of pulmonary hypertension in Eisenmenger physiology

Pregnancy
Dehydration or acute vasodilation (eg, sauna, hot tub)
Increased fluid volume
Worsened renal or hepatic function
Chronic environmental hypoxia
Increased left-sided filling pressure
    Left ventricular diastolic dysfunction
    Obstructive congenital lesion
    Myocardial restriction
    Systemic hypertension with increased left ventricular afterload
Erythrocytosis and increased blood viscosity; anemia
Hypercoagulability: thrombosis
Acute infection
Arrhythmias

Pregnancy carries extreme risk for persons who have Eisenmenger physiology, with case series reporting high maternal and fetal mortality rates (both up to 50%), particularly in the first several days after delivery [33]. Therapeutic termination of pregnancy during the second and third trimesters precipitates fluid volume and hormonal fluctuations and is similarly risky. Although some modern case series have reported successful pregnancy, labor, and delivery with use of intensive medical therapies (see later discussion), there are no reliable ways to predict mortal or morbid outcomes. In all congenital centers that care for patients who have Eisenmenger physiology, pregnancy remains absolutely contraindicated for adults who have Eisenmenger physiology. Birth control counseling is strongly advised, although the preferred method of contraception has not been established. Maternal sterilization carries a risk of mortality, hormonal therapies increase the risk for thrombosis, barrier methods have a higher failure rate than other methods, and intrauterine device implantation may carry infection risk. Double barrier methods, such as condoms with spermicidal foam, may reduce failure rates, but comparative studies between the various methods have not been performed in patients who have Eisenmenger physiology.

The improving understanding of PAH and subpulmonary ventricular failure in patients who have Eisenmenger physiology has led to recognition that therapy should include efforts to modulate pulmonary vascular inflammation and its ramifications. Until recently, therapies for adults with shunt-associated pulmonary hypertension have consisted of supplemental oxygen, anticoagulation, diuretics, high-dose calcium channel blocker therapy, and lung or lung/heart transplantation. The benefit of supplemental oxygen administration in patients who have Eisenmenger physiology has been debated. Patients with large shunts often remain severely hypoxemic, even with high-flow supplemental oxygen. The same guidelines used to provide oxygen to patients who have chronic obstructive pulmonary disease are applied to individuals who have Eisenmenger physiology, but clinical trials to systematically assess benefit of oxygen supplementation in these patients have not been conducted [34,35].

Likewise, treatment with calcium channel blockers and prostacyclin has shown limited benefit or even subjective deterioration [36]. Transplant-free survival in Eisenmenger physiology is difficult to predict, with some patients having long periods of survival despite severe hypoxemia. Perioperative transplant mortality also is higher in this cohort of patients, although some individuals fare well after transplantation [37].

Anticoagulation with warfarin is widely used in patients who have CHD-PAH. In adults who have Eisenmenger physiology, increasing recognition of in vivo prothrombotic states [38] and in vitro abnormalities of coagulation in persons with cyanosis [39] has supported the anticoagulation of patients despite the lack of randomized studies to support the practice.

The medical therapy of Eisenmenger physiology has raised concerns about worsening of right-to-left shunting and the safety of using pulmonary arterial modulating therapies that also have systemic vasodilator potential. Some of these agents (intravenous prostacyclin, subcutaneously administered treprostinil, inhaled iloprost, and oral beraprost, bosentan, or sildenafil) have improved hemodynamics and exercise capacity in case series of patients who have CHD-PAH [40–46]. Randomized, controlled trials showing benefit of many of these agents in patients who have PAH (intravenous prostacyclin, subcutaneously administered treprostinil, and oral beraprost and sitexsantan) have included smaller numbers of persons who have Eisenmenger physiology. The use of these trials in guiding therapy for persons who have Eisenmenger physiology is limited, however, because the trials were not designed prospectively to test hypotheses within the CHD subgroup [44–48].

The BREATHE-5 trial of bosentan for CHD was the first randomized, controlled trial of an agent specifically for individuals affected by Eisenmenger physiology. It compared oral bosentan to placebo and found that in short-term (16-week) follow-up, bosentan was not only safe but also led to improvement in pulmonary hemodynamics and to 6-minute walk distance and WHO/NYHA functional class (Fig. 1) [18]. The positive findings of this trial justify the use of bosentan as a first-line therapy for patients who have CHD-PAH to improve functional capacity and potentially prolong survival. In view of this favorable response to medical therapy, further studies of pulmonary vasoactive agents—alone and in combination—in individuals who have CHD-PAH are strongly encouraged.

Immediate postoperative reactive pulmonary hypertension

Pulmonary vascular reactivity may be heightened in the immediate postoperative phase of cardiopulmonary surgery, which can precipitate marked increases in pulmonary vascular resistance and lead to acute subpulmonary ventricular failure, with attendant decrease in cardiac output, systemic hypotension, metabolic acidemia, and cardiac ischemia. Peribronchial edema and bronchoconstriction may lead to increase in airway resistance and alteration in gas exchange because of worsening ventilation/perfusion matching [49]. These perioperative acute increases in pulmonary resistance that precipitate a crisis tend to occur in individuals with more dynamic and less fixed resistance.

Perioperative endothelial cell dysfunction is thought to be central in the pathogenesis of immediate postoperative pulmonary hypertension, leading to an imbalance in eicosanoid production [50,51] and impaired nitric oxide synthesis [52], favoring vasoconstriction and vascular proliferation. Increased synthesis and decreased clearance of endothelin are also thought to contribute [53].

The increasing knowledge of such processes has led to management strategies aimed at lowering PA pressure and reducing right ventricular afterload while optimizing fluid balance. Reduction of adrenergic tone also may be helpful. Enhancing

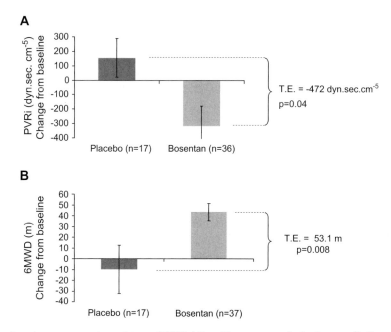

Fig. 1. Decrease in pulmonary vascular resistance (PVRi) (*A*) and improvement in 6-minute walk distance (6MWD) (*B*) were noted after short-term (4-month) therapy with bosentan, as compared with placebo, in double-blind, randomized, controlled trial in patients with Eisenmenger physiology. T.E. = treatment effect. (From Galie N, Beghetti M, Gatzoulis MA, et al. Bosentan therapy in patients with Eisenmenger syndrome: a multicenter, double-blind, randomized, placebo-controlled study. Circulation 2006;114:51; with permission.)

postoperative right ventricular function and atrio-ventricular valve function and optimizing medical management (including use of appropriate sedation agents and treatment of painful stimuli, avoidance of respiratory or metabolic acidosis, overcoming alveolar hypoxia or mechanical atelectasis, and correcting anemia or myocardial demand abnormalities) may reverse the crisis, but potential residual anatomic abnormalities that could be corrected surgically also should be sought.

Standard vasodilator agents, such as angiotensin-converting enzyme inhibitors or beta blockers, are rarely helpful in this situation because they are not pulmonary selective, and calcium channel blockers should be avoided because of their negative inotropic effects. Newer vasodilators, such as epoprostenol and phosphodiesterase inhibitors (III and V), have been tried with some success, and inhaled vasodilators, such as inhaled nitric oxide or inhaled epoprostenol, have piqued particular interest because they are more pulmonary selective than systemically administered vasodilators and may improve gas exchange by improving ventilation/perfusion matching [54–59].

Support of systemic blood pressure is critically important to maintain coronary perfusion in

acute right heart syndrome, necessitating use of agents such as norepinephrine. Low cardiac output states may be treated with the addition of dobutamine or similar agents. An aggressive approach such as that described has nearly eliminated mortality related to postoperative pulmonary hypertension in most large centers, but morbidity and duration of mechanical ventilation, intensive care unit stay, and hospitalization are all still increased [49,60].

Normal to mildly abnormal pulmonary vascular resistance states

Nearly unique to CHD (although somewhat analogous to acute right ventricular failure caused by myocardial infarction) are states that require lowest possible PVR for continued survival. Examples in CHD include individuals who have tricuspid atresia or similar single ventricle physiologies who undergo surgical creation of cavopulmonary anastomoses (Glenn shunt and its variants or Fontan palliation and its variants). These surgeries create unique pulmonary circulations that lack pulsatile flow and connect directly to the systemic venous circulation. With the Glenn shunt, the superior vena cava communicates directly with the pulmonary arteries, whereas with the Fontan anastomosis, the inferior vena cava is likewise connected to the pulmonary arteries along with the superior vena cava, typically via construction of an intra- or extracardiac baffle. Because the right ventricle has been bypassed and circulation of blood relies solely on left ventricular function, any increase in pulmonary vascular impedance can interfere with left ventricular filling. Maintenance of a low PVR is critically important.

An interesting physiologic aspect of these anastomoses between systemic and pulmonary circulations is that blood flow patterns might not be considered intuitive (because responses of the systemic and pulmonary circulations to modulators can be different or even opposite in degree) [61,62].

Although effective in unloading a single ventricular chamber and better separating pulmonary and systemic circulations, the Glenn and Fontan procedures are still associated with functional impairment because of limitations of a single ventricular system. Whether long-term pulmonary vasoactive therapy to maintain low PVR improves outcomes in these patients remains controversial [63–65].

Similar controversy exists regarding the potential benefits of administering pulmonary vasoactive agents to individuals with defects such as Ebstein's anomaly or tetralogy of Fallot, which depend on the functional status of the right ventricle. Because of increasing morbidities seen with aging in patients with these defects, further study of such potential therapies would be welcomed.

Summary

CHD-PAH, although common (15%–30%) in all-comers with CHD, is variable in terms of clinical manifestations, severity of associated PAH, and response to therapy and outcomes (depending on lesion anatomy, pulmonary circulation flows and pressures, and presence and timings of surgeries). Genetic abnormalities inherent in some of these circumstances require further study. Evaluation of patients who have CHD-PAH includes imaging and catheterization in centers with particular expertise in CHD-PAH so as to most safely characterize the severity, nature, and potential for treatment of pulmonary

hemodynamic abnormalities. Surgical correction may be desirable after rigorous preinterventional assessment. Patients who are not surgical candidates or who fail to improve early or late after surgery may have the potential to respond to idiopathic PAH therapies. Lung or heart/lung transplantation remains an option for selected recalcitrant patients.

References

[1] Friedman WF. Proceedings of National Heart, Lung and Blood Institute pediatric cardiology workshop: pulmonary hypertension. Pediatr Res 1986;20: 811–24.

[2] Kidd L, Driscoll DJ, Gersony WM, et al. Second natural history study of congenital heart defects: results of treatment of patients with ventricular septal defects. Circulation 1993;87:138–51.

[3] Diller GP, Dimopoulis K, Okonko D, et al. Exercise intolerance in adult congenital heart disease: comparative severity, correlates, and prognostic implication. Circulation 2005;112:828–35.

[4] Simonneau G, Galie N, Rubin LJ, et al. Clinical classification of pulmonary hypertension. J Am Coll Cardiol 2004;43(Suppl):5S–12S.

[5] Galie N. Classification of patients with congenital systemic-to-pulmonary shunts associated with pulmonary arterial hypertension: current status and future directions. In: Beghetti M, editor. Pulmonary arterial hypertension related to congenital heart disease. Munich (Germany): Elsevier GmbH; 2006. p. 11–7.

[6] Wood P. The Eisenmenger syndrome or pulmonary hypertension with reversed central shunt. Br Med J 1958;46:701–9.

[7] Rabinovitch M, Haworth SG, Castaneda AR, et al. Lung biopsy in congenital heart disease: a morphometric approach to pulmonary vascular disease. Circulation 1978;58:1107–22.

[8] Fratz S, Geiger R, Kresse H, et al. Pulmonary blood pressure, not flow, is associated with net endotehlin-1 production in the lungs of patients with congenital heart disease and normal pulmonary vascular resistance. J Thorac Cardiovasc Surg 2003;126:1724–9.

[9] van Albada ME, Shoemaker RG, Kemna MS, et al. The role of increased pulmonary blood flow in pulmonary arterial hypertension. Eur Respir J 2005; 26:487–93.

[10] Black SM, Bekker JM, Johengen MJ, et al. Altered regulation of the ET-1 cascade in lambs with increased pulmonary blood flow and pulmonary hypertension. Pediatr Res 2000;47:97–106.

[11] Van Beneden R, Rondelet B, Kerbaul F, et al. Ang-1/ BMPR2 signalling and the expression of MCP-1 and ICAM in overcirculation-induced experimental pulmonary hypertension. Eur Respir J 2004;24:533S.

[12] Mata-Greenwood E, Meyrick B, Soifer SJ, et al. Expression of VEGF and its receptors Flt-1 and Flk-1/KDR is altered in lambs with increased pulmonary blood flow and pulmonary hypertension. Am J Physiol Lung Cell Mol Physiol 2003;285: L222–31.

[13] Cornfield DN, Resnik ER, Herron JM, et al. Pulmonary vascular K+ channel expression and vasoreactivity in a model of congenital heart disease. Am J Physiol Lung Cell Mol Physiol 2002;283:L1210–9.

[14] Black SM, Sanchez LS, Mata-Greenwood E, et al. sGC and PDE5 are elevated in lambs with increased pulmonary blood flow and pulmonary hypertension. Am J Physiol Lung Cell Mol Physiol 2001;281: L1051–7.

[15] Fratz S, Meyrick B, Ovadia B, et al. Chronic endothelin A receptor blockade in lambs with increased pulmonary blood flow and pressure. Am J Physiol Lung Cell Mol Physiol 2004;287:L592–7.

[16] Rondelet B, Kerbaul F, Motte S, et al. Bosentan for the prevention of overcirculation-induced experimental pulmonary arterial hypertension. Circulation 2003;107:1329–35.

[17] Rondelet B, Kerbaul F, Van Beneden R, et al. Signalling molecules in overcirculation-induced pulmonary hypertension in piglets: effects of sildenafil therapy. Circulation 2004;110:2220–5.

[18] Galie N, Beghetti M, Gatzoulis MA, et al. Bosentan therapy in patients with Eisenmenger syndrome: a multicenter, double-blind, randomized, placebo-controlled study. Circulation 2006;114:48–54.

[19] Bolger AP, Sharma R, Li W, et al. Neurohormonal activation and the chronic heart failure syndrome in adults with congenital heart disease. Circulation 2002;106:92–9.

[20] Cacoub P, Dorent R, Maistre G, et al. Endothelin-1 in primary pulmonary hypertension and the Eisenmenger syndrome. Am J Cardiol 1993;71:448–50.

[21] Ishikawa S, Miyauchi T, Sakai S, et al. Elevated levels of plasma endothelin-1 in young patients with pulmonary hypertension caused by congenital heart disease are decreased after successful surgical repair. J Thorac Cardiovasc Surg 1995;110: 271–3.

[22] Cacoub P, Dorent R, Nataf P, et al. Endothelin-1 in the lungs of patients with pulmonary hypertension. Cardiovasc Res 1997;33:196–200.

[23] Roberts KE, McElroy JJ, Wong WP, et al. BMPR2 mutations in pulmonary arterial hypertension with congenital heart disease. Eur Respir J 2004;24: 371–4.

[24] Steele PM, Fuster V, Cohen M, et al. Isolated atrial septal defect with pulmonary vascular obstructive disease: long-term follow-up and prediction of outcome after surgical correction. Circulation 1987;76: 1037–42.

[25] Batista RJ, Santos JL, Takeshita N, et al. Successful reversal of pulmonary hypertension in Eisenmenger complex. Arq Bras Cardiol 1997;68(4):279–80.

[26] Daliento L, Somerville J, Presbitero P, et al. Eisenmenger syndrome: factors relating to deterioration and death. Eur Heart J 1998;19:1845–55.

[27] Saha A, Balakrishnan K, Jaiswal P, et al. Prognosis for patients with Eisenmenger syndrome of various aetiology. Int J Cardiol 1994;45:199–207.

[28] Vongpatanasin W, Brickner ME, Hillis LD, et al. The Eisenmenger syndrome in adults. Ann Intern Med 1998;128:745–55.

[29] Cantor WJ, Harrison DA, Moussadji JS, et al. Determinants of survival and length of survival in adults with Eisenmenger syndrome. Am J Cardiol 1999;84:677–81.

[30] Kilner P. Cardiovascular magnetic resonance imaging. In: Gatzoulis MA, Webb GD, Daubeney PEF, editors. Diagnosis and management of adult congenital heart disease. London: Elsevier Limited; 2003. p. 49–56.

[31] Sondel PM, Tripp ME, Ganick DJ, et al. Phlebotomy with iron therapy to correct the microcytic polycythemia of chronic hypoxia. Pediatrics 1981;67:667–70.

[32] Perloff JK, Marelli AJ, Miner PD. Risk of stroke in adults with cyanotic congenital heart disease. Circulation 1993;87:1954–9.

[33] Jones P, Patel A. Eisenmenger's syndrome and problems with anaesthesia. Br J Hosp Med 1996;54(5): 214–9.

[34] Bowyer JJ, Busst CM, Denison DM, et al. Effect of long-term oxygen treatment at home in children with pulmonary vascular disease. Br Heart J 1986;55: 385–90.

[35] Sandoval J, Aguirre JS, Pulido T, et al. Nocturnal oxygen therapy in patients with the Eisenmenger syndrome. Am J Respir Crit Care Med 2001;164: 1682–7.

[36] Gildein HP, Wildberg A, Moellin R. Comparative studies of hemodynamics under prostacyclin and nifedipine in patients with Eisenmenger syndrome. Z Kardiol (Germany) 1995;84:55–63.

[37] Trulock EP. Lung transplantation for primary pulmonary hypertension. Clin Chest Med 2001;22: 583–93.

[38] Silversides CK, Granton JT, Konen T, et al. Pulmonary thrombosis in adults with Eisenmenger syndrome. J Am Coll Cardiol 2003;42:1982–7.

[39] Rosove MH, Hocking WG, Harwig SS, et al. Studies of beta-thromboglobulin, platelet factor 4, fibrinopeptide-A in erythrocytosis due to cyanotic congenital heart disease. Thromb Res 1983;29:225–35.

[40] Rosenzweig EB, Kerstein D, Barst RJ. Long-term prostacyclin for pulmonary hypertension with associated congenital heart defects. Circulation 1999;99: 1858–65.

[41] McLaughlin VV, Genthner DE, Panella MM, et al. Compassionate use of continuous prostacyclin in the management of secondary pulmonary hypertension: a case series. Ann Intern Med 1999;130:740–3.

[42] Ferndandes SM, Newburger JW, Lang P, et al. Usefulness of epoprostenol therapy in the severely ill

adolescent/adult with Eisenmenger physiology. Am J Cardiol 2003;91:46–9.

[43] Olschewski H, Simonneau G, Galie N, et al. Inhaled iloprost for severe pulmonary hypertension. N Engl J Med 2002;347:322–9.

[44] Barst RJ, Rubin LJ, Long WA, et al. A comparison of continuous intravenous epoprostenol (prostacyclin) with conventional therapy for primary pulmonary hypertension: The Primary Pulmonary Hypertension Study Group. N Engl J Med 1996;334:296–302.

[45] Simonneau G, Barst RJ, Galie N, et al. Continuous subcutaneous infusion of treprostinil, a prostacyclin analogue, in patients with pulmonary arterial hypertension: a double-blind, randomized, placebo-controlled trial. Am J Respir Crit Care Med 2002;165:800–4.

[46] Galie N, Humbert M, Vachiery JL, et al. Effects of beraprost sodium, an oral prostacyclin analogue, in patients with pulmonary arterial hypertension: a randomized, double-blind, placebo-controlled trial. J Am Coll Cardiol 2002;39:1496–502.

[47] Rubin LJ, Badesch DB, Barst RJ, et al. Bosentan therapy for pulmonary arterial hypertension. N Engl J Med 2002;346:896–903.

[48] Barst RJ, Langleben D, Frost A, et al. Sitaxsentan therapy for pulmonary arterial hypertension. Am J Respir Crit Care Med 2004;169:441–7.

[49] Bando K, Turrentine MW, Sharp TG, et al. Pulmonary hypertension after operations for congenital heart disease: analysis of risk factors and management. J Thorac Cardiovasc Surg 1996;112:1600–7.

[50] Wessel D, Adatia I, Giglia TM, et al. Use of inhaled nitric oxide and acetylcholine in the evaluation of pulmonary hypertension and endothelial dysfunction after cardiopulmonary bypass. Circulation 1993;88:2128–38.

[51] Adatia I, Barrow S, Stratton P, et al. Effect of intracardiac repair on biosynthesis of thromboxane A2 and prostacyclin in children with a left to right shunt. Br Heart J 1994;72:452–6.

[52] Schulze-Nieck I, Penny DJ, Rigby ML, et al. L-arginine and substance P reverse the pulmonary endothelial dysfunction caused by congenital heart surgery. Circulation 1999;100:749–55.

[53] Hiramatsu T, Imai Y, Takanishsi Y, et al. Time course of endothelin-1 and nitrate anion levels after cardiopulmonary bypass in congenital heart defects. Ann Thorac Surg 1997;63:648–52.

[54] Carroll CL, Backer CL, Mavroudis C, et al. Inhaled prostacyclin following surgical repair of congenital

heart disease: a pilot study. J Card Surg 2005;20:436–9.

[55] Ivy DD, Kinsella JP, Ziegler JW, et al. Dipyridamole attenuates rebound pulmonary hypertension after inhaled nitric oxide withdrawal in postoperative congenital heart disease. J Thorac Cardiovasc Surg 1998;115:875–82.

[56] Atz AM, Lefler AK, Fairbrother DL, et al. Sildenafil augments the effect of inhaled nitric oxide for postoperative pulmonary hypertensive crises. J Thorac Cardiovasc Surg 2002;124:628–9.

[57] Schulze-Neick I, Li J, Reader JA, et al. The endothelin antagonist BQ123 reduces pulmonary vascular resistance after surgical intervention for congenital heart disease. J Thorac Cardiovasc Surg 2002;124:435–41.

[58] Miller OI, Tang SF, Keech A, et al. Inhaled nitric oxide and prevention of pulmonary hypertension after congenital heart surgery: a randomised double-blind study. Lancet 2000;356:1464–9.

[59] Smith HA, Canter JA, Christian KG, et al. Nitric oxide precursors and congenital heart surgery: a randomized controlled trial of oral citrulline. J Thorac Cardiovasc Surg 2006;132:58–65.

[60] Schulze-Neick I, Li J, Penny DJ, et al. Pulmonary vascular resistance after cardiopulmonary bypass in infants: effect on postoperative recovery. J Thorac Cardiovasc Surg 2001;121:1033–9.

[61] Bradley SM, Simsic JM, Mulvihill DM. Hypoventilation improves oxygenation after bidirectional superior cavopulmonary connection. J Thorac Cardiovasc Surg 2003;126:1033–9.

[62] Hoskote A, Li J, Hickey C, et al. The effects of carbon dioxide on oxygenation and systemic, cerebral and pulmonary vascular hemodynamics after the bidirectional superior cavopulmonary anastomosis. J Am Coll Cardiol 2004;44:1501–9.

[63] Guadagni G, Bove EL, Migliavacca F, et al. Effects of pulmonary afterload on the hemodynamics after the hemi-Fontan procedure. Med Eng Phys 2001;23:293–8.

[64] Ikai A, Shirai M, Nishimura K, et al. Hypoxic pulmonary vasoconstriction disappears in a rabbit model of cavopulmonary shunt. J Thorac Cardiovasc Surg 2004;127:1450–7.

[65] Simsic JM, Bradley SM, Mulvihill DM. Sodium nitroprusside after bidirectional superior cavopulmonary connection: preserved cerebral blood flow velocity and systemic oxygenation. J Thorac Cardiovasc Surg 2003;126:186–90.

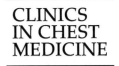

Clin Chest Med 28 (2007) 255–269

Chronic Thromboembolic Pulmonary Hypertension

William R. Auger, MD*, Nick H. Kim, MD, Kim M. Kerr, MD,
Victor J. Test, MD, Peter F. Fedullo, MD[1]

*Division of Pulmonary and Critical Care Medicine, University of California, San Diego,
9300 Campus Point Drive, La Jolla, CA 92037, USA*

The description of organized thrombus in major pulmonary arteries can be found in autopsy reports dating back to the late nineteenth and early twentieth centuries, typically in association with other diseases, such as tuberculosis, lung cancer, and congenital heart disease, and rarely in the absence of another pathologic condition [1]. Not until the 1950s was the antemortem diagnosis and clinical syndrome of chronic thrombotic obstruction of the major pulmonary arteries better characterized [1–4]. Carroll [4] was the first to use cardiac catheterization and pulmonary angiography in detailing features of this unusual disease. In 1958, Hurwitt and colleagues [5] reported the first surgical attempt to remove the adherent thrombus from the vessel wall. Although the patient died, this operation provided the conceptual foundation for the distinction between acute and chronic thromboembolic disease of the pulmonary vascular bed, and established that an endarterectomy, and not an embolectomy, would be necessary if a surgical remedy for this disease was to be successful.

The first bilateral pulmonary thromboendarterectomy (PTE) performed through a transverse sternotomy using cardiopulmonary bypass is credited to Houk and colleagues [6] in 1963. Over the following 2 decades, reports describing the natural history and clinical characteristics of chronic thromboembolic disease, and small, anecdotal series of surgical successes in the treatment of this disorder appeared with increasing frequency [7–14]. A review of the world's experience with PTE up to 1985 showed an overall perioperative mortality rate of 22% in 85 patients who underwent the procedure [15]. With improvements in diagnostic capabilities, surgical techniques, endarterectomy instrumentation, and postoperative management, Moser and colleagues [16] at the University of California, San Diego (UCSD) published results of a study of 42 patients who had chronic thromboembolic pulmonary hypertension (CTEPH) and underwent surgery at a single medical center, showing in-hospital mortality of 16.6%. This publication further documented the considerable postoperative improvements in pulmonary hemodynamics and functional capabilities experienced by these patients, which were sustained a year or more beyond surgery.

Over the past 2 decades, the number of programs worldwide dedicated to the diagnosis and management of patients who have chronic thromboembolic pulmonary vascular disease has increased steadily. At UCSD, nearly 2000 patients from national and international referral sources underwent PTE between 1989 and 2006 [17]. During this same period, programs in North America, Europe, Japan, and Australia were developed to manage an increasing medical need [18–25]. Worldwide interest has been fueled by the rise in physician recognition of this treatable form of pulmonary hypertension, the appreciation that medical management of CTEPH is minimally effective in altering prognosis, declining perioperative mortality rates, and the knowledge that thromboendarterectomy can dramatically improve pulmonary hemodynamic status, functional outcome, and long-term survival.

---

* Corresponding author.

[1] Present address: Division of Pulmonary and Critical Care Medicine, University of California, San Diego, 200 West Arbor Drive, San Diego, CA 92103.

E-mail address: bauger@ucsd.edu (W.R. Auger).

Epidemiology and risk factors

Available evidence suggests that CTEPH is an extension of the natural history of acute pulmonary embolic disease, although it occurs in a minority of individuals who survive a pulmonary embolism. The actual incidence of CTEPH, however, has been difficult to define. Based on patients diagnosed with CTEPH and the rate of patients known to survive pulmonary embolic events each year in the United States, an estimated 0.1% to 0.5% of survivors later develop symptomatic CTEPH [26,27]. This estimate would equate to an annual incidence between 500 to 2500 cases in the United States alone. Because limited information has been available from centers in the United States specializing in the treatment of patients who have pulmonary hypertension, these projections markedly exceed the number of patients diagnosed with symptomatic CTEPH each year. Consequently, these estimates are either overstated or CTEPH is significantly underdiagnosed, the latter of which seems most likely given the results of recent publications.

In a prospective study of 78 patients surviving an acute pulmonary embolus, Ribeiro and colleagues [28] examined echocardiographic findings for a year, and performed clinical follow-up for 5 years. Four patients (5.1%) developed clinically significant CTEPH, three of which underwent PTE for progressive right ventricular failure. In a more recent prospective longitudinal study, Pengo and colleagues [29] evaluated the incidence of symptomatic CTEPH in consecutive patients after an acute pulmonary embolic event. Median follow-up was 94.3 months in 223 patients who had no history of prior venous thromboembolism. Seven patients developed CTEPH within the first 2 years, for a cumulative incidence of 3.8%. No additional patients developed CTEPH beyond this 2-year period. CTEPH occurred more frequently in patients who experienced a prior venous thromboembolism: 11 of 82 patients (13.4%) compared with 3 of 58 (5.2%) patients who experienced a prior deep vein thrombosis and 8 of 24 (33.0%) patients who had a previous pulmonary embolus. Another prospective study reported a CTEPH incidence of 1.3%, in a group of 320 patients who had an acute pulmonary embolism who were followed up for a minimum of 1 year [30].

Currently, limited information is available regarding what factors might predispose patients to developing CTEPH. Links between observed associations and the pathophysiologic mechanisms leading to chronic thromboembolic disease are similarly unknown. However, growing experience with this disease entity has provided several insights about potential risk factors. In the Pengo study, not only did a history of multiple pulmonary embolic events place patients at a greater risk for developing CTEPH, but a younger age at presentation, larger perfusion defects at diagnosis, and idiopathic pulmonary embolic disease were found to be significant risk factors [29]. In patients who have an acute pulmonary embolism, Ribeiro and colleagues [28] reported that pulmonary artery systolic pressures higher than 50 mm Hg at presentation were associated with persistent pulmonary hypertension after 1 year. However, in contrast to the Pengo study, Rebeiro and colleagues [28] found that age older than 70 years at presentation was statistically linked to a higher risk for developing CTEPH. The size of the initial thrombus burden may also be important. In a study where massive pulmonary embolism was defined as greater than 50% obstruction of the pulmonary vascular bed, the incidence of CTEPH was 20.2% despite the use of thrombolytic therapy [31].

Although hereditary thrombophilic states (deficiencies of antithrombin III, protein C or protein S, or factor II and factor V Leiden mutations) represent risk factors for venous thromboembolism, their prevalence in patients who have established CTEPH was shown to be no different than in patients who have primary pulmonary hypertension or control subjects [32,33]. The presence of antiphospholipid antibodies (with or without an accompanying lupus anticoagulant) has been found to be one of the most common hypercoagulable states associated with the development of CTEPH. The antiphospholipid antibodies can be found in up to 21% of patients who have CTEPH [32]. Bonderman and colleagues [34] also showed increased levels of factor VIII in 41% of 122 patients who had CTEPH, levels that were substantially higher compared with patients who had nonthromboembolic pulmonary arterial hypertension. Additionally, the factor VIII levels remained elevated after successful PTE surgery, which would suggest a genetic basis for this finding. In one series of only 24 patients, hyperhomocysteinemia was shown in 7 of 14 patients who had CTEPH, whereas 12 of 24 patients were reported to have antiphospholipid antibodies [33].

An association between several medical conditions and CTEPH has been reported. In a case-control study, Bonderman and colleagues [35] compared 109 consecutive patients who had CTEPH with 187 patients who did not develop chronic thromboembolic disease after experiencing an acute pulmonary embolism. Multivariate analysis showed that prior splenectomy, the presence of a ventriculoatrial shunt to treat hydrocephalus, and chronic inflammatory disorders (such as osteomyelitis and inflammatory bowel disease) were associated with an increased risk for CTEPH. A link between CTEPH and splenectomy was also reported in a retrospective study by Jais and colleagues [36]. Over a 10-year period, 257 patients who had CTEPH were compared with patients who had idiopathic pulmonary hypertension (n = 276) and with patients who had other chronic pulmonary conditions evaluated for lung transplantation (n = 180). The prevalence of prior splenectomy in patients who had CTEPH was found to be 8.6%, compared with 2.5% in the idiopathic pulmonary arterial hypertension group and 0.56% in patients who had other pulmonary disorders. Additionally, in the CTEPH group, the chronic thromboembolic disease was generally more distal, and therefore these patients were less likely to be surgical candidates (8 of 22 patients). The pathophysiologic basis for this association is not entirely clear; a prothrombotic state related to the loss of filtering abnormal erythrocytes by the spleen has been postulated [37].

Pathogenesis of chronic thromboembolic pulmonary hypertension

Clinical observation and what is known about the natural history of acute pulmonary embolism would suggest that incomplete resolution of pulmonary emboli rather than in situ thrombosis of the pulmonary arteries is the inciting event in chronic thromboembolic disease [38–40]. However, the aberrant mechanisms through which thromboembolic material undergoes incomplete thrombolysis and is then incorporated into the pulmonary arterial wall remain elusive. In normal subjects, Rosenhek and associates [41] showed that, under physiologic conditions, the pulmonary artery has increased fibrinolytic capabilities compared with the aorta. This finding seems to be based on higher levels of tissue plasminogen activator (TPA) expression versus plasminogen activator-inhibitor (PAI-1). However, in patients who had CTEPH, Olman and colleagues [42] and Lang and colleagues [43] were unable to show a reversal in the TPA–PAI-1 relationship

that would favor incomplete thrombus dissolution. Although this same group was able to show a greater expression of PAI-1 and factor VIII on the surface of neovessels within organized thromboemboli, the exact role this played in sustaining thrombus within the pulmonary vascular bed is unclear [44]. More recently, in a small group of patients who had this disease, fibrin itself was shown to be resistant to plasmin-mediated lysis [45], seemingly because of an alteration in fibrin(ogen) structure. Additional investigation in a larger group of patients who have CTEPH is required to validate this aberration as a common pathway in the organization of acute pulmonary thromboemboli.

Even more incomplete is the understanding of the hemodynamic evolution to pulmonary hypertension after an acute pulmonary embolic event. In otherwise healthy individuals, the degree of hemodynamic impairment after an acute pulmonary embolus tends to correlate with the degree of pulmonary vascular obstruction. More than 3 decades ago, McIntyre and Sasahara [46] studied 20 healthy patients who had newly diagnosed pulmonary embolism. Obstruction of at least 25% to 30% of the pulmonary vascular bed was required to significantly raise pulmonary vascular pressures, although a mean pulmonary artery pressure higher than 40 mm Hg was not observed despite angiographically massive obstruction. As the degree of pulmonary arterial obstruction increased to 40% to 50%, cardiac index declined, reflecting a normal right ventricular response to an abrupt and significant rise in pulmonary vascular resistance. The frequency at which hemodynamic impairment was witnessed was notable in this study. Of these 20 patients, 70% exhibited a mean pulmonary artery pressure higher than 25 mm Hg. Similar observations regarding the hemodynamic impact of acute pulmonary emboli have been more recently reported. Although no correlation with thrombus burden was seen, Grifoni and colleagues [47] showed echocardiographic evidence of right ventricular dysfunction in 53% of 209 patients presenting with acute symptomatic pulmonary embolism. Of the patients with right ventricular compromise, 58% were normotensive and clinically stable (31% of 209). In the setting of existing cardiopulmonary disease, the degree of obstruction necessary to cause pulmonary hypertension is likely to be considerably less [40,46].

However, for most patients undergoing antithrombotic therapy, pulmonary perfusion scan abnormalities and echocardiographic abnormalities steadily improve and typically stabilize over 4 to 6 weeks [48,49]. However, incomplete resolution of perfusion scan defects can be seen and is more common than is generally appreciated. In a review of four clinical studies, normalization of perfusion scan defects occurred in less than 50% of patients when evaluated 6 months after the acute event [50]. In 244 patients who survived a year after an acute pulmonary embolism, Miniati and colleagues [30] showed an improving but incomplete restoration of pulmonary blood flow during this period. At diagnosis, median pulmonary vascular obstruction as assessed by perfusion scans was 42.3% (range, 8.2%–72.9%). After 1 month of antithrombotic therapy, 90% of patients had a residual vascular obstruction of 30% or less; after 1 year, residual pulmonary vascular obstruction was 15% or less in 75% of patients and 5% or less in 75%. Only in 153 of 235 patients (65.1%) was the lung scan assessed as normal. However, because the incidence of CTEPH in this same study was 1.3% (four patients), the fact that chronic thrombotic residual may be common after acute pulmonary emboli strengthens prior observations that they are typically of little hemodynamic consequence [27].

For patients who develop CTEPH, the pathophysiologic mechanisms to explain the progression to pulmonary hypertension remain unclear, although an apparent deviation exists from the normal events described earlier. A large percentage of patients who have established CTEPH—up to 40% to 50% in some series [19,51]—have not been previously diagnosed with acute venous thromboembolic disease, and therefore have not benefited from antithrombotic therapy. One can argue that recurrent, asymptomatic pulmonary emboli [52], or asymptomatic pulmonary emboli whose initial hemodynamic impact failed to resolve [28], may be operative in the development of clinically significant CTEPH in this group of patients. However, another plausible explanation is based on clinical observations in patients diagnosed with acute pulmonary embolic disease who undergo anticoagulant therapy and ultimately develop CTEPH. Two distinct processes seem to occur: (1) nonresolution and organization of the acute thrombus burden in the proximal pulmonary vascular bed, and (2) the gradual development of a peripheral vasculopathy, indistinguishable from that seen in idiopathic pulmonary arterial hypertension, in the vascular bed unencumbered by thrombus. Several observations

support this theory: (1) pulmonary hypertension is seen to progress in the absence of recurrent thromboembolic events or in situ thrombosis, as judged by stable perfusion scan defects over time [30]; (2) a poor correlation exists between the extent of proximal vessel involvement and the degree of pulmonary hypertension, suggesting a component of pulmonary vascular resistance (PVR) in the distal, unobstructed vascular bed; (3) histopathology showing hypertensive arteriopathic changes in the resistive vessels of patients who have CTEPH [53] in the obstructed and unobstructed lung regions; (4) persistent post–PTE pulmonary hypertension despite chronic proximal thrombus removal and reestablishment of perfusion to the previously obstructed lung regions.

The reasons for the development of this vasculopathy are being investigated. It has been hypothesized to be secondary to high pressures and sheer stress, although these vessel changes would be expected to occur only in the unobstructed vascular bed [53]. Other possibilities, including genetic factors, have been examined. Bone morphogenetic protein receptor type 2 (BMPR-2) down-regulation has been associated with the development of idiopathic and familial pulmonary arterial hypertension, but has not been observed in patients who have CTEPH [54,55]. Angiopoetin-1, a protein molecule involved in the recruitment of smooth muscle cells around blood vessels, is upregulated in CTEPH and has been associated with other forms of pulmonary hypertension [55]. As is the case in idiopathic pulmonary hypertension, the endothelin system may also be upregulated in patients who have CTEPH [56,57].

Clinical presentation

Patients who have CTEPH typically complain of exertional dyspnea and a gradual decrease in exercise tolerance over months to years. Numerous factors are likely to affect the progression of these symptoms and, therefore, the timing of patient presentation. For example, patient age, previous physical health, state of conditioning, residence at altitude, and comorbid medical conditions (eg, parenchymal lung disease) seem to influence the clinical impact of chronic thromboembolic disease on patients. Although individual tolerances vary, the physiologic basis for these complaints relates to limitations in cardiac performance caused by an elevated PVR, and increased minute ventilatory needs from an elevated alveolar dead space.

Other symptoms are reported with varying frequencies, such as a nonproductive cough (especially with exertion), hemoptysis, and palpitations. A change in voice quality or hoarseness may result from vocal cord dysfunction caused by compression of the left recurrent laryngeal nerve between the aorta and an enlarged left main pulmonary artery. Chest discomfort is often pleuritic in nature, presumptively because of peripherally infarcted lung. However, exertion-related chest pain can also occur, often prompting evaluation for coronary artery disease. This complaint typically occurs late in CTEPH, as does exertion-related presyncope, syncope, and resting dyspnea, with resting dyspnea indicating that right ventricular function is unable to accommodate normal resting metabolic needs.

The nonspecific nature of these complaints undoubtedly contributes to the diagnostic delay experienced by most patients who have chronic thromboembolic disease. Another confounder is that fact that patients who have CTEPH may not provide a history of prior acute symptomatic pulmonary embolism or deep vein thrombosis. Reports indicate that the average delay from the onset of cardiopulmonary symptoms to establishment of the correct diagnosis can range from 2 to 3 years [19,27]. Consequently, many patients are improperly labeled with alternative diagnoses during the course of their illness, such as physical deconditioning, mild chronic obstructive pulmonary disease, congestive heart failure, or, occasionally, psychogenic dyspnea.

Physical examination findings similarly reflect the stage of pulmonary vascular disease at which a patient presents for evaluation. In the absence of right-sided cardiac dysfunction, physical signs attributable to CTEPH may be subtle or absent. Even in the setting of severe pulmonary hypertension, patients can appear relatively well. The examination findings of pulmonary hypertension, such as a right ventricular lift, fixed splitting of the second heart sound with an accentuated pulmonic component, a right ventricular S_4 gallop, and a tricuspid regurgitation murmur, must be carefully discerned. In the absence of coexisting parenchymal lung disease or airflow obstruction, pulmonary auscultation is typically unremarkable. In approximately 30% of patients who have CTEPH, pulmonary flow murmurs can be appreciated [58]. Jugular venous distention, a right ventricular S_3 gallop, severe tricuspid regurgitation, hepatomegaly, ascites, and peripheral edema suggest more advanced right-heart dysfunction. The

presence of cyanosis may suggest right-to-left shunting through a patent foramen ovale in patients who have pulmonary hypertension. Lower-extremity examination may also disclose superficial varicosities and venous stasis skin discoloration in patients who have experienced prior venous thrombosis.

Diagnostic evaluation

Patients who have unexplained exertional dyspnea should be carefully evaluated, and pulmonary vascular disease considered. Even some of the more standard diagnostic tests, such as chest radiography and pulmonary function tests, may provide clues to the presence of pulmonary hypertension and chronic thromboembolic disease.

In CTEPH, chest radiography is often unremarkable in the early stages, but several radiographic abnormalities may be apparent as the disease progresses. With significant pulmonary hypertension, dilatation of the central pulmonary arteries often occurs, and patients who have CTEPH frequently exhibit irregularly shaped and asymmetrically enlarged proximal vessels [59]. This finding may be mistaken for hilar adenopathy. With the increasing afterload placed on the right ventricle, radiographic signs of chamber enlargement, such as obliteration of the retrosternal space and prominence of the right heart border, may become apparent. In the absence of coexisting parenchymal lung disease, the lung fields are free of alveolar–interstitial markings, although hypo- and hyperperfused lung regions may be present. In poorly perfused lung regions, peripheral alveolar opacities, linear scar-like lesions, and localized pleural thickening can be observed and often represent sequelae of prior infarctions.

Electrocardiographic findings are similarly dependent on the hemodynamic severity of the disease. Right axis deviation, right ventricular hypertrophy, right atrial enlargement, right bundle-branch block, ST segment displacement, and T-wave inversions in anterior precordial and inferior limb leads can be seen in CTEPH, although they are not specific to this condition.

Pulmonary function testing, commonly performed during an evaluation for dyspnea, is most useful for excluding coexisting parenchymal lung disease or airflow obstruction. For patients who have CTEPH alone, spirometry is generally unremarkable, although in some patients lung volume measurements may disclose a mild to moderate restrictive defect believed to be related to parenchymal scarring from prior lung infarction [60]. Similarly, a mild to moderate reduction in single-breath diffusing capacity for carbon monoxide (DL_{CO}) can be present in CTEPH, but a normal value does not exclude the diagnosis [61]. A severe reduction in DL_{CO}, however, should prompt consideration of an alternative pulmonary process significantly affecting the distal pulmonary vascular bed.

Even in the setting of significant pulmonary hypertension caused by chronic thromboembolic disease, resting arterial blood gas analysis may show a normal oxygen level (Pao_2), although when measured, dead-space ventilation will frequently be elevated. When exercising, patients who have CTEPH will often exhibit a decline in Pao_2 levels and an inappropriate increase in dead-space ventilation. These findings reflect ventilation–perfusion (V/Q) inequalities and an inappropriate cardiac output response to exercise resulting in a low mixed venous oxygen saturation [62]. Hypoxemia at rest implies very severe right ventricular dysfunction or the presence of a right-to-left shunt, as through a patent foramen ovale.

Transthoracic echocardiography has become a valuable noninvasive tool for evaluating the presence of pulmonary hypertension in patients who have unexplained exertional dyspnea. Currently available technologies allow for an estimate of pulmonary artery systolic pressures using Doppler analysis of the tricuspid regurgitant envelope, and an estimate of cardiac output. Right heart chamber enlargement, abnormal right ventricular systolic function, paradoxical interventricular septal motion, and the impact of an enlarged right ventricle on left ventricular filling are additional echocardiographic findings in the setting of significant pulmonary hypertension [63]. The echocardiogram is also useful for the excluding left ventricular dysfunction, valvular disease, or complex cardiac malformations as possible causes for pulmonary hypertension. Contrast echocardiography after the venous injection of agitated saline is useful in detecting a patent foramen ovale or a previously unsuspected septal defect. In symptomatic patients with echocardiographic evidence of only minimally elevated pulmonary artery pressures or right ventricular compromise at rest, obtaining a study during exercise may document a substantial rise in pulmonary artery pressures along with an increase in right heart size.

With the diagnosis of pulmonary hypertension, radioisotopic V/Q scanning plays a pivotal role in distinguishing between large-vessel occlusive disease and small-vessel pulmonary vascular disease. Patients who have CTEPH will invariably show one or more segmental or larger perfusion defects in lung regions with normal ventilation. This finding contrasts with the normal or subsegmental mottled perfusion pattern observed in idiopathic pulmonary arterial hypertension or other forms of small-vessel pulmonary vascular disease [64,65]. Experts have also observed that the magnitude of perfusion defects in chronic thromboembolic disease often understates the actual degree of vascular obstruction determined with angiography or at surgery [66]. During organization, proximal vessel thromboemboli may recanalize or narrow the vessel in such a manner that radiolabeled macroaggregated albumin may pass beyond the region of partial obstruction to a limited degree, thereby creating *gray zones*, or areas of relative hypoperfusion on the perfusion scan. Furthermore, mismatched segmental or larger defects in patients who have pulmonary hypertension are not specific for chronic thromboembolic disease. Extrinsic vascular compression from mediastinal adenopathy or fibrosis; primary pulmonary vascular tumors such as angiosarcoma; pulmonary venoocclusive disease; and large-vessel pulmonary arteritis may result in a V/Q appearance indistinguishable from CTEPH [67–69]. Consequently, additional imaging studies are needed to define the vascular abnormality and establish the diagnosis.

Largely because of recent improvements in the speed, quality, and resolution of thoracic imaging afforded by the ongoing refinements in multidetector CT, this modality has assumed an increasingly important role in diagnosing and managing thromboembolic disease. CT findings in chronic thromboembolic disease include mosaic perfusion of the lung parenchyma; central pulmonary artery enlargement; right atrial and right ventricular enlargement; variations in the size of lobar and segmental-level vessels (often diminutive in lung regions most involved with chronic thrombi); peripheral, scar-like densities in hypoattenuated lung regions; and the presence of mediastinal collateral vessels arising from the systemic arterial circulation [70–72]. CT imaging is also valuable in providing information on the status of the lung parenchyma in patients who have coexisting emphysematous or restrictive lung disease and in detecting mediastinal pathology that might account for occlusion of the central pulmonary arteries [73]. This last capability is particularly important in patients who have unilateral occlusion of a main pulmonary artery [74,75].

With well-timed contrast enhancement of the pulmonary vasculature during CT imaging, organized thrombus will often seem to line the larger pulmonary vessels in either a concentric or eccentric manner. Abrupt narrowing and tapering of pulmonary arteries, web-like strictures, pouch defects, and other irregularities of the intimal surface may also be appreciated. These findings should be distinguished from the intraluminal filling defects and abrupt vessel cutoff seen in acute thromboembolic disease. Although the equivalence, if not superiority, of CT to pulmonary angiography for detecting chronic central vascular lesions has been established [72], the ability of the newer multislice scanners to evaluate segmental and subsegmental vessels now seems to be approaching that of pulmonary angiography [76]. Clinicians must recognize, however, that thromboemboli may organize and become endothelialized along the vessel wall in such a manner that their presence on CT angiography may not be apparent. Consequently, the absence of lining thrombus visualized within the central pulmonary vessels on CT scan does not exclude the diagnosis of chronic thromboembolic disease or the possibility of surgical intervention. Conversely, the demonstration of central thrombus has been described in primary pulmonary hypertension and other end-stage lung disorders [77,78]. Surgical endarterectomy in these cases not only involves a substantial perioperative mortality risk but also is unlikely to mitigate the existing pulmonary hypertension.

For patients who have suspected CTEPH, pulmonary angiography represents the gold standard and, when properly performed, remains a safe and reliable way to define the extent and proximal location of organized thromboemboli [79]. Several angiographic patterns have been found to correlate with the presence of chronic thromboembolic material at surgery [80], including vascular webs or band-like narrowings, intimal irregularities, pouch defects, abrupt and often angular narrowing of major pulmonary arteries, and proximal obstruction of pulmonary vessels (Fig. 1). As with CT findings, the angiographic appearance of chronic thromboembolic disease is distinct from the intraluminal filling defects observed after acute pulmonary embolism.

In most patients who have CTEPH, two or more of these angiographic findings are present and distributed bilaterally. From a technical standpoint, the diagnostic usefulness of the pulmonary angiogram depends on an appropriately sized and time-contrast bolus and minimization of any chest movement. At UCSD, simultaneous frontal and lateral views are routinely obtained, because the extent of disease may be significantly underappreciated from a single projection.

Cardiac catheterization may be performed at pulmonary angiography, providing valuable information for assessing perioperative risk in patients who have CTEPH. Right heart catheterization defines the severity of the pulmonary hypertension and degree of cardiac dysfunction. Measurements of oxygen saturation in the vena cava, right-sided cardiac chambers, and pulmonary artery can occasionally document left-to-right shunts undetected by echocardiography. Left heart catheterization and coronary arteriography supply essential supplemental information in patients at risk for coronary artery disease or believed to have left heart dysfunction or valvular disease.

Management of chronic thromboembolic pulmonary hypertension: surgical therapy

The evaluation of patients who are believed to have CTEPH is intended to establish whether a PTE (ie, the surgical removal of organized thrombus from the pulmonary vascular bed) is possible and appropriate. An absolute criterion for surgery is the presence of accessible chronic thromboembolic disease. Current surgical techniques allow organized thrombi to be removed from the main, lobar, and proximal segmental vessels. With an accurate determination of surgical accessibility, the clinical prediction that the removal of these lesions will reduce right ventricular afterload and pulmonary pressures is essential to the decision to perform surgery. In this assessment, the clinician must consider the extent of surgically accessible disease in relation to the degree of pulmonary hypertension. The increase in PVR associated with chronic thromboembolic disease seems to arise not only from the central, surgically accessible lesions but also from a distal, small vessel arteriopathy. PTE relieves only the portion of the overall PVR arising from the surgically accessible component of the chronic thromboembolic disease.

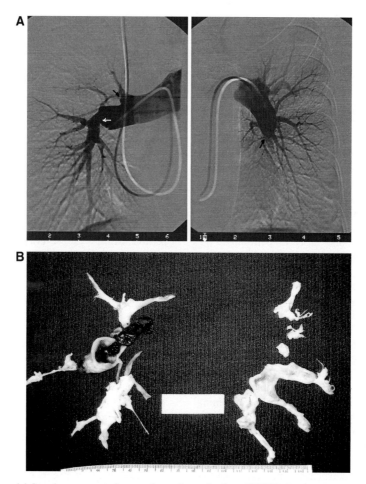

Fig. 1. (*A*) Right and left pulmonary arteriogram in patient who has CTEPH. Dark arrows depict near occlusive "pouch" defects; white arrow indicates vascular narrowing from chronic thrombus in the right interlobar vessel. (*B*) Thromboendarterectomy specimen from patient whose angiogram in shown in Fig. 1A.

When patients have a significant amount of coexisting distal vascular disease, an endarterectomy of the proximal lesions may not substantially reduce the PVR, placing them at risk for hemodynamic instability and death in the early postoperative period. Therefore, a key focus of the preoperative workup is to partition vascular resistance into proximal and distal components. Currently, this determination remains part of the art of the PTE evaluation. When the PVR seems elevated disproportionately to the degree of proximal disease as visualized by CT scan, angiography, or angioscopy [81,82], this information should be considered in discussions of perioperative risks with the patient. Several more quantitative techniques are being investigated with the goal of partitioning "upstream and downstream" components of PVR in patients who have CTEPH

[83,84]. Using a pulmonary artery occlusion technique, Kim and colleagues [84] showed a strong negative correlation between the preoperative upstream (or proximal) resistance and postoperative measures of PVR, with all postoperative deaths occurring in patients whose preoperative upstream resistance was less than 60%.

When determining whether PTE surgery is appropriate, the individual patient's symptoms and the personal impact of the disease on functional capabilities and survivorship must be considered. Patients presenting for evaluation typically exhibit significant limitations from the hemodynamic or ventilatory compromise caused by the pulmonary vascular obstruction. Most patients who ultimately undergo surgery have preoperative PVRs greater than 300 dynes/s/cm^{-5}, generally in the range of 700 to 1100 dynes/s/cm^{-5} [17,19–25]. With this degree of vascular resistance, patient impairment at rest and with exercise can be debilitating and, in the absence of surgical intervention, prognosis is poor [85,86]. For patients who have less severe pulmonary hypertension, surgery is considered based on individual circumstances. Included in this category are patients who have chronic thromboemboli involving one main pulmonary artery, those who have particularly vigorous lifestyle expectations (eg, professional athletes), and those who live at altitude. In such cases, surgery would be performed to alleviate the exercise impairment associated with high dead space and minute ventilatory demands. Surgery is also occasionally offered to patients who have normal pulmonary hemodynamics or mild pulmonary hypertension at rest who have documented pulmonary pressure elevation with exertion. This group of patients has received greater attention because of growing concerns that their pulmonary hypertension will likely progress without surgical intervention.

An assessment of the comorbid conditions that could adversely affect perioperative mortality or morbidity should also be considered when discussing PTE candidacy with patients and their families. Coexisting coronary artery disease, parenchymal lung disease, renal insufficiency, hepatic dysfunction, or the presence of a hypercoagulable state may complicate patient management during the postoperative period. Correction of pulmonary hypertension and right ventricular dysfunction with PTE surgery will often improve hepatic and renal function postoperatively. For patients who have coronary artery or valvular heart disease, coronary artery bypass grafting or valve replacement can be performed at thromboendarterectomy without increased surgical risk [87]. Similarly, advanced age and morbid obesity are not absolute contraindications to PTE, although they impact risk assessment and postoperative management strategies. One exception seems to be the presence of severe parenchymal or obstructive lung disease. The postoperative course in these patients is frequently complicated by prolonged ventilatory support, and once successfully weaned, patients may experience only minimal symptomatic improvement given their underlying pulmonary disease.

A detailed description of the PTE procedure is beyond the scope of this article, although several articles can be referenced [17,88,89]. However, several features of the procedure can be highlighted. Surgical success is founded on the concept that a true endarterectomy to remove the organized thrombi is to be accomplished, not an embolectomy. The chronic thromboembolic material is fibrotic and incorporated into the native vascular wall. An endarterectomy involves identification of the "pseudo-intima" and creation of a dissection plane to adequately free the thrombotic residua from the central pulmonary vascular bed. Removal of nonadherent, partially organized thrombus within the lumen of the central pulmonary arteries without the full endarterectomy is ineffective in reestablishing blood flow and reducing right ventricular afterload. Cardiopulmonary bypass with periods of circulatory arrest is essential to ensure optimal exposure of the pulmonary vascular intima in a bloodless field. The significant back-bleeding created by bronchial arterial blood flow is mitigated through interrupting cardiopulmonary bypass (circulatory arrest periods). This exposure allows the circumferential dissection of thromboembolic residua from the involved lobar, segmental, and subsegmental vessels.

Safeguards to ensure tissue integrity therefore become an integral component of this surgical procedure, allowing circulatory arrests to be accomplished without adverse consequences. Although standard flow for cardiopulmonary bypass is used, the patient is systemically cooled to 20°C. Hemodilution to a hematocrit in the range of 18% to 25% is performed to decrease blood viscosity during hypothermia and to optimize capillary blood flow. Additional cerebral protection is provided by surrounding the head with ice and a cooling blanket, and phenytoin is administered intravenously during the cooling period to reduce the risk for perioperative seizure activity. When the patient's temperature reaches 20°C, the aorta is cross-clamped and a single dose of cold cardioplegic solution is administered. Further myocardial protection is achieved with the use of a cooling jacket wrapped around the heart. After the aorta is cross-clamped, thiopental is administered until the electroencephalogram becomes isoelectric. When the patient is cooled to the optimal level of hypothermia, periods of circulatory arrest can be initiated. The endarterectomy can proceed at this point, usually first on the right side, then on the left. After the endarterectomy is completed, cardiopulmonary bypass is resumed and rewarming commenced. Given the high incidence of sinus arrest within the first 24 hours postendarterectomy, atrial and ventricular epicardial wires are placed. Mediastinal chest tubes also are left in place to evacuate any accumulated blood during the first two to three postoperative days. After rewarming and successful defibrillation of the heart, cardiopulmonary bypass is discontinued and mechanical ventilation resumed.

The short-term and long-term hemodynamic outcomes have been favorable in most patients who have CTEPH who undergo thromboendarterectomy surgery. With restoration of blood flow to previously occluded lung segments, an immediate reduction in right ventricular afterload occurs, resulting in a decline in pulmonary artery pressures and an augmentation in cardiac output. Since 1997, several groups have reported this improvement in pulmonary hemodynamics after surgery [17,22–25,90–92]. Furthermore, studies have reported this hemodynamic improvement to be sustained months to years postendarterectomy, accompanied by substantial gains in functional status, gas exchange, and quality of life [20,93–97]. However, not all patients who have CTEPH experience normalization or near-normalization of their pulmonary hemodynamics after undergoing endarterectomy surgery; approximately 10% to 15% of patients are left with a residual PVR more than 500 dynes/s/cm^{-5}. Although the postoperative hemodynamic improvement is significant in two thirds of these patients, approximately 3% to 5% of patients experience minimal to no hemodynamic benefit from surgery. This finding is based the presence of a distal vasculopathy, with PVR, pulmonary arterial pressures, and cardiac function unaffected by whatever amount of proximal vessel chronic thromboembolic material was removed. If the patient survives the immediate postoperative period, long-term pulmonary vasodilator therapy, such as the use of intravenous epoprostenol or an endothelin antagonist, should be considered.

In patient series reported since 1996, operative mortality rates range from 4.4% to 24% [17,21–25,90–92,98]. Factors contributing to perioperative mortality risks have not been completely elucidated, although New York Heart Association (NYHA) class IV functional status, age older than 70 years, the presence of right ventricular failure (correlated with high right atrial pressures), morbid obesity, and the duration of pulmonary hypertension have been to reported to impact postoperative survivorship [17,21,90,99,100]. Several studies have also suggested that more severe preoperative pulmonary hypertension correlates with higher postoperative mortality rates. In a report by Hartz and associates [21], a preoperative PVR more than 1100 dynes/s/cm^{-5} and a mean pulmonary artery pressure more than 50 mm Hg

predicted a significantly higher operative mortality. Similarly, Tscholl and colleagues [90] showed that a preoperative PVR more than 1136 dynes/s/cm^{-5} adversely influenced postoperative survivorship. Furthermore, in a report of 500 patients who had PTE, Jamieson and colleagues [17] showed that a preoperative PVR of more than 1000 dynes/s/cm^{-5} was associated with an significantly higher operative mortality rate of 10.1% compared with only 1.3% in those who had a lower preoperative PVR. Causes of death after PTE surgery are variable, and include cardiac arrest, multiorgan failure, uncontrollable mediastinal bleeding, sepsis syndrome, and massive pulmonary hemorrhage [21,23–25,90]. However, a series involving 1500 patients showed that severe reperfusion lung injury and residual pulmonary hypertension and right ventricular dysfunction were the leading contributors to perioperative mortality [17]. Results from this same group have also shown that long-term survivorship after hospital discharge is dramatically improved relative to the expected longevity if these patients had forgone surgical intervention. In a cohort of 532 patients followed up postoperatively for up to 19 years, Archibald and colleagues [96] showed a 75% probability of survivorship beyond 6 years.

Management of chronic thromboembolic pulmonary hypertension: medical therapy

Pharmacotherapy for treating pulmonary hypertension may be beneficial in select patients who have chronic thromboembolic disease. Four distinct patient groups to consider include (1) patients who have surgically accessible CTEPH who elect not to undergo PTE surgery because of personal choice or in whom comorbidities are so significant that surgery is contraindicated; (2) patients who have severe pulmonary hypertension and right ventricular dysfunction who exhibit distal chronic thromboembolic disease or a limited amount of resectable chronic thrombus, and therefore are unlikely to benefit from attempted PTE surgery; (3) patients who have not yet undergone PTE who have severe pulmonary hypertension and right heart failure, in whom pharmacotherapy would be a "stabilizing bridge" to surgery to reduce the postoperative mortality risk; and (4) patients who have undergone PTE and have residual pulmonary hypertension. Data examining the use of pulmonary vasodilator therapy in each one of these groups are limited.

However, based on the pathophysiologic mechanisms explaining the evolution of pulmonary hypertension in chronic thromboembolic disease, the use of vasodilator therapy in select patients warrants careful evaluation.

For inoperable CTEPH, Ono and colleagues [101] evaluated the use of beraprost (an oral prostacyclin analog) and conventional therapy in a small group of patients (N = 20) compared with a matched group (N = 23) undergoing conventional therapy alone. Fifty (50%) percent of patients in the beraprost group experienced an improvement in functional class during a follow-up period of 2 ± 1 month, and no functional class improvement was seen in patients only undergoing conventional therapy. During this same period, hemodynamic measurements were performed in a small number of patients (n = 10). Overall, the decline in mean PA pressure and total peripheral resistance was modest, although statistically significant, an no significant rise in cardiac output occurred. Throughout the extended follow-up period, improved survivorship was also seen in the patients treated with beraprost.

More recently, the use of bosentan, an endothelin receptor antagonist, has been studied in patients who have inoperable CTEPH. Bonderman and colleagues [102] evaluated 16 patients treated with bosentan for 6 months, showing an improvement in NYHA functional status in 11 patients, a reduction in pro-brain natriuretic peptide levels (pro-BNP), and an improvement in 6-minute walk distance. In a retrospective study, Hughes and colleagues [103] reported on 47 patients who had CTEPH treated with bosentan for a year (39 patients who had distal chronic thromboembolic disease and 8 patients who had post-PTE pulmonary hypertension), and obtained hemodynamic data on 28 patients at 1 year. Overall, an improvement was seen in 6-minute walk distance, functional classification, cardiac index, and total pulmonary resistance. The greatest improvement was observed in patients who had pulmonary hypertension after undergoing endarterectomy surgery. In an open-label pilot trial evaluating 3 months of bosentan therapy in 19 patients who had inoperable CTEPH, Hoeper and colleagues [104] showed that a significant reduction in pulmonary vascular resistance, an increase in 6-minute walk distance, and an improvement in pro-BNP levels occurred.

Sildenafil, a PDE-5 inhibitor, has also been studied to a limited extent in patients who have inoperable CTEPH. Ghofrani and colleagues [105] treated 12 patients who had CTEPH with sildenafil for 6 months. Baseline hemodynamics showed severe pulmonary hypertension (PVR index, 1935 ± 228 dyn/s/cm^{-5}; cardiac index, 2.0 L/min^{-1}/m^{-2}), with acute pulmonary vasoreactivity documented at initial right heart catheterization (inhaled nitric oxide and sildenafil). After 6 months, 6-minute walk distance substantially increased, PVR index was markedly improved, and cardiac index significantly increased. Sheth and coworkers [106] examined the effects of sildenafil in six patients who had severe inoperable CTEPH and left ventricular dysfunction. At 6 weeks, an improvement was seen in mean pulmonary artery pressure, mean pulmonary capillary wedge pressure, dyspnea scores, and NYHA functional class.

Given the greater perioperative mortality rates seen in patients who have operable chronic thromboembolic disease with severe pulmonary hypertension [17,21,90], experts hypothesize that using pulmonary vasodilator therapy preoperatively may have beneficial effects on early postoperative survival. Using intravenous prostacyclin for a period of 46 ± 12 days before surgery, Nagaya and colleagues [107] showed a preoperative decrease in PVR of 28% (1510 + 53 dynes/s/cm^{-5} to 1088 + 58 dynes/s/cm^{-5}) and a reduction in BNP levels in 12 patients who ultimately underwent pulmonary thromboendarterectomy. Postoperative mortality in this group was 8.3% compared with no deaths in the 21 patients who had CTEPH with a preoperative PVR of 1200 dynes/s/cm^{-5} or less. Postoperative hemodynamic improvement was comparable between the groups. Although this study was able to show a hemodynamic benefit of prostacyclin in a small number of patients who had severe pulmonary hypertensive CTEPH, the effect of pulmonary vasodilator pretreatment as a bridge to PTE and its effects on postoperative outcome remain unknown. As a result, the use of pulmonary vasodilator therapy in patients who have CTEPH who are likely to have operable chronic thromboembolic disease should not inappropriately delay surgical intervention.

References

[1] Ball KP, Goodwin JF, Harrison CV. Massive thrombotic occlusion of the large pulmonary arteries. Circulation 1956;14:766–83.

[2] Owen WR, Thomas WA, Castleman B, et al. Unrecognized emboli to the lungs with subsequent cor pulmonale. N Engl J Med 1953;249:919–26.

[3] Hollister LE, Cull VL. The syndrome of chronic thrombosis of the major pulmonary arteries. Am J Med 1956;21:312–20.

[4] Carroll D. Chronic obstruction of major pulmonary arteries. Am J Med 1950;9:175–85.

[5] Hurwitt ES, Schein CJ, Rifkin H, et al. A surgical approach to the problem of chronic pulmonary artery obstruction due to thrombosis or stenosis. Ann Surg 1958;147:157–65.

[6] Houk VN, Hufnagel CH, McClenathan JE, et al. Chronic thrombotic obstruction of major pulmonary arteries: report of a case successfully treated by thromboendarterectomy and a review of the literature. Am J Med 1963;35:269–82.

[7] Synder WA, Kent DC, Baisch BF. Successful endarterectomy of chronically occluded pulmonary artery: clinical report and physiologic studies. J Thorac Cardiovasc Surg 1963;45:482–9.

[8] Castleman B, McNeeley BU, Scannell G. Case records of the Massachusetts General Hospital, Case 32-1964. N Engl J Med 1964;271:40–50.

[9] Moser KM, Houk VN, Jones RC, et al. Chronic, massive thrombotic obstruction of pulmonary arteries: analysis of four operated cases. Circulation 1965;32:377–85.

[10] Nash ES, Shapiro S, Landau A, et al. Successful thromboembolectomy in long-standing thromboembolic pulmonary hypertension. Thorax 1966;23:121–30.

[11] Moor GF, Sabiston DC Jr. Embolectomy for chronic pulmonary embolism and pulmonary hypertension: case report and review of the problem. Circulation 1970;41:701–8.

[12] Cabrol C, Cabrol A, Acar J, et al. Surgical correction of chronic postembolic obstructions of the pulmonary arteries. J Thorac Cardiovasc Surg 1978;76:620–8.

[13] Sabiston DC Jr, Wolfe WG, Oldham HN Jr, et al. Surgical management of chronic pulmonary embolism. Ann Surg 1977;185:699–712.

[14] Utley JR, Spragg RG, Long WB, et al. Pulmonary endarterectomy for chronic thromboembolic obstruction: recent surgical experience. Surgery 1982;92:1096–102.

[15] Chitwood WR, Sabiston DC Jr, Wechsler AS. Surgical treatment of chronic unresolved pulmonary embolism. Clin Chest Med 1984;5:507–36.

[16] Moser KM, Daily PO, Peterson K, et al. Thromboendarterectomy for chronic, major-vessel thromboembolic pulmonary hypertension: immediate and long-term results in 42 patients. Ann Intern Med 1987;107:560–5.

[17] Jamieson SW, Kapelanski DP, Sakakibara N, et al. Pulmonary endarterectomy: experience and lessons learned in 1,500 cases. Ann Thorac Surg 2003;76:1457–64.

[18] Zund G, Pretre R, Niederhauser U, et al. Improved exposure of the pulmonary arteries for thromboendarterectomy. Ann Thorac Surg 1998;66:1821–3.

[19] Simonneau G, Azarian R, Brenot F, et al. Surgical management of unresolved pulmonary embolism: a personal series of 72 patients. Chest 1995;107:52S–5S.

[20] Mayer E, Dahm M, Hake U, et al. Mid-term results of pulmonary thromboendarterectomy for chronic thromboembolic pulmonary hypertension. Ann Thorac Surg 1996;61:1788–92.

[21] Hartz RS, Byme JG, Levitsky S, et al. Predictors of mortality in pulmonary thromboendarterectomy. Ann Thorac Surg 1996;62:1255–9.

[22] Nakajima N, Masuda M, Mogi K. The surgical treatment for chronic pulmonary thromboembolism—our surgical experience and current review of the literature. Ann Thorac Cardiovasc Surg 1997;3:15–21.

[23] Ando M, Okita Y, Tagusari O, et al. Surgical treatment for chronic thromboembolic pulmonary hypertension under profound hypothermia and circulatory arrest in 24 patients. J Card Surg 1999;14:377–85.

[24] Rubens F, Wells P, Bencze S, et al. Surgical treatment of chronic thromboembolic pulmonary hypertension. Can Respir J 2000;7:49–57.

[25] D'Armini AM, Cattadori B, Monterosso C, et al. Pulmonary thromboendarterectomy in patients with chronic pulmonary hypertension: hemodynamic characteristics and changes. Eur J Cardiothorac Surg 2000;18:696–702.

[26] Dalen JE, Albert JS. Natural history of pulmonary embolism. Prog Cardiovasc Dis 1975;17:259–70.

[27] Fedullo PF, Auger WR, Kerr KM, et al. Chronic thromboembolic pulmonary hypertension. Semin Resp Crit Care Med 2003;24:273–85.

[28] Ribeiro A, Lindmarker P, Johnsson H, et al. Pulmonary embolism: one-year follow-up with echocardiography Doppler and five-year survival analysis. Circulation 1999;99:1325–30.

[29] Pengo V, Lensing AWA, Prins MH, et al. Incidence of chronic thromboembolic pulmonary hypertension after pulmonary embolism. N Engl J Med 2004;350:2257–64.

[30] Miniati M, Simonetta M, Bottai M, et al. Survival and restoration of pulmonary perfusion in a long-term follow-up of patients after pulmonary embolism. Medicine 2006;85:253–62.

[31] Liu P, Meneveau N, Schiele F, et al. Predictors of long-term clinical outcome in patients with acute massive pulmonary embolism after thrombolytic therapy. Chin Med J (Engl) 2003;116:503–9.

[32] Wolf M, Boyer-Neumann C, Parent F, et al. Thrombotic risk factors in pulmonary hypertension. Eur Respir J 2000;15:395–9.

[33] Colorio CC, Martinuzzo ME, Forastiero RR, et al. Thrombophilic factors in chronic thromboembolic pulmonary hypertension. Blood Coagul Fibrinolysis 2001;12:427–32.

[34] Bonderman D, Turecek PL, Jakowitsch J, et al. High prevalence of elevated clotting factor VIII in

chronic thromboembolic pulmonary hypertension. Thromb Haemost 2003;90:372–6.

[35] Bonderman D, Jakowitsch J, Adlbrecht C, et al. Medical conditions increasing the risk of chronic thromboembolic pulmonary hypertension. Thromb Haemost 2005;93:512–6.

[36] Jais X, Ioos V, Jardim C, et al. Splenectomy and chronic thromboembolic pulmonary hypertension. Thorax 2005;60:1031–4.

[37] Lang I, Kerr K. Risk factors for chronic thromboembolic pulmonary hypertension. Proc Am Thorac Soc 2006;3:568–70.

[38] Egermayer P, Peacock AJ. Is pulmonary embolism a common cause of pulmonary hypertension? Limitations of the embolic hypothesis. Eur Respir J 2000;15:440–8.

[39] Fedullo PF, Rubin LJ, Kerr KM, et al. The natural history of acute and chronic thromboembolic disease: the search for the missing link. Eur Respir J 2000;15:435–7.

[40] Peterson KL. Acute pulmonary embolism: has its evolution been redefined? Circulation 1999;99: 1280–3.

[41] Rosenhek R, Korschineck I, Gharehbaghi-Schnell E, et al. Fibrinolytic balance of the arterial wall: pulmonary artery displays increased fibrinolytic potential compared with the aorta. Lab Invest 2003;83:871–6.

[42] Olman MA, Marsh JJ, Lang IM, et al. Endogenous fibrinolytic system in chronic large-vessel thromboembolic pulmonary hypertension. Circulation 1992;86:1241–8.

[43] Lang IM, Marsh JJ, Olman MA, et al. Parallel analysis of tissue-type plasminogen activator and type 1 plasminogen activator inhibitor in plasma and endothelial cells derived from patients with chronic pulmonary thromboemboli. Circulation 1994;90:706–12.

[44] Lang IM, Marsh JJ, Olman MA, et al. Expression of type 1 plasminogen activator inhibitor in chronic pulmonary thromboemboli. Circulation 1994;89: 2715–21.

[45] Morris TA, Marsh JJ, Chiles PG, et al. Fibrin derived from patients with chronic thromboembolic pulmonary hypertension is resistant to lysis. Am J Respir Crit Care Med 2006;173(11):1270–5.

[46] McIntyre KM, Sasahara AA. The hemodynamic response to pulmonary embolism in patients without prior cardiopulmonary disease. Am J Cardiol 1971,28.288–94.

[47] Grifoni S, Olivotto I, Cecchini P, et al. Sort-term clinical outcome of patients with acute pulmonary embolism, normal blood pressure, and echocardiographic right ventricular dysfunction. Circulation 2000;101:2817–22.

[48] Wolfe MW, Lee RT, Feldstein ML, et al. Prognostic significance of right ventricular hypokinesis and perfusion lung scan defects in pulmonary embolism. Am Heart J 1994;127:1371–5.

[49] Wartski M, Collignon M-A. Incomplete recovery of lung perfusion after 3 months in patients with acute pulmonary embolism treated with antithrombotic agents. J Nucl Med 2000;41:1043–8.

[50] Nijleuter M, Hovens MMC, Davidson BL, et al. Resolution of thromboemboli in patients with acute pulmonary embolism. A systematic review. Chest 2006;129:192–7.

[51] Fedullo PF, Auger WR, Kerr KM, et al. Chronic thromboembolic pulmonary hypertension. N Engl J Med 2001;345:1465–72.

[52] Ryu JH, Olson EJ, Pellikka PA. Clinical recognition of pulmonary embolism: problem of unrecognized and asymptomatic cases. Mayo Clin Proc 1998;73:873–9.

[53] Moser KM, Bloor CM. Pulmonary vascular lesions occurring in patients with chronic major vessel thromboembolic pulmonary hypertension. Chest 1993;103:685–92.

[54] Deng Z, Morse JH, Slager SL, et al. Familial pulmonary hypertension is caused by mutations in the bone morphogenetic protein receptor-II gene. Am J Hum Genet 2000;67:737–44.

[55] Du L, Sullivan CC, Chu D, et al. Signaling molecules in nonfamilial pulmonary hypertension. N Engl J Med 2003;348(6):500–9.

[56] Bauer M, Wilkens H, Langer F, et al. Selective upregulation of endothelin B receptor gene expression in severe pulmonary hypertension. Circulation 2002;105(9):1034–6.

[57] Kim H, Yung GL, Marsh JJ, et al. Endothelin mediates pulmonary vascular remodeling in a canine model of chronic thromboembolic pulmonary hypertension. Eur Respir J 2000;15(4):640–8.

[58] Auger WR, Moser KM. Pulmonary flow murmurs: a distinctive physical sign found in chronic pulmonary thromboembolic disease [abstract]. Clin Res 1989;37:145A.

[59] Woodruff WW III, Hoeck BE, Chitwood WR Jr, et al. Radiographic findings in pulmonary hypertension from unresolved embolism. AJR Am J Roentgenol 1985;144:681–6.

[60] Morris TA, Auger WR, Ysrael MZ, et al. Parenchymal scarring is associated with restrictive spirometric defects in patients with chronic thromboembolic pulmonary hypertension. Chest 1996;110:399–403.

[61] Steenhuis LH, Groen HJM, Koeter GH, et al. Diffusion capacity and haemodynamics in primary and chronic thromboembolic pulmonary hypertension. Eur Respir J 2000;16:276–81.

[62] Kapitan KS, Buchbinder M, Wagner PD, et al. Mechanisms of hypoxemia in chronic thromboembolic pulmonary hypertension. Am Rev Respir Dis 1989;139:1149–54.

[63] Dittrich HC, McCann HA, Blanchard DG. Cardiac structure and function in chronic thromboembolic pulmonary hypertension. Am J Card Imaging 1994;8:18–27.

[64] Lisbona R, Kreisman H, Novales-Diaz J, et al. Perfusion lung scanning: differentiation of primary from thromboembolic pulmonary hypertension. AJR Am J Roentgenol 1985;144:27–30.

[65] Powe JE, Palevsky HI, McCarthy KE, et al. Pulmonary arterial hypertension: value of perfusion scintigraphy. Radiology 1987;164:727–30.

[66] Ryan KL, Fedullo PF, Davis GB, et al. Perfusion scan findings understate the severity of angiographic and hemodynamic compromise in chronic thromboembolic pulmonary hypertension. Chest 1988;93:1180–5.

[67] Bailey CL, Channick RN, Auger WR, et al. "High probability" perfusion lung scans in pulmonary venoocclusive disease. Am J Respir Crit Care Med 2000;162:1974–8.

[68] Cook DJ, Tanser PH, Dobranowski J, et al. Primary pulmonary artery sarcoma mimicking pulmonary thromboembolism. Can J Cardiol 1988;4: 393–6.

[69] Palevsky HI, Cone L, Alavi A. A case of "false-positive" high probability ventilation-perfusion lung scan due to tuberculous adenopathy with a discussion of other causes of "false-positive" high probability ventilation-perfusion lung scans. J Nucl Med 1991;32:512–7.

[70] King MA, Bergin CJ, Yeung D, et al. Chronic pulmonary thromboembolism: detection of regional hypoperfusion with CT. Radiology 1994;191: 359–63.

[71] Schwickert HC, Schweden F, Schild HH, et al. Pulmonary arteries and lung parenchyma in chronic pulmonary embolism: preoperative and postoperative CT findings. Radiology 1994;191:351–7.

[72] Tardivon AA, Musset D, Maitre S, et al. Role of CT in chronic pulmonary embolism: comparison with pulmonary angiography. J Comput Assist Tomogr 1993;17:345–52.

[73] Berry PF, Buccigrossi D, Peabody J, et al. Pulmonary vascular occlusion and fibrosing mediastinitis. Chest 1986;89:296–301.

[74] Bergin CJ, Hauschildt JP, Brown MA, et al. Identifying the cause of unilateral hypoperfusion in patients suspected to have chronic pulmonary thrombo-embolism: diagnostic accuracy of helical CT and conventional angiography. Radiology 1999; 213:743–9.

[75] Cho SR, Tisnado J, Cockrell CH, et al. Angiographic evaluation of patients with unilateral massive perfusion defects on the lung scan. Radiographics 1987;7:729–45.

[76] Pitton MB, Kemmerich G, Herber S, et al. Chronic thromboembolic pulmonary hypertension: diagnostic impact of multi-slice CT and selective pulmonary-DSA. Rofo 2002;147:474–9.

[77] Moser KM, Fedullo PF, Finkbeiner WE, et al. Do patients with primary pulmonary hypertension develop extensive central thrombi? Circulation 1995; 91:741–5.

[78] Russo A, De Luca M, Vigna C, et al. Central pulmonary artery lesions in chronic obstructive pulmonary disease. A transesophageal echocardiographic study. Circulation 1999;100:1808–15.

[79] Pitton MB, Duber C, Mayer E, et al. Hemodynamic effects of nonionic contrast bolus injection and oxygen inhalation during pulmonary angiography in patients with chronic major-vessel thromboembolic pulmonary hypertension. Circulation 1996; 94:2485–91.

[80] Auger WR, Fedullo PF, Moser KM, et al. Chronic major-vessel thromboembolic pulmonary artery obstruction: appearance at angiography. Radiology 1992;182:393–8.

[81] Shure D, Gregoratos G, Moser KM. Fiberoptic angioscopy: role in the diagnosis of chronic pulmonary arterial obstruction. Ann Intern Med 1985; 103:844–50.

[82] Sompradeekul S, Fedullo PF, Kerr KM, et al. The role of pulmonary angioscopy in the preoperative assessment of patients with thromboembolic pulmonary hypertension (CTEPH) [abstract]. Am J Respir Crit Care Med 1999;159:A456.

[83] Fesler P, Kim HS, Channick RN, et al. Partition of pulmonary vascular resistance in chronic thromboembolic pulmonary hypertension. Am J Respir Crit Care Med 2002;165:A332.

[84] Kim HS, Fesler P, Channick RN, et al. Preoperative partitioning of pulmonary vascular resistance correlates with early outcome after thromboendarterectomy for chronic thromboembolic pulmonary hypertension. Circulation 2004;109:18–22.

[85] Riedel M, Stanek V, Widimsky J, et al. Longterm follow-up of patients with pulmonary thromboembolism: late prognosis and evolution of hemodynamic and respiratory data. Chest 1982;81: 151–8.

[86] Lewczuk J, Piszko P, Jagas J, et al. Prognostic factors in medically treated patients with chronic pulmonary embolism. Chest 2001;119:818–23.

[87] Thistlethwaite PA, Auger WR, Madani MM, et al. Pulmonary thromboendarterectomy combined with other cardiac operations: indications, surgical approach, and outcome. Ann Thorac Surg 2001;72: 13–9.

[88] Daily PO, Dembitsky WP, Jamieson SW. The evolution and the current state of the art of pulmonary thromboendarterectomy. Semin Thorac Cardiovasc Surg 1999;11:152–63.

[89] Mayer E, Klepetko W. Techniques and outcomes of pulmonary endarterectomy for chronic thromboembolic pulmonary hypertension. Proc Am Thorac Soc 2006;3(7):589–93.

[90] Tscholl D, Langer F, Wendler O, et al. Pulmonary thromboendarterectomy—risk factors for early survival and hemodynamic improvement. Eur J Cardiothorac Surg 2001;19:771–6.

[91] Mayer E, Kramm T, Dahm M, et al. Early results of pulmonary thromboendarterectomy in chronic

thromboembolic pulmonary hypertension. Z Kardiol 1997;86:920–7.

[92] Masuda M, Nakajima N. Our experience of surgical treatment for chronic pulmonary thromboembolism. Ann Thorac Cardiovasc Surg 2001;7: 261–5.

[93] Kramm T, Mayer E, Dahm M, et al. Long-term results after thromboendarterectomy for chronic pulmonary embolism. Eur J Cardiothorac Surg 1999;15:579–84.

[94] Kapitan KS, Clausen JL, Moser KM. Gas exchange in chronic thromboembolism after pulmonary thromboendarterectomy. Chest 1990;98:14–9.

[95] Tanabe N, Okada O, Nakagawa Y, et al. The efficacy of pulmonary thromboendarterectomy on long-term gas exchange. Eur Respir J 1997;10: 2066–72.

[96] Archibald CJ, Auger WR, Fedullo PF, et al. Long-term outcome after pulmonary thromboendarterectomy. Am J Respir Crit Care Med 1999;160: 523–8.

[97] Zoia MC, D'Armini AM, Beccaria M, and the Pavia Thromboendarterectomy Group. Mid-term effects of pulmonary thromboendarterectomy on clinical and cardiopulmonary functional status. Thorax 2002;57:608–12.

[98] Mares P, Gilbert TB, Tschernko EM, et al. Pulmonary artery thromboendarterectomy: a comparison of two different postoperative treatment strategies. Anesth Analg 2000;90:267–73.

[99] Daily PO, Dembitsky WP, Iversen S, et al. Risk factors for pulmonary thromboendarterectomy. J Thorac Cardiovasc Surg 1990;99:670–8.

[100] Moser KM, Auger WR, Fedullo PF. Chronic major vessel thromboembolic pulmonary hypertension. Circulation 1990;81:1735–43.

[101] Ono F, Nagaya N, Okumura H, et al. Effect of orally active prostacyclin analogue on survival in patients with chronic thromboembolic pulmonary hypertension without major vessel obstruction. Chest 2003;123:1583–8.

[102] Bonderman D, Nowotny R, Skoro-Sajer N, et al. Bosentan therapy for inoperable chronic thromboembolic pulmonary hypertension. Chest 2005;128: 2599–603.

[103] Hughes RJ, Jais X, Bonderman D, et al. The efficacy of bosentan in inoperable chronic thromboembolic pulmonary hypertension: a 1-year follow-up study. Eur Respir J 2006;28:138–43.

[104] Hoeper MM, Kramm T, Wilkens H, et al. Bosentan therapy for inoperable chronic thromboembolic pulmonary hypertension. Chest 2005;128: 2363–7.

[105] Ghofrani HA, Schermuly RT, Rose F, et al. Sildenafil for long-term treatment of nonoperable chronic thromboembolic pulmonary hypertension. Am J Respir Crit Care Med 2003;167:1139–41.

[106] Sheth A, Park JE, Ong YE, et al. Early haemodynamic benefit of sildenafil in patients with coexisting chronic thromboembolic pulmonary hypertension and left ventricular dysfunction. Vascul Pharmacol 2005;42:41–5.

[107] Nagaya N, Sasaki N, Ando M, et al. Prostacyclin therapy before pulmonary thromboendarterectomy in patients with chronic thromboembolic pulmonary hypertension. Chest 2003;123:338–43.

ELSEVIER
SAUNDERS

Clin Chest Med 28 (2007) 271–277

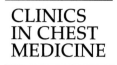

CLINICS
IN CHEST
MEDICINE

Index

Note: Page numbers of article titles are in **boldface** type.

A

Acute respiratory distress syndrome (ARDS), treatment of, prostanoid therapy in, 137

Adrenomedullin (AM), for PAH, 178–179

Adventitial remodeling, pulmonary hypertension and, 32–33

Ambrisentan, in PAH management, clinical trials of, 122

Amiloride, in PAH management, 96

Angiopoitin-1, in PAH management, 179–180

Anorectic agents, PAH and, 12

Anticoagulation, in PAH management, 99–103

Arachidonic acid pathway, epoprostenol and, 127

ARDS. See *Acute respiratory distress syndrome (ARDS).*

Atrial septostomy, in PAH management, 187–190
  described, 187–188
  hemodynamic effects of, 188–190
  long-term effects of, 190
  procedure for, 188
  rationale for, 187–188
  risks associated with, 188

B

Beraprost
  bosentan and, in PAH management, 173
  in PAH management, 133

Biomarker(s), plasma, as surrogate end point in PAH, 80–81

BMPR2 mutations
  FPAH due to, 46
    prevalence of, 46
  in disease states, 49–50
  in sporadic PAH or IPAH, 46–47

BMPR2 signaling pathway, in PAH, 48–49

Bosentan
  beraprost and, in PAH management, 173
  epoprostenol and, in PAH management, 172
  iloprost and, in PAH management, 172–173
  in PAH management, clinical trials of, 118–119
  sildenafil and, in PAH management, 173–174
  treprostinil and, in PAH management, 173

Bosentan Randomized Trial of Endothelin Antagonist Therapy (BREATHE), 118–119

Brain natriuretic peptide, in pulmonary hypertension in respiratory disease diagnostic evaluation, 224

BREATHE. See *Bosentan Randomized Trial of Endothelin Antagonist Therapy (BREATHE).*

Breathing, sleep-disordered, pulmonary hypertension in, 223

C

Calcium channel blockers, in PAH management, 103–109

Cardiac catheterization, in PAH, 67

Cardiac defects, congenital, prostanoid therapy for, 135

Cardiac imaging, as surrogate end point in PAH, 81

Cardiac surgery, prostanoid therapy and, 137–138

Cardiopulmonary exercise testing, as surrogate end point in PAH, 172–83

Catheterization
  cardiac, in PAH, 67
  heart, right, in pulmonary hypertension in respiratory disease diagnostic evaluation, 225

CHD-PAH. See *Congenital heart disease associated with pulmonary arterial hypertension (CHD-PAH).*

Chest radiography, in PAH, 60–62